a LANGE medical book

Gastrointestinal Physiology

Second Edition

D1603281

Kim E. Barrett, PhD
Professor of Medicine
Dean of Graduate Studies
University of California, San Diego
La Jolla, California

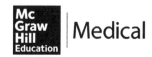 Medical

New York   Chicago   San Francisco   Lisbon   London   Madrid   Mexico City
Milan   New Delhi   San Juan   Seoul   Singapore   Sydney   Toronto

Gastrointestinal Physiology, Second Edition

Copyright © 2014 by McGraw-Hill Education. Printed in the United States of America. Except as permitted under the United States Copyright Act of 1976, no part of this publication may be reproduced or distributed in any form or by any means, or stored in a data base or retrieval system, without prior written permission of the publisher.

1 2 3 4 5 6 7 8 9 0   DOC/DOC   18 17 16 15 14 13

ISBN 978-0-07-177401-7
MHID 0-07-177401-7
ISSN 0-07-142310-9

This book was set in Adobe Garamond Pro by Thomson Digital.
The editors were Michael Weitz and Christina M. Thomas.
The production supervisor was Richard Ruzycka.
Project management was provided by Ritu Joon, Thomson Digital.
RR Donnelley was printer and binder.

This book is printed on acid-free paper.

McGraw-Hill Education books are available at special quantity discounts to use as premiums and sales promotions, or for use in corporate training programs. To contact a representative please e-mail us at bulksales@mcgraw-hill.com.

To my loving husband, Peter H. Pierce
whose care and patience make all things possible

Contents

Preface

When I set out originally to write this volume, it was my hope primarily to introduce medical and pharmacy students to the functioning of the gastrointestinal system in the context of a classical physiology curriculum. By using examples of common digestive disease states and their treatment, I sought to illuminate the normal functioning of what is, in my opinion, a supremely elegant system. It is not difficult to grasp the basic design requirements for the gut. Indeed, I have often begun my lectures with a slide of a baby's romper and arrows pointing to the two extremes of the alimentary canal labeled "in" and "out." However, the overlapping layers of regulatory controls, the many systemic redundancies, and the existence of extensive, bidirectional signaling between the various segments of the gut and the organs that drain into it all make for a complex body of knowledge that can be challenging, sometimes, for students to master. My intent, mainly, was to generate an accessible reference that could be used to review this material, perhaps as a supplement to a more general physiology course text. I have certainly been very gratified by the positive response to the text from both students and colleagues, and surmise that it filled a need.

However, the period that has intervened since I first designed this text has seen dramatic changes in the approach to medical education in many, if not most, institutions, at least in North America. Many medical schools, including my own, have moved away from stand-alone courses in physiology as well as other preclinical subjects, and have implemented integrated curricula that examine many medically-relevant facets of body systems, including anatomy, pathophysiology, and therapeutics, in concert with physiological information. I was fortunate (I especially cannot claim any prescience) that my original template for the book actually is well-suited for an organ- or systems-based curriculum, since I had intentionally already included much of the framing material surrounding physiology in my plan for the volume. Thus, while the volume retains only the word "physiology" in its title, I believe from experience that it also represents a useful resource for the GI block of a broader course.

The second edition is not unchanged, of course. First, I am grateful to students and colleagues from both within and outside my own institution who alerted me to minor errors in the original text. While some mistakes are almost inevitable in a project of this scope, no many how many pairs of eyes pass over it, it is certainly nice to correct as many as possible. Second, I have inserted new information on emerging topics, such as the communication between the intestine and central nervous system that controls food intake, the myriad roles newly ascribed to the intestinal microbiota, contemporary approaches to therapy for a number of GI maladies, and the role of the gut in obesity. Finally, I have overhauled a substantial number of the original illustrations, both to provide a more consistent style within and between chapters, and to clarify key concepts. Illustrations that summarize new topics have also been added.

With all the changes, however, the basic premise and goal of the book remain the same as in the original edition—to convince medical students and other trainees of the beauty of the design of the GI system, so vital to life and also the source of both human pleasure and suffering. As before, I take responsibility for any errors, and encourage readers to bring them to my attention. I also thank Michael Weitz at McGraw-Hill, my editor on this and other projects, especially for his encouragement, pep talks, cajoling, and forbearance.

Kim E. Barrett, PhD
La Jolla, California

Functional Anatomy of the GI Tract and Organs Draining into It

1

OBJECTIVES

- ▶ *Understand the basic functions of the gastrointestinal system and the design features that subserve these*
- ▶ *Describe the functional layers of the gastrointestinal tract and the specializations that contribute to function*
  - ▶ Glands
  - ▶ Epithelium
  - ▶ Mucosa
  - ▶ Muscle
  - ▶ Sphincters
- ▶ *Identify the segments of the gastrointestinal tract and the specialized functions attributed to each*
- ▶ *Understand the circulatory features of the intestine and variations that occur after meals*
- ▶ *Describe the basic anatomy of the neuromuscular systems of the gut*

OVERVIEW OF THE GASTROINTESTINAL SYSTEM AND ITS FUNCTIONS

Digestion and Absorption

The gastrointestinal system primarily conveys nutrients, electrolytes, and water into the body. In unicellular organisms, metabolic requirements can be met by diffusion or transport of substances from the environment across the cell membrane. However, the greatly increased scale of multicellular organisms, along with the fact that most such organisms are terrestrial, and thus not normally swimming in a soup of nutrients, means that specialized systems have evolved to convey nutrients into and around the body. Thus, the gastrointestinal system and liver work in concert with the circulatory system to ensure that the nutritional requirements of cells distant from the exterior of the body can be met.

1

Most nutrients in a normal human diet are macromolecules and thus cannot readily permeate across cell membranes. Likewise, nutrients are not usually taken predominantly in the form of solutions, but rather as solid food. Thus, in addition to the physical process of food uptake, the intestines serve to physically reduce the meal into a suspension of small particles mixed with nutrients in solution. These are then chemically altered resulting in molecules capable of traversing the intestinal lining. These processes are referred to as *digestion*, and involve gastrointestinal motility as well as the influences of pH changes, biological detergents, and enzymes.

The final stage in the assimilation of a meal involves movement of digested nutrients out of the intestinal contents, across the intestinal lining, and into either the blood supply to the gut or the lymphatic system, for transfer to more distant sites in the body. Collectively, this directed movement of nutrients is referred to as *absorption*. The efficiency of absorption may vary widely for different molecules in the diet as well as those supplied via the oral route with therapeutic intent, such as drugs. The barriers to absorption encountered by a given nutrient will depend heavily on its physicochemical characteristics, and particularly on whether it is hydrophilic (such as the products of protein and carbohydrate digestion) or hydrophobic (such as dietary lipids). For the main substances vitally required by the body, the gastrointestinal tract does not rely solely on diffusion across the lining to provide for uptake, but rather has evolved active transport mechanisms that take up specific solutes with high efficiency.

There is significant excess capacity in the systems for both digestion and absorption of a meal, including an excess of enzymes and other secreted products as well as an excess in the surface area available for absorption in healthy individuals. Thus, assimilation of nutrients is highly efficient, assuming adequate amounts are presented to the lumen. In former times, this doubtlessly assisted our ancestors in surviving under circumstances where food was not always plentiful. On the other hand, in modern times, and in developed countries, this excess capacity for nutrient uptake may contribute to high rates of obesity.

Excretion

The gastrointestinal system also serves as an important organ for excretion of substances out of the body. This excretory function extends not only to the obvious nonabsorbable residues of the meal, but also to specific classes of substances that cannot exit the body via other routes. Thus, in contrast to the excretory function of the renal system, which handles predominantly water-soluble metabolic waste products, the intestine works together with the biliary system to excrete hydrophobic molecules, such as cholesterol, steroids, and drug metabolites. As we will see later, the intestine also harbors a complex ecosystem of symbiotic bacteria known as commensals, even in the healthy state, and many members of this community die on a daily basis and are lost through the stool. Finally, the cells of the intestinal lining themselves turn over rapidly, and the stool also contains residues of these dead cells that are shed from the lining after their function has been fulfilled.

Host Defense

The intestine is a long tube, stretching from the mouth to the anus, whose inner surface exists in continuity with the exterior of the body. This, of course, is essential to its function of bringing nutrients from the environment into the body: however, this also implies that the intestine, like the skin, is a potential portal into the body for less desirable substances. Indeed, we exploit this property to deliver drugs via the oral route. In addition, the intestine is potentially vulnerable to infectious microorganisms that can enter the gut with the ingestion of food and water. To protect itself and the body, the intestine has evolved a sophisticated system of immune defenses. In fact, the gastrointestinal tract represents the largest lymphoid organ of the body, with significantly more lymphocytes than are found in the circulating immune system. The gastrointestinal immune system is also characterized by specific functional capabilities, most notably by being able to distinguish between "friend" and "foe," mounting immune defenses against pathogens while being tolerant of dietary antigens and the beneficial commensal bacteria.

ENGINEERING CONSIDERATIONS

Given the functions of the gastrointestinal system discussed earlier, we turn now to a consideration of anatomic features needed to support these functions. In this discussion, the gastrointestinal system can be thought of as a machine (Figure 1–1) in which distinct portions conduct the various processes needed for assimilation of a meal without uptake of significant quantities of harmful substances or microorganisms.

Design of Hollow Organs

The gastrointestinal tract itself is a long muscular tube stretching from the mouth to the anus. Within the lining of this tube, blind-ended glandular structures invaginate into the wall of the gut and empty their secretions into the gut *lumen*, defined as the cavity within the intestine. At various points along the length of the gastrointestinal tract, more elaborate glandular organs are also attached to the intestine and are connected to the intestinal lumen via ducts, also allowing secretions to drain into the intestine where they can be mixed with intestinal contents. Examples of such organs include the pancreas and salivary glands. Glands in general can be considered as structures that convert raw materials from the bloodstream into physiologically useful secretions, such as acid and enzyme solutions. The function of these hollow organs is closely coordinated with that of the intestine itself to provide optimal processing of the meal following ingestion.

In general, the hollow organs that drain secretions into the gut have a common structure. Specialized secretory cells form structures known as acini where a primary secretion is produced at the blind end of the gland. Clusters of such acini, which can be likened to a bunch of grapes, then empty into tube-like ductular structures; with larger ducts collecting the secretions from a group of smaller ones until a main collecting duct is reached that connects directly into the gut

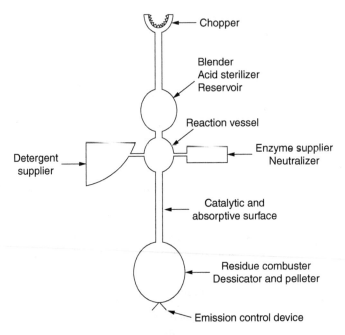

Figure 1–1. The gastrointestinal system as a machine that conducts digestive, absorptive, immune, and excretory functions. (Based on a figure originally designed by Alan F. Hofmann and used with permission.)

lumen. The *branching morphogenesis* that results in these structures during development amplifies the functional surface area of the gland and its capacity for secretion. The liver, which will be considered in this volume as a critical participant in gastrointestinal function overall, has a highly specialized structure that will be discussed in detail in a later chapter. For now, it suffices to say that the liver is designed not only to secrete substances into the gastrointestinal lumen via the biliary system, but also to receive absorbed substances from the intestine that travel first to the liver via the portal circulation before being processed and then distributed to the body as a whole.

Cellular Specialization

The tube that comprises the gastrointestinal tract is made up of functional layers comprised of specialized cell types (Figure 1–2). The first layer encountered by an ingested nutrient is the epithelium, which forms a continuous lining of the entire gastrointestinal tract as well as the lining of the glands and organs that drain into the tube. The epithelium is a critical contributor to intestinal function since it must provide for the selective uptake of nutrients, electrolytes, and water while rejecting harmful solutes. The surface area of the intestinal epithelium is amplified by being arranged into crypt and villus structures (Figure 1–3). The former are analogous to the glands discussed earlier,

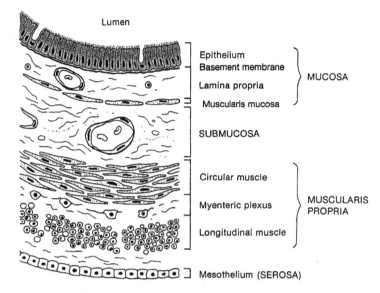

Figure 1–2. Organization of the wall of the intestine into functional layers. (Adapted from Madara and Anderson, in: *Textbook of Gastroenterology.* 4th ed. 151–165, copyright Lippincott Williams and Wilkins, 2003, and used with permission.) The submucosal plexus is not shown in this diagram (see Figure 1–8).

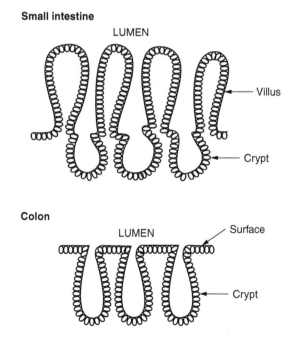

Figure 1–3. Comparison of the morphology of the epithelial layers of the small intestine and colon.

whereas villi are finger-like projections that protrude into the intestinal lumen and which are covered by epithelial cells. In the large intestine, only crypts are seen, interspersed with surface epithelium between the crypt openings.

The majority of the gastrointestinal epithelium is columnar in nature, where a single layer of tall, cylindrical cells separates the gut lumen from the deeper layers of the wall of the gut. The structure of the columnar epithelium can be compared to a six-pack of soda cans, with the cans representing the cells and the plastic holder that links them as a series of intercellular junctions that provide a barrier to passive movement of solutes around the cells.

An exception to the rule that the gut epithelium is columnar in nature is found in the first part of the intestinal tube, known as the esophagus, where the epithelial lining is referred to as a stratified squamous epithelium. At this site, the epithelium forms a multilayer reminiscent of the structure of the skin, with cells migrating toward the lumen from a basal germinal layer.

Indeed, the epithelium of the gut as a whole is subject to constant renewal, unlike the majority of tissues in the adult body. We can speculate that this continuous turnover may be designed to prevent the accumulation of genetic mutations in the epithelial compartment produced by luminal toxins, although this protection may also confer an increased risk of malignancy. Gastrointestinal epithelial cells turn over every 3 days or so in humans, undergoing a cycle of division and differentiation before succumbing to programmed cell death (or apoptosis) and being shed into the lumen or engulfed by their neighbors. Epithelial cells arise from stem cells that are anchored permanently in specific positions in the gut lining, located at the base of crypts in the intestine and in the middle of gastric glands in the stomach. Following several cycles of division, epithelial cells also differentiate into specialized cell types with specific functions in the digestive process.

In the stomach, some epithelial cells migrate downwards, deeper into the gland, and become chief or parietal cells that contribute specific products to the gastric juice, or endocrine cells that regulate the function of the latter secretory cell types. The remainder of the gastric epithelial cells migrate upwards to become cells capable of secreting mucus and bicarbonate ions.

In the small intestine, a few cells migrate downwards into the base of the crypt, where they become long-lived Paneth cells, which secrete antimicrobial peptides that are important components of the host defense system of the gut. Paneth cells (or a Paneth-like cell in the colon) also appear to supply critical factors that maintain the stem cell niche. The majority of the daughter cells that arise from stem cells and their subsequent divisions migrate upwards toward the villus (or surface epithelium in the colon), and of these, most are destined to differentiate into absorptive epithelial cells with the capacity for the final steps of nutrient digestion, and uptake of the resulting products. A few cells, however, differentiate into goblet cells, which produce mucus, or enteroendocrine cells that respond to luminal conditions and regulate the functions of the other epithelial cell types as well as those of more distant organs. The proportions of the different lineages remain constant via mechanisms that have yet to be fully elucidated, although signals from mesenchymal cells surrounding the crypt, such as myofibroblasts, are known to regulate the differentiation programs.

Beneath the epithelium is a basement membrane, overlying a layer of loose connective tissue known as the lamina propria. This contains nerve endings and blood vessels, as well as a rich assortment of immune and inflammatory cells that contribute to host defense as well as to the control of normal gut physiology. Taken together, the epithelium and lamina propria are referred to as the mucosa. The mucosa also contains a thin layer of smooth muscle known as the muscularis mucosae, which may be important in providing for villus movement. Beneath this layer, there is a plexus of nerve cell bodies known as the submucous (or submucosal) plexus, designed to relay information to and away from the mucosa, including the epithelial cells. Then, beyond the mucosa are the smooth muscle layers that provide for overall gut motility. These are arranged circumferentially around the outer side of the intestinal tube.

Closest to the mucosa is a layer of circular muscle that reduces the diameter of the intestinal lumen when it contracts. On the outer side of the gut, a layer of smooth muscle in which the fibers are arranged longitudinally along the axis of the tube provides for intestinal shortening. Working together, these two outer muscle layers can provide for complex motility patterns that subserve specific gut functions, as will be described in more detail later. Sandwiched between the circular and longitudinal muscle layers, the myenteric plexus of nerves regulates their function.

Division of Intestine into Functional Segments

Movement of the meal constituents along the length of the intestine is a regulated process, and involves selective retention at specific sites to promote optimal digestion and absorption. This is accomplished by specialized smooth muscular structures known as sphincters, whose function is also coordinated with that of the system as a whole (Figure 1–4). For example, the pylorus, which controls outflow from the stomach, retains the bulk of the meal in the gastric lumen and releases it slowly to more distal segments in order to match the availability of nutrients to the capacity of the enzymes required for digestion and the absorptive surface area. Similarly, the ileocecal valve retains the majority of the gastrointestinal microbiota within the lumen of the colon, opening only intermittently to permit the residues of the digested meal, along with water and cellular debris, to enter the large intestine. Finally, the sphincter of Oddi relaxes in conjunction with a meal to allow the outflow of both biliary and pancreatic secretions into the lumen.

Figure 1–4 shows the location of the major gastrointestinal sphincters and the gastrointestinal segments that they delineate. Most gastrointestinal sphincters are under involuntary control, and perform their normal cycles of relaxation and contraction without conscious input, in response to signals released during the progress of meal ingestion and digestion. Many may also function in a manner that is largely autonomous of the central nervous system, being controlled instead by

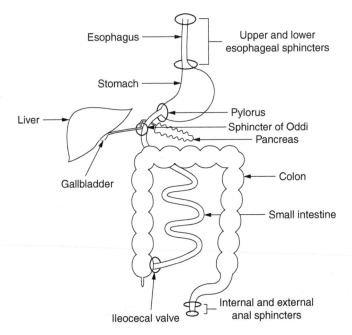

Figure 1–4. Overall anatomy of the gastrointestinal system and division of the GI tract into functional segments by sphincters and valves.

the enteric nervous system. On the other hand, the external anal sphincter can be controlled voluntarily, a skill learned during toilet training in infancy and sometimes used to comic effect to selectively expel flatus. The esophageal sphincters are regulated by the central nervous system.

ORGANS AND SYSTEMS INVOLVED IN THE RESPONSE TO A MEAL

Several intestinal and extraintestinal tissues cooperate to respond appropriately to the ingestion of a meal. Collectively, these tissues can sense, signal, and respond to meal ingestion with altered function (Chapter 2). Moreover, the tissues and their functions are interactive and highly efficient, and redundancy exists among the majority of GI-regulatory mechanisms. We turn now to a tour along the length of the gastrointestinal system, introducing the functions of each segment of the gastrointestinal tract and the structural features that underlie these. More detailed discussions of the function of each segment will be provided in subsequent chapters. Specific features of the circulatory systems designed to carry absorbed nutrients away from the gut, and the neuromuscular system that provides for motility and regulation, will also be considered.

Oral Cavity and Esophagus

The oral cavity is concerned with initial intake of food and with shaping and lubricating a smooth bolus of ingested materials such that it can be swallowed. The teeth, via the action of chewing, reduce large portions of food into sizes suitable for passage through the esophagus. Salivary glands, which drain into the oral cavity at several points, supply an aqueous environment and also mucus that coats the surface of the bolus and thus aids in swallowing. This also minimizes the risk that small particles will be aspirated into the lungs. The environment of the oral cavity also contributes to the control of food intake, since the aqueous environment permits diffusion of taste molecules to specific receptors on the tongue that relay information centrally as to whether the meal is palatable. Salivary secretions also reduce microbial contamination of the oral cavity.

The structures of the oral cavity are also intimately involved in swallowing. As is the case throughout the gastrointestinal tract, the contents of the oral cavity are moved from one location to another by the formation of a pressure gradient. At the beginning of a swallow, the tip of the tongue separates a bolus from the bulk of the contents of the mouth and moves it backwards toward the oropharyngeal cavity. The palate is moved upwards to seal off the nasal cavity, which, under normal circumstances, prevents pressure generated in the mouth from being dissipated through the nose. With the mouth shut, the tongue propels the bolus backwards into the oropharynx, with the larynx rising and the glottis closing to seal off the laryngeal airway. The bolus also forces the epiglottis backwards to act as a lid over the closed glottis, and the bolus is then forced into the proximal esophagus. After the bolus moves below the level of the clavicle, the larynx descends, the glottis opens, and respiration resumes.

The esophagus is a muscular tube that serves to transfer the bolus from the mouth to the stomach. The upper third of the esophagus is surrounded by striated muscle overlaid by a thick submucous elastic and collagenous network. This network contributes to obliteration of the esophageal lumen via mucosal folds, until these are smoothed out by the passage of a swallowed bolus. The muscle then transitions to smooth muscle that works in concert with the swallowing reflex to propel the bolus toward the stomach.

This function of the esophagus is independent of gravity. A food bolus can be moved from the mouth to the stomach even if a person is standing on his or her head. Toward the lowest portion of the esophagus, the smooth muscle gradually thickens and interacts with neurogenic and hormonal factors, as well as the diaphragm, to serve functionally as the lower esophageal sphincter. The raised pressure in this final segment of the esophagus prevents excessive backflow, or reflux, of the gastric contents into the esophageal lumen. Failure of this process leads to gastroesophageal reflux disease, or GERD. The refluxed contents of the stomach can cause damage to the esophageal epithelium because it is not designed to withstand prolonged exposure to the injurious mixture of acid and pepsin (see below). GERD is one of the most common gastrointestinal disorders.

Stomach

The stomach is a muscular bag that functions primarily as a reservoir, controlling the rate of delivery of the meal to more distal segments of the gastrointestinal tract. It also participates in digestion and partially sterilizes the meal, although these functions are dispensable. Anatomically, it is divided into three regions, the cardia (which overlaps with the lower esophageal sphincter), fundus, and antrum, each with distinctive structures that subserve specific functions (Figure 1–5).

The cardia begins at the Z line, where the squamous epithelium of the esophagus gives way to the columnar epithelium of the remainder of the gastrointestinal tract; it mostly secretes mucus and bicarbonate to protect the surface from the corrosive gastric contents. The surface of the stomach overall is thrown into folds known as rugae, which can readily be observed by the naked eye. At the microscopic level, the surface area of the stomach is further amplified by pits, which represent the entrances to deep gastric glands. The specific structures of these glands differ in the three regions of the stomach; they are shallowest in the cardia, intermediate (though with deep pits) in the antrum, and deepest in the fundus.

The fundic (or gastric) glands are further specialized in that they contain specific secretory cells that produce the characteristic components of gastric juice—acid and pepsin—which are products of parietal and chief cells, respectively. Thus, the predominant function of the fundus is to serve as a secretory region. On the other hand, the antrum (also referred to as the pyloric zone) engages in extensive motility patterns, mixing the gastric contents and grinding and sieving ingested particles. Eventually, the meal is gradually emptied into the small intestine via the pylorus.

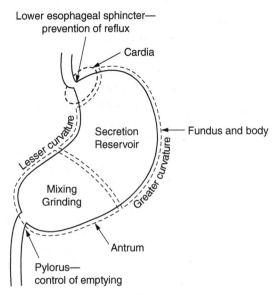

Figure 1–5. Functional regions of the stomach.

The motility functions of the stomach include one important additional feature known as receptive relaxation. This provides for relaxation of the gastric musculature as its walls are stretched during filling, ensuring that the pressure in the stomach does not increase significantly as its volume expands. This response is vital to ensure that the meal is not forced back into the esophagus under normal conditions, and is integral to the reservoir function of the stomach. The stomach is not essential to digestion of a mixed meal and large portions can be resected, if necessary due to disease, or as a way to counteract morbid obesity. However, an individual lacking a significant portion of their stomach will not be able to tolerate large meals due to the loss of this reservoir function.

Duodenal Cluster Unit

The first segment of the small intestine, approximately 12 in. in length, is referred to as the duodenum, and begins as a bulb-shaped structure immediately distal to the pylorus. Together with the pancreas and biliary system, the proximal duodenum makes up the duodenal cluster unit, with the tissues arising from a common embryological progenitor. This segment of the gastrointestinal system acts as a critical regulator of digestion and absorption. Endocrine cells within the wall of the duodenum, as well as chemo- and mechanosensitive nerve endings, monitor the characteristics of the luminal contents and emit signals that coordinate the functions of more distant regions of the gastrointestinal tract to ready them for the arrival of the meal, or to retard the flow of contents from the stomach. As noted previously, the products of the exocrine pancreas and bile from the gallbladder eventually drain into the duodenum with egress of secretions controlled by opening of the sphincter of Oddi.

Small Intestine

The remainder of the small intestine consists of the jejunum and ileum. The jejunum serves as the site of absorption of the majority of nutrients in the healthy individual, and has a markedly amplified surface area due to the presence of surface folds (known as folds of Kerckring) and tall, slender villi. The surface area of the jejunum is also amplified considerably by an abundance of microvilli on the apical surface of villus epithelial cells. More distally, the ileum has fewer folds and shorter, sparser villi, and is less actively engaged in nutrient absorption with the exception of that of specific solutes such as conjugated bile acids, which are exclusively salvaged by transporters expressed in the terminal ileum. However, if jejunal absorption is impaired, such as in the setting of maldigestion, the ileum represents an anatomic reserve that can be called on for absorption. As a result, the small intestine has excess capacity for both digestion and absorption, and thus malabsorption is a relatively rare event.

Colon

The colon, or large intestine, serves as a reservoir for the storage of wastes and indigestible materials prior to their elimination by defecation. In general, the

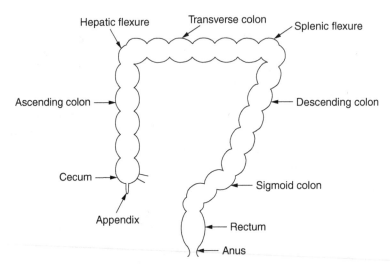

Figure 1–6. Anatomy of the large intestine comprising the cecum, colon, rectum, and anus.

colonic epithelial cells (or colonocytes) do not express absorptive transporters for conventional nutrients such as monosaccharides, peptides, amino acids and vitamins but may be actively involved in the uptake of other luminal constituents. As its name implies, the large intestine is of a considerably larger diameter than the small intestine, with a thicker wall and folds known as haustrae.

The colon is divided into several regions: the ascending, transverse, descending, and sigmoid colon, which are defined anatomically but may also subserve different functions (Figure 1–6). For example, in the ascending and transverse colon, there is an emphasis on reclamation of fluid remaining from the process of digestion as well as salvage of other dietary by-products, such as absorption of short-chain fatty acids produced by the bacterial fermentation of carbohydrates, including dietary fiber. The more distal parts of the colon, on the other hand, are mostly a region through which the fecal material is propelled without major modifications of its composition. Some luminal solutes, such as bile acids and bilirubin, are modified in the colon by bacterial metabolism. In fact, the colon contains an abundant commensal ecosystem comprised primarily of anaerobic bacteria in a healthy individual, and these symbionts are important contributors to whole-body nutritional status. Each individual develops a characteristic microbiome, which may account for variable propensity to obesity.

The smooth muscle of the colon, under the influence of the enteric nervous system, produces mixing motility patterns that maximize the time for reabsorption of fluid and other useful solutes. The descending colon, on the other hand, serves primarily as the storage reservoir for fecal wastes. When these are propelled through the sigmoid colon into the rectum via mass peristalsis (usually in response to reflexes such as the orthocolic reflex, on arising, or the gastrocolic reflex, initiated by signals from food in the stomach), stretch receptors initiate a reflex relaxation of the internal anal sphincter and also send afferent impulses to the central nervous system indicating a need to defecate. Defecation can, however, be postponed to a convenient time by contraction of the external anal sphincter and levator ani muscles, which are under voluntary control. Compared with other segments of the gastrointestinal tract, propulsive motility in the colon is relatively sluggish until a reflex sufficient to trigger mass peristalsis and defecation occurs, and components of the colonic contents may remain in the colon for days.

Splanchnic Circulation and Lymphatics

Blood supply to the intestines is vitally important in providing oxygen to the gut, and for carrying away absorbed nutrients, particularly those that are water-soluble, to sites of usage elsewhere in the body. Conversely, most lipids enter the lymphatic drainage of the gut initially because they are packaged in particles (chylomicrons) too large to pass through the junctions linking capillary endothelial cells. Lymph fluid containing absorbed lipids is thereafter emptied into the bloodstream via the thoracic duct.

The circulation of the gastrointestinal tract is unusual because of its anatomy (Figure 1–7). Unlike venous blood draining from other organs of the body, which returns directly to the heart, blood flow from the intestine flows first to the liver via the portal vein. Conversely, the liver is unusual in receiving a considerable portion of its blood supply not as arterial blood, but as blood that has first perfused the splanchnic capillary beds of the intestine. This anatomic arrangement of the

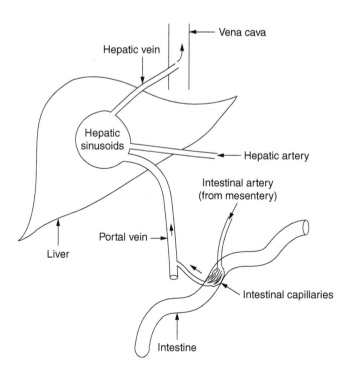

Figure 1–7. Schematic anatomy of the splanchnic circulation.

intestinal and hepatic blood supply ensures that substances absorbed from the gut flow first to the hepatocytes where they can be detoxified if needed. This line of defense may also reduce the bioavailability of orally-administered drugs if they are susceptible to a high degree of such "first-pass" metabolism. Any particulates are also filtered from the blood by specialized liver macrophages known as Kupffer cells.

Gastrointestinal blood flow is also notable for the range of its dynamic regulation. Even in the fasting state, the splanchnic circulation receives blood flow (25% of cardiac output) that is disproportionate to the mass of the organs perfused (5%). Under these circumstances, the liver receives approximately 65% of its blood flow via the portal system. In the post-prandial period, furthermore, blood is diverted from the skeletal muscles and other body systems and blood flow through specific vessels perfusing the intestine can increase more than fivefold. Under these circumstances, the liver receives more than 85% of its blood supply via the portal system. These dramatic changes in blood distribution are produced by hormonal and neurogenic stimuli occurring secondary to the ingestion of a meal. They are also the origin of warnings from mothers to their children about the dangers of swimming immediately after lunch, and perhaps the sleepiness that sometimes occurs in the post-prandial period. On the other hand, redistribution of blood flow to the muscles during intense, prolonged exercise (such as running a marathon) can result in intestinal ischemia and injury.

Neuromuscular System

The motility functions of the gastrointestinal tract are essential to propel ingested nutrients along the length of the alimentary canal, and also to control the length of time available for digestion and absorption. As outlined above, the motility patterns of the intestine are brought about by the integrated control of the contraction and relaxation of the circular and longitudinal muscle layers, under the influence of both hormones released in response to the meal, as well as nervous impulses supplied by the autonomic and enteric nervous systems.

Extrinsic innervation of the gut occurs via both sympathetic and (more prominently) parasympathetic pathways. Sympathetic innervation primarily involves postganglionic adrenergic nerves originating in prevertebral ganglia. These nerves synapse mainly with others in the enteric nervous system, discussed later, but a few may directly innervate secretory cells in various glands (especially the salivary glands) or the smooth muscle cells of blood vessels, leading to vasoconstriction. Parasympathetic innervation, on the other hand, is via preganglionic nerve fibers that synapse with cell bodies in the myenteric plexus. Many of these fibers are contained in the vagus nerve, which follows blood vessels to innervate the stomach, small intestine, cecum, and ascending and transverse colon. The remainder of the colon receives parasympathetic innervation via the pelvic nerve.

Many of the parasympathetic nerves that end in the myenteric plexus are cholinergic and excitatory, but there is also substantial evidence for nerves that mediate their effects via other non-adrenergic, non-cholinergic neurotransmitters, and which are inhibitory. These latter nerves, for example, may mediate relaxation of the internal anal sphincter and pylorus.

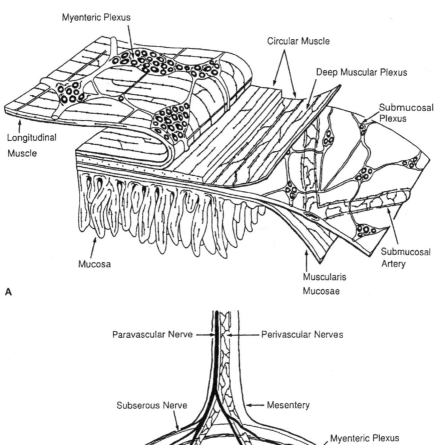

Myenteric Plexus

Circular Muscle

Deep Muscular Plexus

Submucosal
Plexus

Longitudinal
Muscle

Mucosa

Submucosal
Artery

Muscularis
Mucosae

A

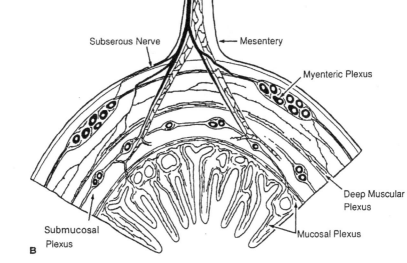

Paravascular Nerve

Perivascular Nerves

Subserous Nerve

Mesentery

Myenteric Plexus

Deep Muscular
Plexus

Submucosal
Plexus

Mucosal Plexus

B

Figure 1–8. Plexuses of the enteric nervous system and their relationship to the other functional layers of the gut wall. Panel **A** shows intact tissue, while Panel **B** is a transverse section. (Adapted from Furness and Costa, *Neuroscience* 5:1–20, copyright Pergamon Press, 1980, and used with permission.)

The most striking aspect of intestinal neurophysiology, however, is the *enteric nervous system* contained wholly within the gut wall. The enteric nervous system consists predominantly of neurons with their cell bodies in the myenteric or submucosal plexuses, and is comprised of several morphologically distinct classes of neurons, with the different morphologies thought to correspond to different chemical "coding," that is to say, a different complement of neurotransmitters. The anatomy of the enteric nervous system and its relationship to other gut structures is shown in Figure 1–8.

The enteric nervous system serves as a relay station to conduct and interpret information supplied by extrinsic autonomic afferents carrying impulses that originate centrally, and also to pass information from sensory efferents that have their endings in the epithelium or smooth muscle. Thus, the enteric nervous system controls the activity of secretomotor neurons that ultimately cause changes in motility and/or secretory behavior of the intestine and organs draining into it in response to centrally-mediated signals. The enteric nervous system can also function autonomously and mediate reflexes that do not involve the central nervous system at all. It is thought that many of the stereotypic motility functions of the gut arise predominantly from such intrinsic regulatory pathways. The autonomy of the enteric nervous system in many situations has led some to refer to it as the "little brain."

KEY CONCEPTS

 The GI system fulfills the functions of digestion and absorption, excretion, and host defense.

 The GI system represents a complex and cooperative network of various organs.

 Cellular specialization underlies the various functional responses required of the GI system.

 The GI system is highly efficient, interactive, and redundant.

 The circulatory features of the GI tract and liver set them apart from other organs.

 Many functions of the GI tract are governed by the enteric nervous system, or the "little brain".

STUDY QUESTIONS

1–1. A patient who is being treated for long-standing osteoarthritis with a non-steroidal anti-inflammatory drug (NSAID) also takes a daily proton pump inhibitor to reduce the toxicity of her NSAID treatment. She comes to her physician complaining of recurrent bouts of diarrhea during a series of business trips to Guatemala. The apparent increase in her sensitivity to infections acquired by the oral route is most likely due to reduced secretory function of which of the following?

A. Stomach

B. Pancreas

C. Gallbladder

D. Salivary glands

E. Lymphocytes

1–2. A medical student is reviewing histological sections of the human small intestine using a light microscope. She notes that the apical surface of the enterocytes appears "fuzzy." This is ascribable to which ultrastructural feature(s) of the epithelial cells?

A. Tight junctions

B. Microvilli

C. Adherens junctions

D. Lateral cell spaces

E. Mitochondria

1–3. A patient receiving chemotherapy for a prostate tumor develops severe abdominal pain and diarrhea. Following the treatment, his gastrointestinal symptoms subside. The resolution of his symptoms most likely reflects repair of which of the following cell types?

A. Lymphocytes

B. Smooth muscle

C. Epithelial cells

D. Enteric nerves

E. Paneth cells

1–4. A patient being treated for depression comes to his physician complaining that he has difficulty swallowing his food. He also reports that he has recently been treated by his dentist for several cavities and that he has a chronic feeling of "heartburn." The patient's symptoms can most likely be ascribed to an effect of his anti-depressant medication on secretion of which of the following?

A. Pancreatic juice

B. Gastric juice

C. Bile

D. Immunoglobulin A

E. Saliva

1-5.   *A pharmaceutical scientist trying to develop a new drug for hypertension gives a candidate compound orally to rats. He determines that the drug is adequately absorbed from the intestine, but levels in the systemic circulation remain below the therapeutic range. The drug is most likely metabolized by which organ?*

   A. *Small intestine*

   B. *Kidney*

   C. *Lung*

   D. *Liver*

   E. *Spleen*

SUGGESTED READINGS

Poole DP, Furness JB. Enteric nervous system structure and neurochemistry related to function and neuropathology. In: Johnson LR, Ghishan FK, Kaunitz JD, Merchant JL, Said HM, Wood JD, eds. *Physiology of the Gastrointestinal Tract*. 5th ed. San Diego: Academic Press; 2012:557–581.

Turner JR, Madara JL. Epithelia: biologic principles of organization. In: Yamada T, Alpers DH, Kalloo AN, Kaplowitz N, Owyang C, Powell DW, eds. *Textbook of Gastroenterology*. 5th ed. Chichester: Wiley-Blackwell; 2009:151–165.

Makhlouf GM, Murthy KS. Smooth muscle of the gut. In: Yamada T, Alpers DH, Kalloo AN, Kaplowitz N, Owyang C, Powell DW, eds. *Textbook of Gastroenterology*. 5th ed. Chichester: Wiley-Blackwell; 2009:103–132.

Medema JP, Vermeulen L. Microenvironmental regulation of stem cells in intestinal homeostasis and cancer. *Nature*. 2011;474:318–326.

Neurohumoral Regulation of Gastrointestinal Function

2

OBJECTIVES

- ▶ *Understand the integrated response to a meal and the need for mechanisms that regulate the function of the gastrointestinal tract as a whole*
- ▶ *Describe modes of communication in the gastrointestinal tract*
  - ▶ General features of neurohumoral regulation
  - ▶ Characteristics of chemical signals
- ▶ *Understand principles of endocrine regulation*
  - ▶ Definition of a hormone
  - ▶ Identify established and candidate GI hormones and their mechanisms of action
- ▶ *Understand the design of the enteric nervous system and neurocrine regulation*
- ▶ *Describe immune and paracrine regulatory pathways*
- ▶ *Understand how the GI tract and the brain cooperate to regulate food intake*

REQUIREMENT FOR INTEGRATED REGULATION

As we have learned from the previous chapter, the gastrointestinal system subserves several functions that are critical for whole-body homeostasis. For nutrient assimilation in particular, specific tissues and regions of the gastrointestinal system must sense, signal, and respond to the ingestion of a meal (Figure 2–1). By cooperating with the central nervous system, the gastrointestinal system is also intimately involved in the control of food intake. To conduct the business of the gastrointestinal system most efficiently, the various segments must communicate. Thus, the activities of the gastrointestinal tract and the organs that drain into it are coordinated temporally via the action of a series of chemical mediators, with the system being referred to collectively as *neurohumoral regulation*, implying the combined action of soluble and neuronal pathways. The integrated regulation of gastrointestinal function underlies the efficiency of the system as described in Chapter 1, and its ability to provide for the effective uptake of nutrients even when they are in short supply.

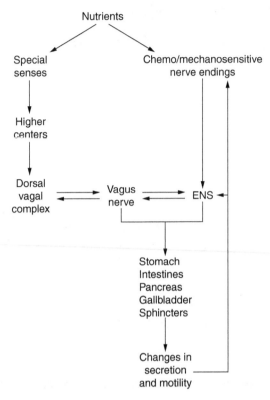

Figure 2-1. Overview of neural control of the gastrointestinal system. Nutrients activate both special senses (smell, taste) as well as specific sensory nerve endings that exist within the wall of the gut. These responses are conveyed via the autonomic nervous system and enteric nervous system (ENS) to alter the function of the gastrointestinal tract and organs draining into it, resulting in changes in secretion and motility. Such functional changes may additionally feedback on neural control to allow for appropriate homeostasis of the system.

COMMUNICATION IN THE GI TRACT

General Features of Neurohumoral Regulation

The gastrointestinal tract stretches from mouth to anus, implying that communication that rests simply on diffusion of locally released signals will not be adequate for the timely transfer of information from one segment to another. Likewise, the gastrointestinal tract also needs to communicate its status to organs that drain into it, such as the pancreas and gallbladder, and to distant organs, such as the brain. Thus, the system has evolved mechanisms for communication over significant distances, although local messengers also play a role in fine-tuning information delivery or, in some cases, amplifying or antagonizing it. Overall, information is carried between the various sites by chemical entities possessing specific physicochemical properties. Another general principle underlying communication in the gastrointestinal system is that of functional redundancy. Several different mediators may often produce the same physiologic response, and single mediators may alter the function of more than one system.

CHARACTERISTICS OF CHEMICAL SIGNALS

Neurohumoral regulation is effected by several classes of chemical messengers—peptides, derivatives of amino acids such as histamine and nitric oxide, small molecule neurotransmitters, and lipid mediators such as prostaglandins and steroids. The gastrointestinal tract is a rich source of unique peptides that are synthesized by enteroendocrine cells as well as packaged in nerve endings. In fact, all five of the known gastrointestinal hormones are peptides, but it does not always follow that any gastrointestinal peptide is a hormone. Major gastrointestinal messengers that have definitely been assigned physiologic roles are listed in Table 2–1.

Overproduction of gastrointestinal messengers and their release in an uncontrolled fashion can lead to disease states. For example, Zollinger–Ellison syndrome is the result of a secreting gastrinoma, and results in pathologic increases in gastric acid secretion among other symptoms. Likewise, carcinoid tumors overproduce the paracrine/neurotransmitter 5-hydroxytryptamine (5-HT), also known as serotonin.

Finally, the kinetics of information transfer by any given molecule will also depend on its stability and/or the rate of its reuptake. Several of the gastrointestinal messengers that are designed to act over long distances incorporate structural features that retard their metabolism. Conversely, mediators that act only in the

Table 2–1. Major physiologic neurohumoral regulators of gastrointestinal function

Endocrine	Neurocrine	Paracrine	Immune/ Juxtacrine
Gastrin	Acetylcholine	Histamine	Histamine
Cholecystokinin	Vasoactive intestinal polypeptide	Prostaglandins	Cytokines
Motilin	Substance P	Somatostatin	Reactive oxygen species
Secretin	Nitric oxide	5-hydroxytryptamine	Adenosine
Glucose-dependent insulinotropic peptide	Cholecystokinin		
Ghrelin	5-hydroxytryptamine		
	Somatostatin		
	Calcitonin-gene related peptide		

immediate vicinity of their site of release are rapidly degraded and/or actively taken back into nerves for repackaging into secretory vesicles.

GENERAL MECHANISMS OF ACTION

Hydrophobic messengers, such as steroids and nitric oxide, can readily traverse cell membranes and thus can interact with intracellular targets. Hydrophilic messengers, such as peptides, many small molecule neurotransmitters, and prostaglandins, on the other hand, use classical receptor/second messenger pathways to mediate their effects.

The majority of the hydrophilic messengers that are relevant to gastrointestinal physiology bind to receptors linked to G-proteins, with consequent increases in intracellular calcium or cyclic AMP (cAMP). The use of different second messengers also provides for potentiation, or synergism, when a given cell is acted on by more than one mediator simultaneously. An example of such synergy is found in the control of acid secretion by gastric parietal cells, as will be covered in detail in Chapter 3. And at least one chemical mediator in the gastrointestinal tract, somatostatin, acts at receptors linked to inhibitory G proteins. These can antagonize increases in cAMP produced by other mediators.

Specific Modes of Communication

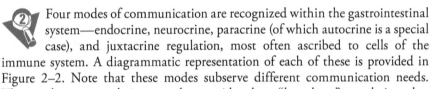

Four modes of communication are recognized within the gastrointestinal system—endocrine, neurocrine, paracrine (of which autocrine is a special case), and juxtacrine regulation, most often ascribed to cells of the immune system. A diagrammatic representation of each of these is provided in Figure 2–2. Note that these modes subserve different communication needs. Thus endocrine regulation can be considered as "broadcast" regulation that impacts the function of several systems simultaneously. The specificity of this mode of communication is determined by the distribution of receptors for the endocrine messenger, or, to carry forward the broadcast analogy, to those who have their radio receiver tuned in to the specific station carrying the data.

Neurocrine communication, on the other hand, can also transmit information over long distances, but is analogous to communication by telephone rather than radio; the specificity is determined by spatial delimitation of the site(s) at which the message is ultimately delivered, based on synapses at target cells. Of course, the target cell is also required to bear an appropriate receptor for the neurotransmitter that is delivered, but in general, nerves do not innervate cells that are unable to respond to the former's messengers.

Finally, paracrine and immune regulation are usually only effective in the immediate vicinity of mediator release. Thus, these can be considered as modes of communication that are analogous to live conversations between a few individuals.

ENDOCRINE COMMUNICATION

Because of its ability to regulate multiple sites in an essentially simultaneous fashion, endocrine regulation is critical to the integrated function of the gastrointestinal tract and organs that drain into it in response to a meal. The intestine is

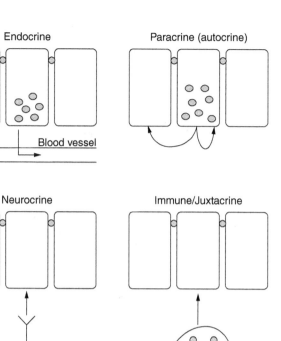

Figure 2–2. Modes of communication in the gastrointestinal system. Information is conveyed by endocrine, neurocrine, paracrine, and immune/juxtacrine routes. Autocrine regulation is a special class of paracrine regulation.

extremely well supplied with cell types responsible for the synthesis and release of endocrine mediators, known as *hormones*; in fact, if all of the endocrine cells within the gut were assembled as a single structure, they would make up the largest endocrine organ in the body. The gastrointestinal hormones were also the first to be discovered, with the identification of secretin by Bayliss and Starling in 1902. We define gastrointestinal hormone here as an endocrine messenger that both is released by and acts upon the gastrointestinal system. However, the intestine also produces other hormones with targets outside the GI system. An example is ghrelin, a stomach peptide that affects feeding behavior via the central nervous system.

Endocrine hormones are packaged within the secretory granules of distinct cell types within the wall of the intestinal tract, and released in response to nervous activity as well as chemical and mechanical signals coincident with food ingestion. The endocrine cells of the gut have been identified with letters to denote their hormonal contents; gastrin, secretin, cholecystokinin, glucose-dependent insulinotropic peptide (also referred to as gastric inhibitory peptide, or GIP), motilin and ghrelin are stored in G, S, I, K, M (or Mo) and A/X cells, respectively. Some endocrine cells may have processes that contact the luminal contents and are activated to release their mediators in response to specific features of luminal composition, such as acidity, osmolarity, or nutrients such as amino acids and free fatty acids. Direct neural control of hormone release by neurotransmitters is also important in some cases. In other cases, hormone release in response to changes in luminal composition can also be activated by a reflex arc that first involves activation of a sensory enteric nerve ending, with subsequent release of specific neurotransmitters close to the surface of the endocrine cell to stimulate exocytosis. Yet other endocrine cells are designed to respond to conditions existing in the interstitium.

Endocrine cells that contact the lumen are referred to as having an "open" morphology; those that do not are called closed. An electron micrograph showing a typical open enteroendocrine cell is shown in Figure 2–3. Note how the apical pole of the cell is in contact with the lumen, and how the secretory granules are toward the base of the cell, strategically located to release their contents into the lamina propria and thence into the bloodstream.

The hormones that are released from these endocrine cells diffuse into the lamina propria and thence into the portal circulation. From there, they travel to target organs and modify secretion, motility, and cell growth. Most hormones signal to segments of the gastrointestinal tract that are distal to their site of release, but feedback signaling can also occur. For example, cholecystokinin, released from the duodenal mucosa, can signal back to the stomach to retard its emptying. Some hormones additionally act by binding to receptors on nerves such as, for example, on vagal afferents. In this way, their action can be amplified by the simultaneous recruitment of neurocrine regulation as discussed below.

All of the currently known GI hormones are peptides, but not all peptides isolated from the gastrointestinal tract are hormones. In fact, the GI tract is a very rich source of biologically active peptides, comparable to the central nervous system, but thus far, only five have fulfilled all of the criteria to be considered a hormone, despite intense scrutiny. The criteria that must be fulfilled to define a hormone are listed in Table 2–2. Of these, the structural criterion seems relatively trivial in the days of automated peptide sequencers and synthesizers, but represented a technical *tour de force* in the early twentieth century when most of the GI hormones were discovered. Other gastrointestinal peptides that have not yet fulfilled all of the criteria listed, yet which are suspected to have physiologic functions following their release, are considered to be "candidate hormones" and several have attracted the interest of the pharmaceutical industry on the basis of their specific properties, as will be discussed below.

The GI hormones are synthesized in various segments of the gastrointestinal tract (Figure 2–4), but only gastrin appears to be present in the stomach of healthy individuals. The stomach is also the major source of ghrelin, contributing about two-thirds of the body's production of this hormone. The remaining hormones are present in greatest amounts in the duodenum and jejunum, with tapering

Table 2–2. Criteria that define a gastrointestinal hormone

A physiologic event in one segment of the gastrointestinal system alters the activity of another

The effect persists after neural connections have been severed

A substance isolated from the site of stimulation must reproduce the effect of the physiologic stimulus following injection into the bloodstream at levels seen physiologically

The hormone must be identified chemically and its structure confirmed by synthesis

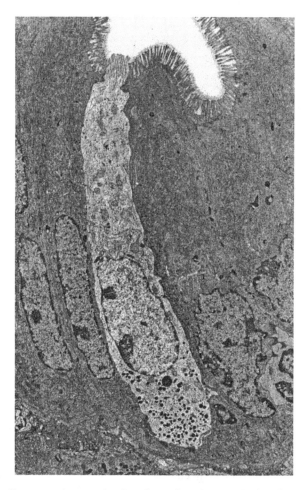

Figure 2–3. Electron micrograph of an "open" gastrointestinal endocrine cell in the human jejunum amid several enterocytes. Secretory granules are localized to the basolateral pole of the endocrine cell. (Reproduced with permission from Solcia et al. Endocrine cells of the digestive system. In: Johnson LR, ed. *Physiology of the Gastrointestinal Tract.* 2nd ed. New York: Raven Press; 1987.)

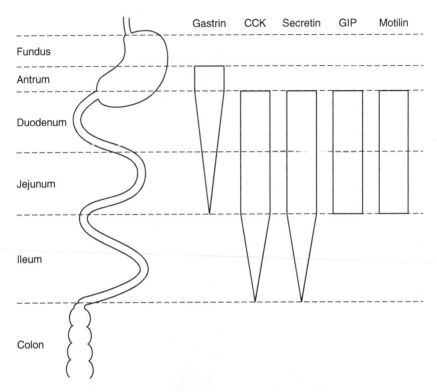

Figure 2-4. Sites of production of the five gastrointestinal hormones along the length of the gastrointestinal tract. The width of the bars reflects the relative abundance at each location.

expression of cholecystokinin and secretin into the ileum in addition. However, under normal conditions, most of the release of gastrin occurs in the stomach, and of the other hormones in the duodenum and, to some extent, the jejunum. Ileal expression of some hormones, therefore, represents another example of the "reserve capacity" of the intestine that can be called upon to regulate gastrointestinal function if required. Further, in health, there appears to be little if any expression of gastrointestinal hormones in the colon. However, because the endocrine cells that secrete these peptides arise from multipotential stem cells in the gut epithelium, when colonic epithelial tumors also arise, sometimes one or more gastrointestinal hormones are aberrantly expressed. This may have clinical significance in that several of the GI hormones are known to have trophic or growth-promoting effects, and thus may contribute to the unregulated growth of some colon cancers in an autocrine fashion.

NEUROCRINE REGULATION

As described above, neurocrine regulation of gastrointestinal function is mediated by specific nerve endings of both the enteric and central nervous system.

Neurotransmitters stored in these nerve endings are released on receipt of an electrical signal, and diffuse across synaptic clefts to alter secretomotor function in the gastrointestinal tract as well as in related organs, such as the pancreas and biliary system. These neurotransmitters thus provide information exchange that is exquisitely spatially specific, and because of their relative instability, there is very little spillover of information conveyed by neurotransmitters even to immediately adjacent sites, and certainly essentially none is conveyed via the circulation.

PARACRINE COMMUNICATION

Some substances are designed to act only in the immediate area of their release, and yet are released from cell types other than nerves. Communication via such pathways is referred to as *paracrine*, and provides an important additional layer of control for gastrointestinal secretomotor function, particularly in response to changes in local conditions. Paracrine regulators, like neurotransmitters, are readily metabolized or retaken up to limit the duration of their activity. A special case of paracrine regulation is labeled autocrine, which involves the release of a substance that then acts back on its cell of origin. Intestinal epithelial cells may engage in autocrine regulation since they are capable of releasing growth factors that influence their proliferation and/or migration along the crypt–villus axis.

IMMUNE COMMUNICATION

A final class of communication in the gastrointestinal system that has emerged in importance in recent years is that mediated by the release of substances by cells of the mucosal immune system. These cells are activated by antigenic substances or products of pathogenic microorganisms, and release a variety of chemical mediators including amines (such as histamine), prostaglandins, and cytokines. Immune regulation is important in changing the function of the secretomotor systems of the gastrointestinal tract during times of threat, for example, invasion of the mucosa by pathogens. Immune mediators may also be responsible for intestinal dysfunction in the setting of inflammation or conditions such as food allergies, where inappropriate immune responses to substances that would normally be innocuous may be deleterious for the host. Finally, immune cell types, especially mast cells, which are abundant in the lamina propria, may be activated by endogenous substances such as bile acids in the lumen, or by specific peptide neurotransmitters. Thus, there is at least the potential that immune regulation contributes to gastrointestinal regulation not only under pathological circumstances, but also in response to normal physiologic events.

PRINCIPLES OF ENDOCRINE REGULATION

Established GI Hormones

As noted above, five gastrointestinal peptides have fulfilled the criteria to be named as gastrointestinal hormones (Table 2–3). These fall into three groups based on structural and signaling similarities, as described in this section.

Table 2–3. Factors influencing release of gastrointestinal hormones

	Gastrin	CCK	Secretin	GIP	Motilin
Proteins/amino acids	↑	↑	↔	↔	↓*
Fatty acids	↔	↑	↑	↑	↓*
Glucose	↔	↔	↔	↑	↓*
Acid	↓	↔	↑	↔	↔
Neural stimulation	↑	↑	↔	↔	↑
Stretch	↑	↔	↔	↔	↔
Luminal peptide releasing factors	↔	↑	↔	↔	↔

*Motilin release is reduced by feeding, but the precise mechanism is unclear.

GASTRIN/CCK FAMILY

Gastrin and cholecystokinin (CCK) occur in the gastrointestinal system in various forms, and are structurally related peptides that also bind to closely related receptors known as CCK_1 and CCK_2 receptors. In common with most other biologically-active peptides, both gastrin and CCK are synthesized initially as long propeptides that are sequentially cleaved to generate active forms, which are then stored for release in response to physiologic stimuli. The intermediate products may share biological activity with the final cleavage products but may possess different abilities to be transported widely throughout the body. For example, short forms of CCK are effectively cleared from the portal circulation during a first pass through the liver, whereas longer forms may persist to enter the systemic circulation and thus affect the function of sites more distant from the gut. However, all forms of both CCK and gastrin share a common C-terminal pentapeptide, which is amidated as a final step in processing in I and G cells, respectively.

Amidation is believed to increase the stability of these structures by blocking carboxypeptidase activity. The structure of the C-termini of gastrin and CCK is shown in Figure 2–5. The major biologically active forms of gastrin are 17- and 34-amino acid peptides, which may or may not be sulfated; this post-translational modification is of unknown function, because sulfated and unsulfated forms appear to have equivalent stability and potency. However, G-34 has a longer half-life than G-17, so despite the fact that greater quantities of the fully-processed G-17 are released from G cells in response to a meal, G-34 is the predominant form that can be measured in the circulation. CCK also occurs as a family of peptides of decreasing length (CCK-58, CCK-39, CCK-33, and CCK-8), but unlike gastrin, all of the released peptides are sulfated. The sulfation of CCK peptides appears critical for their high-affinity interaction with their receptor, as will be discussed in greater detail below.

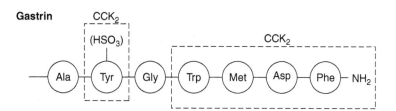

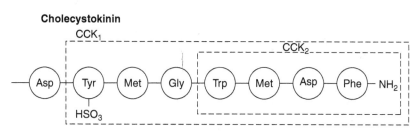

Figure 2–5. Comparison of the C-termini of gastrin and cholecystokinin. Note the C-terminal amidation. The boxes denote the structural features that define enhanced affinity for CCK$_1$ versus CCK$_2$ receptors.

As for gastrin, the shortest form of CCK, CCK-8, is more rapidly cleared from the circulation and indeed the majority is probably lost after a single pass through the liver. CCK is also interesting for the diversity of its biological effects. Although it was named for its ability to contract (-kinin) the gallbladder (cholecysto-), it affects the function of numerous other tissues and cell types, and can be considered as the master regulator of the duodenal cluster unit. CCK has also been shown to signal the central nervous system via vagal afferents to indicate satiety, or fullness, resulting in considerable efforts to discover small molecule analogues that could be used as appetite suppressants to treat obesity (although as yet without success). CCK and gastrin bind to two closely related receptors—CCK$_1$ and CCK$_2$—that are G-protein coupled receptors that signal via increases in cytoplasmic calcium. Both the receptors and their ligands are believed to have each developed from single ancestral precursors via gene duplications, yet it is unknown whether the receptors or ligands diverged earliest. The specificity of CCK and gastrin for these receptors is defined by their structures. Activity at CCK$_1$ receptors requires a sulfated tyrosine at position 7 of the C-terminus, as well as the amidated C-terminus heptapeptide, meaning that only the various CCK peptides possess significant activity at these receptors. Gastrin binds with approximately 1000-fold lower affinity. CCK$_2$ receptors, on the other hand, have a broader specificity with gastrin and CCK being essentially equipotent, because the receptor requires only the amidated C-terminus tetrapeptide for high-affinity binding and activation. Nevertheless, they respond predominantly to gastrin *in vivo* under normal conditions, since this hormone circulates at levels approximately five to tenfold higher than those of CCK.

SECRETIN FAMILY

The secretin family of gastrointestinal peptides includes not only the GI hormones, secretin and GIP, but also a systemic hormone, glucagon, as well as a neuropeptide, vasoactive intestinal polypeptide. The latter is an important inhibitory neurotransmitter causing relaxation of the gastrointestinal smooth muscle to permit specific motility responses, such as peristalsis. Several other systemic peptides also fall into this group, but are not believed to be directly relevant for gastrointestinal physiology and so will not be discussed further here.

Although there is some homology among the amino-acid sequences of these peptides, each is believed to bind to distinct receptors on target cells. Unlike the close relationship and overlapping specificities of CCK_1 and CCK_2 receptors, the receptors for secretin family members do not appear to recognize a short peptide sequence. While the N-terminus of each peptide is most critical for receptor binding, the three-dimensional structure of these peptide ligands also plays a major role in defining specificity. All of the receptors for these family members, however, share the common property of signaling predominantly via associated G proteins of the G_s class, and thus via increasing intracellular levels of cAMP.

Secretin itself is a 27 amino acid peptide that holds the distinction of being the first of any of the hormones in the body to be identified, including classical hormones like insulin. Secretin is synthesized by S cells located predominantly in the duodenal mucosa, and is released in response to a low intraluminal pH. This accords nicely with the major known biological action of secretin, which is to stimulate secretion of bicarbonate by the cells lining the pancreatic and biliary ducts, as well as the duodenal epithelial cells themselves. Up to 80% of the bicarbonate secretory response that occurs in the course of digesting and absorbing a meal is likely due to the direct influence of secretin.

GIP, or glucose-dependent insulinotropic peptide (formerly known as gastric inhibitory peptide, which fortuitously has the same initials) is released from intestinal K cells predominantly in response to the lipid components of a meal. Its primary physiologic actions are to inhibit gastric acid secretion and to stimulate the release of insulin from the endocrine pancreas. The former action represents an example of a feedback regulatory event that contributes to the termination of gastric secretory function once the bulk of the meal has moved into the small intestine. The latter action accounts for the fact that glucose absorbed across the wall of the gastrointestinal tract is cleared from the circulation more rapidly than an equivalent amount of glucose infused intravenously; thus, the gut augments normal systemic mechanisms of glucose homeostasis to ensure that the body is not overwhelmed during the rapid absorption of glucose originating from a meal rich in sugar.

MOTILIN FAMILY

Human motilin is a 22-amino acid linear peptide that is released cyclically from the gut in the fasting state, and is responsible for stimulating a specific pattern of gastrointestinal motility known as the migrating motor complex, which will be discussed in detail in a subsequent chapter. The motilin receptor is also recognized as an important target of pharmacotherapy, binding a number of so-called pro-kinetic agents that can be used clinically to stimulate the motility of the bowel. Cloning of the receptor also led to the discovery of ghrelin as a peptide related to motilin that is a second endogenous ligand. Ghrelin is unusual in that it is post-translationally modified by covalent addition of an octanoyl moiety, which is important for its biological activity. It is involved in the regulation of food intake, as discussed below.

Candidate GI Hormones

As mentioned earlier, the gastrointestinal tract is a rich source of stored peptides and several have received attention for their potential physiologic roles. The most compelling evidence exists for three such peptides—enteroglucagon, pancreatic polypeptide, and peptide YY (tyrosine–tyrosine, indicating a structural feature). Enteroglucagon is a member of the secretin family whereas the other two peptides are related to each other, but not to any of the other hormone families thus far discussed. While none of these peptides have yet fulfilled all of the criteria needed to classify them as a hormone, it is possible that they may do so in the future.

Intestinal L cells make peptides that are closely related to pancreatic glucagon, and arise from differential processing of the same gene. One of these peptides, glucagon-like peptide-1, is a 30-amino acid peptide that inhibits gastric secretion and emptying, and also potently stimulates the release of insulin. The enteroglucagons are released in response to luminal sugars, and thus may contribute to the axis by which circulating glucose concentrations are regulated during the period of glucose absorption after a meal, by coordinating the activities of the intestine and endocrine pancreas. As such, these presumed enteroglucagons act in concert with GIP.

Cells of the pancreatic islets synthesize pancreatic polypeptide as a 36-amino acid linear peptide, which has a globular three-dimensional structure. It is released in response to ingestion of a meal, likely by several constituents including protein, fat, and carbohydrate, although the molecules that mediate signaling between the gut and the pancreas have not been defined. Likewise, although the peptide can be shown to inhibit pancreatic enzyme and bicarbonate secretion, the physiologic significance of this is unclear because infusion of an antibody to neutralize the actions of pancreatic polypeptide during meal digestion and absorption had no effect on the extent of pancreatic secretion. Thus, the precise role of this peptide remains elusive. Indeed, its most useful property at present appears to be that of a clinical diagnostic marker. Many islet cell-derived neoplasms release high levels of this peptide and elevations in the plasma are thus a marker of a possible islet cell tumor.

Finally, a peptide related to pancreatic polypeptide, peptide YY, is synthesized and released by enteroendocrine cells in the distal small intestine and colon in response to the presence of fat in the ileal lumen. Its actions are largely inhibitory, reducing gastrointestinal motility as well as gastric acid secretion and secretion of chloride by the intestinal epithelium. Some have therefore proposed that peptide YY can be considered an *ileal brake*, that is, a substance that acts to slow propulsive motility and reduce luminal fluidity if nutrients remain unabsorbed by the time the meal reaches the ileum, thereby maximizing contact time and the ability to absorb nutrients. Like CCK, moreover, PYY is also implicated in signaling satiety.

PRINCIPLES OF NEUROCRINE REGULATION

"Little Brain" Model of the Enteric Nervous System

 The enteric nervous system is often referred to as the "little brain" (as opposed to the "big brain" of the central nervous system) because many of its responses are autonomous of central input. In fact, the enteric nervous system contains as many nerves as the spinal cord, and the gastrointestinal system is unique in being the only organ system of the body with such an extensive system of intrinsic neural circuits. The various neurons of the enteric nervous system can be considered to perform functions in two primary areas (Figure 2–6). First, program circuits receive inputs regarding the physiologic status of the intestine, and translate these into appropriate changes in function of the smooth muscle, mucosa, glandular structures, and vasculature. Second, integration circuits additionally relay such information to the central nervous system, and in turn integrate information derived from the central nervous system (CNS) with that supplied from intrinsic circuits to modify functional outcomes.

As discussed in Chapter 1, the intrinsic nerves of the gastrointestinal system are arranged into two main plexuses—myenteric and submucosal. Within these plexuses, the neurons can be subdivided according to their

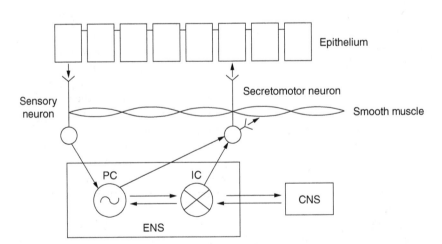

Figure 2–6. Schematic diagram of the enteric nervous system (ENS) and its interactions with the central nervous system (CNS). PC, program circuit; IC, integration circuit.

Table 2–4. Classification of enteric nerves

Type	Primary neurotransmitters
Myenteric neurons	
Stimulatory motor neurons	Acetylcholine
Inhibitory motor neurons	Nitric oxide
Ascending and descending interneurons	Acetylcholine, 5-hydroxytryptamine
Sensory neurons	Substance P
Submucosal neurons	
Noncholinergic secretomotor neurons	Vasoactive intestinal polypeptide
Cholinergic secretomotor neurons	Acetylcholine
Sensory neurons	Substance P

functions (Table 2–4). In the myenteric plexus, inhibitory and excitatory nerves control the function of the circular and longitudinal muscle layers. There are also ascending and descending interneurons that relay information through the myenteric plexus along the length of the gastrointestinal tract. In the submucosal plexus, secretomotor neurons, some of which also innervate blood vessels to promote vasodilatation, regulate the secretion of fluid and electrolytes and contractions of the muscularis mucosa. The plexuses also contain cell bodies of primary afferent nerves with projections to the mucosa that are designed to sense the physiologic environment. Thus, "mechanosensitive" nerves have their cell bodies in the submucosal plexus whereas those responding to specific chemical characteristics of the lumen, or to stretch, have cell bodies in myenteric ganglia.

Enteric Neurotransmitters

The various neurons of the enteric nervous system can be classified into various subtypes on the basis of their morphology, and these appear also to correspond to chemical coding and to function. Most, if not all, enteric neurons store multiple neurotransmitters, but not all of the transmitters in a given nerve may be equally important in terms of information transfer. Some general patterns are also apparent. Excitatory nerves depend largely on cholinergic neurotransmission, with the acetylcholine released from such nerves acting via muscarinic receptors. The actions of acetylcholine in stimulatory pathways for either muscle contraction or secretory functions of the mucosal epithelium may be amplified by tachykinins such as substance P and neurokinin A that are coreleased with the cholinergic messenger. Acetylcholine also serves to deliver information from the parasympathetic branch of the autonomic nervous system, largely via the vagus nerve, to the enteric neurons, although in this case it acts via nicotinic receptors.

Inhibitory nerves in the myenteric plexus, on the other hand, exert their effects predominantly via the release of nitric oxide, although several other neurotransmitters also play varying roles depending on the species and the segment of intestine being considered. These additional inhibitory neurotransmitters include vasoactive intestinal polypeptide (VIP), ATP, and pituitary adenylate cyclase activating peptide (PACAP). VIP is also a critical neurotransmitter for non-cholinergic neurons in the submucosal plexus that function to stimulate secretory function as well as vasodilation.

Interneurons in the myenteric plexus utilize various neurotransmitters to deliver information along the vertical axis, but one common transmitter in such nerves is serotonin, or 5-hydroxytryptamine (5-HT). At least in part, this may account for the clinical efficacy of specific 5-HT antagonists in conditions characterized by abnormal gastrointestinal motility, such as irritable bowel syndrome. Other interneurons containing acetylcholine and somatostatin have been implicated in the generation of a motility pattern known as the migrating motor complex, which sweeps through the duodenum to the ileum in the fasted state but does not propagate into the colon. The distribution of this motility event likewise corresponds with that of the interneurons containing the listed transmitters.

Finally, the intrinsic primary afferents that relay information to the enteric program and integration circuits appear to utilize tachykinins for sensory transmission. These neurons ultimately control intestinal movements, blood flow, and secretion in response to distension, luminal chemistry, and mechanical deformation of the mucosal surface. On the other hand, painful sensations are conveyed via spinal afferents, which pass through the dorsal root ganglia.

Vagal communication with the gastrointestinal tract is, as mentioned, largely mediated through the enteric nervous system and involves cholinergic transmission. Parasympathetic vagal input and vago-vagal reflexes play a critical role in regulating numerous gut functions, particularly during the early phases of response to a meal. The pelvic nerve plays an analogous role in the distal colon and rectum. On the other hand, sympathetic innervation to the intestine, mediated by norepinephrine, is relatively limited in its extent and implications under physiologic circumstances. Instead, it seems likely that sympathetic regulation is called upon to override the normal control of gut function, by slowing motility and inhibiting secretion, as a defense mechanism during times of threat to whole body homeostasis, such as in the setting of hemorrhagic shock or a fall in right atrial pressure.

PARACRINE AND IMMUNE REGULATION
Important Mediators

Paracrine and immune regulation of gastrointestinal function both involve the release of substances from non-excitable cell types, including enteroendocrine cells, enterochromaffin and enterochromaffin-like (ECL) cells, and immune elements in the lamina propria, which then act on neighboring cell types in the immediate environment. Important paracrine/immune mediators are summarized, along with their major sources of origin, in Table 2–5.

Table 2–5. Important paracrine and immune mediators in the gastrointestinal tract

Mediator	Major sources	Selected functions
Histamine	1. ECL cells 2. Mast cells	1. Gastric acid secretion 2. Intestinal chloride secretion
5-hydroxytryptamine	Enterochromaffin cells	Response to luminal nutrients
Somatostatin	D cells	Various inhibitory effects throughout GI tract
Prostaglandins	Subepithelial myofibroblasts	Intestinal secretion; vascular regulation
Adenosine	Various cell types	Intestinal secretion; vascular regulation

Note that some paracrines are also stored in nerves, and thus play a dual role in signaling in the gut. For example, somatostatin, an important inhibitory peptide in the gut, is synthesized by enteroendocrine D cells as well as being stored in interneurons of the enteric nervous system. Other paracrines may also derive from multiple cell sources. Thus, histamine is released from ECL cells in the gastric glands as a classic paracrine, but also from mucosal mast cells in response to antigenic stimulation, where it acts as an immune mediator.

Other important paracrines include prostaglandins, 5-HT released from enterochromaffin cells, and adenosine, which is released by various cells in response to oxidative stress or other triggers and has important roles in regulating both blood flow and intestinal secretion.

Mechanisms of Activation

Paracrine and immune regulators are primarily responsible for fine-tuning physiologic responses that are set into motion by hormonal and neural regulation, and as such are usually released in response to triggers that also act in the immediate environment. Thus, both the endocrine and immune cells that release these substances can be considered as the gut equivalent of the taste buds in the tongue that sample various components of ingested food and send information about its palatability. More distally, therefore, enteroendocrine cells are triggered in response to specific meal components, or by potentially injurious solutes in the lumen in the case of immune cells, the latter usually following sensitization of a susceptible host.

However, in some cases the cells responsible for releasing paracrine and/or immune effectors also receive neural input, and/or are sensitive to the actions of circulating gastrointestinal hormones. The gastric ECL cell in the fundic region is an excellent example of this, releasing histamine both in response to acetylcholine released from enteric nerve endings, or gastrin traveling through the bloodstream from its site of origin in G cells located in the gastric antrum. The relative role of paracrines in physiologic responses is also seen in the observation that both basal and meal-stimulated gastric acid secretion can be markedly attenuated when subjects are treated with an antagonist of the histamine H_2 receptor that mediates effects of the amine on parietal cells, despite the fact that the parietal cell also receives other stimulatory inputs as will be discussed in greater detail in the next chapter.

INTEGRATION OF REGULATORY SYSTEMS

There is considerable cross-talk between the regulatory systems discussed in this chapter, as well as functional redundancy. Moreover, communication mediated by one mode, for example, endocrine, may secondarily activate other modes of communication to amplify the eventual physiologic responses in target organs. An example of this is seen with the GI hormone CCK. On release from the gastrointestinal mucosa, CCK not only travels through the bloodstream to activate secretory and motor responses in other segments of the gut as well as the pancreas and biliary system, but also binds to CCK_1 receptors on primary efferent nerve endings within the intestinal wall that can transmit vago-vagal reflexes to propagate additional signaling. Conversely, a neurocrine messenger, gastrin releasing peptide, acts on G cells to release a hormone that then can distribute the signal more broadly.

Finally, the existence of multiple inputs to many of the cell types involved in the integrated response to a meal not only provides functional redundancy, underscoring the importance of gastrointestinal function for whole-body homeostasis, but also permits synergism, or potentiated responses, at the level of the target cell type. Synergism, or a greater than additive physiologic response, can be predicted to occur if the two (or more) messengers in question activate their target cell by different intracellular signaling cascades.

Integration of intestinal responses also involves the transmission of negative or inhibitory signals. Such feedback inhibition controls the rate of delivery of nutrients such that this is matched with digestive and secretory capacity. Feedback mechanisms also terminate gut secretory responses when they are no longer needed to assimilate a meal, to conserve resources and, in some cases, minimize possible adverse consequences of overly prolonged exposure to gastrointestinal secretions.

CONTROL OF FOOD INTAKE

It is increasingly recognized that the intestine participates centrally in the control of whole-body energy balance, by cooperating with the brain to set the timing and size of meals ingested. A full discussion of the complex subject of the regulation of food intake is beyond the scope of this volume, since it involves many aspects of central neurophysiology. Nevertheless, it is clear that ghrelin is released from the stomach during fasting and its levels peak just before

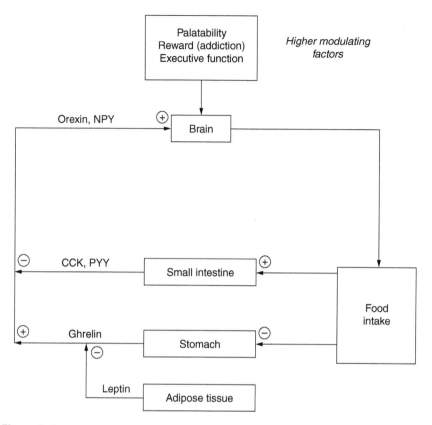

Figure 2–7. Some of the factors involved in the control of food intake via cooperation between the brain and gastrointestinal system. Factors released from intestinal endocrine cells under the influence of luminal nutrients, or a lack thereof, impact central pathways either directly, or by stimulating or inhibiting vagal afferents. CCK, cholecystokinin; NPY, neuropeptide Y; PYY, peptide YY.

eating, after which they are suppressed (Figure 2–7). Ghrelin appears to trigger feeding by a variety of mechanisms, including the stimulation of vagal afferents that in turn trigger the release of signals in the NTS and hypothalamus that promote food intake, such as orexins and neuropeptide Y. Ghrelin release is normally suppressed by the adipokine, leptin, although those who are obese may become desensitized to this effect as well as the direct effect of leptin on vagal afferents. Conversely, CCK and PYY are released from the intestine in response to nutrients and trigger vagal afferent pathways that reduce food intake. Food intake is also importantly modulated by higher brain areas, including those that signal reward and which are involved in addictive behaviors. Clearly, these complex circuits offer many possible targets for drug development to counter the epidemic of obesity, and these are actively being pursued.

KEY CONCEPTS

 Communication between the various segments of the GI tract, as well as the organs that drain into it, is vital for the integrated response to a meal.

 Communication is achieved via the endocrine, neurocrine, paracrine, and immune mediators that act at sites distant from the site of stimulation and locally.

 All GI hormones are peptides, but not all GI peptides are hormones.

 GI hormones can be grouped into families displaying structural homologies and acting via specific second messenger pathways.

 The enteric nervous system serves to regulate the motility and secretory responses of the gut, and to integrate this regulation with information from the central nervous system.

 Stimulatory and inhibitory nerves and neurotransmitters are involved in the communication and regulation of the information.

 Paracrine and immune messengers act locally to modulate endocrine and neurocrine signaling.

 Communication pathways in the gut are both interactive and redundant, and involve the transfer of both positive and negative signals.

 The GI tract produces substances that influence the brain to trigger food intake behaviors, or induce satiety, to maintain body mass during times of different metabolic demands.

STUDY QUESTIONS

2–1.   A scientist isolates a novel peptide from the duodenal mucosa and determines that it inhibits gastric acid secretion when administered intravenously to rats. Based on these experiments, she can conclude that her peptide acts to inhibit acid secretion by which of the following mechanisms?

A. Neurocrine

B. Paracrine

C. Endocrine

D. Juxtacrine

E. None of the above

2–2.   A mouse is genetically engineered to lack CCK_2 receptors. This animal would be expected to display increased circulating levels of which of the following hormones?

A. Gastrin

B. Motilin

C. Secretin

D. Cholecystokinin

E. Insulin

2–3.   An experiment was conducted in which a balloon was inflated inside the stomach of a human volunteer and gastric pressures measured. Despite the increase in gastric volume, gastric pressures remained relatively constant. This remarkable pressure–volume relationship could be abolished by which of the following pharmacological agents?

A. Adrenergic agonist

B. Nitric oxide synthase inhibitor

C. Cholinergic agonist

D. Cholecystokinin

E. An antibody to gastrin

2–4.   From the following list of neurohumoral regulators, identify the substance that does not signal directly via an increase in cAMP.

A. Secretin

B. Gastrin

C. Vasoactive intestinal polypeptide

D. Glucose-dependent insulinotropic peptide

E. Glucagon

2-5.   *In a study of the secretion of gastrointestinal hormones, portal concentrations are measured during luminal perfusion of the small intestine with solutions of various pH levels. Which hormone will increase in the plasma during perfusion with a buffered solution of pH 3?*

   A. Cholecystokinin

   B. Gastrin

   C. Glucose-dependent insulinotropic peptide

   D. Motilin

   E. Secretin

2-6.   *In an experiment, a scientist infuses PYY intravenously in a series of mice. These animals would be expected to display an increase in which of the following:*

   A. Time taken to initiate the next meal

   B. Gastric emptying

   C. Lipid concentrations in the ileal lumen

   D. Levels of orexin in the brain

   E. Plasma leptin

SUGGESTED READINGS

Chao C, Hellmich MR. Gastrointestinal peptides: gastrin, cholecystokinin, somatostatin, and ghrelin. In: Johnson LR, Ghishan FK, Kaunitz JD, Merchant JL, Said HM, Wood JD, eds. *Physiology of the Gastrointestinal Tract.* 5th ed. San Diego: Academic Press; 2012:115–154.

Dockray GJ. The brain–gut axis. In: Yamada T, Alpers DH, Kalloo AN, Kaplowitz N, Owyang C, Powell DW, eds. *Textbook of Gastroenterology.* 5th ed. Chichester: Wiley-Blackwell; 2009:86–102.

Gomez GA, Englander EW, Greeley GH Jr. Postpyloric gastrointestinal peptides. In: Johnson LR, Ghishan FK, Kaunitz JD, Merchant JL, Said HM, Wood JD, eds. *Physiology of the Gastrointestinal Tract.* 5th ed. San Diego: Academic Press; 2012:155–198.

Pandol SJ, Raybould HE, Yee HF. Integrative responses of the gastrointestinal tract and liver to a meal. In: Yamada T, Alpers DH, Kalloo AN, Kaplowitz N, Owyang C, Powell DW, eds. *Textbook of Gastroenterology.* 5th ed. Chichester: Wiley-Blackwell; 2009:3–14.

Sam AH, Troke RC, Tan TM, Bewick GA. The role of the gut/brain axis in modulating food intake. *Neuropharmacology.* 2011;63:46–56.

Wood JD. Enteric neuroimmunophysiology and pathophysiology. *Gastroenterology.* 2004;127:635–657.

Yu LC, Perdue MH. Role of mast cells in intestinal mucosal function: studies in models of hypersensitivity and stress. *Immunol Rev.* 2001;179:61–73.

Gastric Secretion

3

OBJECTIVES

▶ *Understand the physiologic role of gastric acid secretion, as well as that of other gastric secretory products*
  ▶ Identify the regions of the stomach and cell types from which the various gastric secretions originate
▶ *Understand how gastric secretion is initiated in response to anticipation of a meal, and how secretion is amplified once the meal has been ingested*
  ▶ Define cephalic, gastric, and intestinal phases of the secretory response
  ▶ Describe how secretion is terminated once the meal has left the stomach
▶ *Define the cellular basis for acid secretion and the morphologic changes that take place in parietal cells to achieve this*
▶ *Identify clinical correlates of abnormal acid secretion*

BASIC PRINCIPLES OF GASTRIC SECRETION

Role and Significance

The stomach is a muscular reservoir into which the meal enters after being swallowed. While limited digestion may begin in the oral cavity as a result of enzymes contained in saliva, the gastric juices represent the first significant source of digestive capacity. However, the digestive functions of the stomach are not necessary for assimilation of a mixed meal, and indeed, surgical removal of the majority of the stomach because of disease, or in an effort to treat morbid obesity, is not incompatible with adequate nutrition. However, some degree of gastric secretory function is critically required for the absorption of an essential vitamin, B_{12}, and gastric acid may also be important in the absorption of dietary nonheme iron.

Gastric secretions also serve to sterilize the meal. Other than those receiving irradiated meals for medical reasons, humans may ingest significant quantities of microbes with their meals. This is particularly the case in developing countries, where sanitation is inadequate and many do not have access to clean food or water. However, assuming the microbial load ingested is not overwhelming, the secretions of the stomach can kill many of the microorganisms contained therein, and thus maintain the relative sterility of the small intestine.

Table 3–1. Important gastric secretory products

Product	Source	Functions
Hydrochloric acid	Parietal cell	Hydrolysis; sterilization of meal
Intrinsic factor	Parietal cell	Vitamin B_{12} absorption
Pepsinogen	Chief cell	Protein digestion
Mucus, bicarbonate	Surface mucous cells	Gastroprotection
Trefoil factors	Surface mucous cells	Gastroprotection
Histamine	ECL cells	Regulation of gastric secretion
Gastrin	G cells	Regulation of gastric secretion
Gastrin-releasing peptide	Nerves	Regulation of gastric secretion
Acetylcholine (ACh)	Nerves	Regulation of gastric secretion
Somatostatin	D cells	Regulation of gastric secretion

Gastric Secretory Products

The functions outlined in the previous section are subserved by a number of products secreted by the stomach (Table 3–1). The most characteristic secretory product of the stomach is hydrochloric acid, which is not secreted in such large quantities anywhere else in the body. The acidity of the gastric secretions begins the digestive process via simple hydrolysis. This acid also contributes to the ability of the gastric juices to sterilize the meal.

Enzymatic digestion of the meal also occurs as a result of gastric secretions. A proteolytic enzyme, pepsin, is secreted as an inactive precursor, pepsinogen, and auto-catalytically cleaved at the low pH existing in the stomach lumen to yield the catalytically active pepsin. Pepsin is specialized for its role in mediating protein digestion in the stomach by virtue of the fact that it exhibits optimum activity at low pH. The gastric juice also contains a lipolytic enzyme, lipase, which contributes to the initial digestion of triglycerides. Gastric juice also contains a 45 kDa protein synthesized by parietal cells, called intrinsic factor. This binds to vitamin B_{12}, also known as cobalamin, and is required for the eventual absorption of this vitamin more distally in the intestine. Intrinsic factor is specialized for its role by being relatively resistant to degradation by acid and proteolytic enzymes.

The stomach also secretes products important in protecting the mucosa from the harsh effects of the luminal mixture of acid and enzymes. Throughout the stomach, the surface cells are covered with a layer of mucus. Mucus consists of a mixture of mucin glycoproteins, surface phospholipids that endow hydrophobic properties on the surface of the mucus layer, and water. The mucin molecules are cross-linked by disulfide bonds between adjacent molecules, and the oligosaccharides of these structures confer a highly viscoelastic structure that expands considerably upon hydration. The stability of this layer is additionally enhanced by the activity of small peptides, known as trefoil factors, which interact with the carbohydrate side chains of mucin molecules. Bicarbonate ions are also secreted into the base of this mucus layer, which may provide a mechanism whereby the gastric surface is protected from excessively low and potentially injurious pH, via simple neutralization. The mucus layer is considered to provide a substrate in which a pH gradient can be established.

Finally, the stomach secretes a number of products into the mucosa that play critical roles in regulating the secretory and motility functions of the stomach, including gastrin, histamine, and prostaglandins. The roles of these factors will be discussed in more detail later.

ANATOMICAL CONSIDERATIONS

Functional Regions of the Stomach

The stomach is a muscular sac that is described as having a greater and lesser curvature. It lies between the esophagus and the duodenum, and is delimited by the lower esophageal sphincter, and the pylorus, respectively (Figure 1–5). The wall of the stomach contains thick vascular folds known as rugae, and at a microscopic level, the surface epithelium can be seen to be invaginated with a series of gastric pits. Each pit opens to four to five blind-ended gastric glands. The stomach can also be divided into three major regions by both structure and function. Most distally, the cardia represents approximately 5% of the gastric surface area, and is a transitional zone where the stratified squamous epithelium of the esophagus gives way to the columnar epithelium that lines the remainder of the stomach and intestinal tract. The fundus or body of the stomach contains approximately 75% of the gastric glands, which in this region are so-called oxyntic glands that consist of specialized cell types from which arise the characteristic secretions of the stomach (Figure 3–1). Finally, the antrum of the stomach, immediately proximal to the pylorus, contains glands that secrete gastrin, the primary regulator of postprandial gastric secretion. The antrum also fulfills important motility functions that will be described in Chapter 8.

Gastric Cell Types

The oxyntic, or parietal glands found in the gastric fundus contain a variety of specific cell types (Figure 3–1). The most notable are probably the parietal cells, which are specialized to secrete acid and intrinsic factor. More basally in the gland, there are chief cells, which store pepsinogen in apical granules that can release their contents via a process of exocytosis. The glands also contain endocrine cells that are responsible for releasing products that regulate gastric function, particularly the enterochromaffin-like, or ECL, cells, that synthesize histamine via the action of the enzyme histidine decarboxylase on the amino acid, histidine. The glands also contain D cells, which are closely opposed to the parietal cells and contain the inhibitory paracrine, somatostatin. Toward the top of the gland where

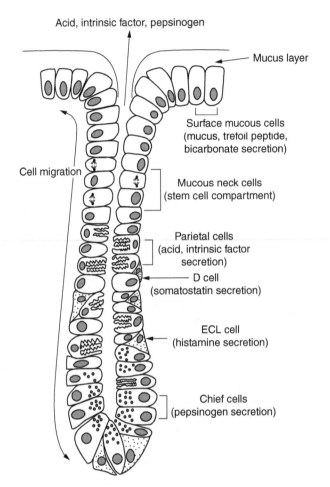

Figure 3–1. Structure of a gastric gland from the fundus and body of the stomach. These acid- and pepsinogen-producing glands are referred to as "oxyntic" glands in some sources.

it joins with the gastric pit, and moving out onto the gastric surface, the gland contains surface mucous cells that secrete mucus, as their name implies. In the isthmus and neck region of the gland lie the mucus neck cells, which are the precursors for all of the other differentiated cell types in the gland. These anchored stem cells give rise to daughter cells, which migrate downward to become parietal, chief, or endocrine cells, or upward to become surface mucous cells. The surface mucous cells turn over every 1–3 days in adult humans.

In the antral mucosa, the glands do not contain parietal or chief cells, but instead are comprised of both mucus-secreting cells and enteroendocrine cells that regulate gastric function. Particularly, the glands contain G cells, which synthesize and

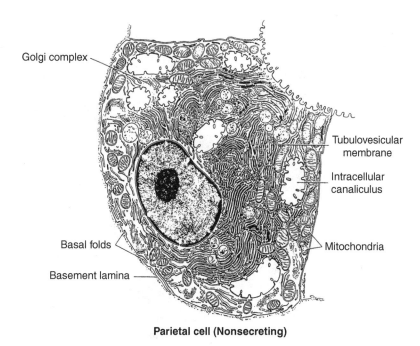

Golgi complex

Tubulovesicular membrane

Intracellular canaliculus

Basal folds

Basement lamina

Mitochondria

Parietal cell (Nonsecreting)

Figure 3–2. Ultrastructural appearance of a resting parietal cell. Note the elaborate system of intracellular membranes and a large number of mitochondria. (Reproduced with permission from Ito. Functional gastric morphology. In: Johnson LR, ed. *Physiology of the Gastrointestinal Tract.* 2nd ed. New York: Raven Press; 1987.)

release gastrin across their basolateral poles, and which have an open morphology implying functionally significant communication with the gastric lumen. Closed endocrine cells are also present, exemplified by D cells.

The parietal cells are remarkable for their secretory capacity and energetic requirements. The capacity for acid secretion in a given individual is directly dependent on the mass of parietal cells. Parietal cell mass is related to body weight, and declines somewhat with age. These cells secrete acid against a concentration gradient of more than 2.5 million fold, from the cytoplasmic pH of 7.2 to a luminal pH of less than 1 when secretion is maximally activated. To sustain such massive rates of secretion, the parietal cell is packed with mitochondria, which are estimated to take up some 30–40% of the cell's volume. The resting parietal cell also contains numerous membranous compartments known as tubulovesicles, as well as a central canaliculus that deeply invaginates the apical membrane (Figure 3–2). This morphology changes dramatically upon cell stimulation (Figure 3–3) as will be described more fully later. Interestingly, parietal cells also appear to provide signals that control the proliferation and differentiation of the other cell types involved in gastric physiology, and especially those of the chief cells.

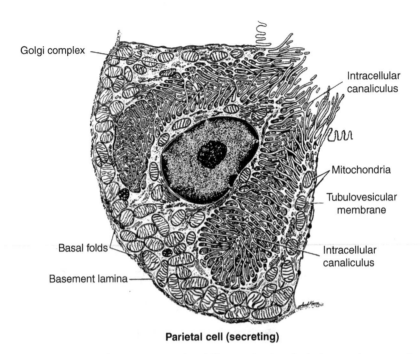

Golgi complex

Intracellular canaliculus

Mitochondria

Tubulovesicular membrane

Intracellular canaliculus

Basal folds

Basement lamina

Parietal cell (secreting)

Figure 3–3. Ultrastructural appearance of a parietal cell during active secretion. The apical membrane is massively amplified by fusion of tubulovesicles and the secretory canaliculi. (Reproduced with permission from Ito. Functional gastric morphology. In: Johnson LR, ed. *Physiology of the Gastrointestinal Tract*. 2nd ed. New York: Raven Press; 1987.)

Innervation

Nerves carried through the parasympathetic vagus nerve, with both efferent and afferent pathways, richly innervate the stomach. Vagal afferents convey information from the dorsal vagal complex, which is integrated with that coming from higher centers, such as the hypothalamus, to set the overall level of secretory function at any given moment. Visceral inputs also contribute to gastric regulation. Notably, the output of taste receptors travels to a brain region called the nucleus tractus solitarius, where this information is again translated into signals that regulate secretion and other gastric functions. A more modest amount of sympathetic innervation is also seen, and activation of sympathetic nerves tends to oppose the actions of the parasympathetic limb. Finally, the enteric nerve plexuses that are seen throughout the gastrointestinal tract encircle the walls of the stomach. These allow for some degree of autonomous function, in addition to transmitting effects of central input. Gastric sensory nerves containing the neurotransmitter calcitonin gene-related peptide (CGRP) are also present, and participate in down-regulation of acid secretion.

The dorsal vagal complex represents an important site where the various influences that can alter gastric secretion are integrated. It receives central input from the hypothalamus, as well as visceral input from the nucleus tractus solitarius. Taste fibers emanating from the oral cavity, and systemic hypoglycemia, represent visceral inputs that can lead to an increase in gastric secretion via vagal pathways originating in the dorsal vagal complex.

REGULATION OF GASTRIC SECRETION

 Control of the secretion of the characteristic products of the cell types lining the stomach represents a paradigm for control of gastrointestinal function as a whole. Thus, the secretory capacity of the stomach is closely integrated with signals coincident with the ingestion of a meal, and modulated as the meal moves through the gastrointestinal tract to provide optimum digestion. Furthermore, the physiological benefits of acid secretion must be balanced with its potential to cause epithelial damage and erosions. There are many mechanisms, therefore, whereby the function of the stomach is controlled.

Regulatory Strata

SHORT AND LONG REFLEXES

Neural input provides an important mechanism for regulation of gastric secretion (Figure 3–4). Reflexes contribute to both the stimulation and inhibition of secretion. For example, distension of the stomach wall, sensed by stretch receptors, activates reflexes that stimulate acid secretion at the level of the parietal cell. These reflexes may be so-called short reflexes, which involve neural transmission contained entirely within the enteric nervous system. In addition, long reflexes also contribute to the control of secretion. These involve the activation of primary afferents that travel through the vagus nerve, which in turn are interpreted in the dorsal vagal complex and trigger vagal outflow via efferent nerves that travel back to the stomach and activate parietal cells or other components of the secretory machinery. These long reflexes are also called *vago-vagal reflexes*. The relative contribution of short and long reflexes to the control of secretion is unknown. However, it is clear that selective gastric vagotomy eliminates some, although not all, of the gastric secretory response to distension as well as a portion of related gastric motor responses.

Acetylcholine is an important mediator of both short and long reflexes in the stomach. It participates in the stimulation of parietal, chief, and ECL cells; the suppression of D cells; and the synapses between nerves within the enteric nervous system. In addition, a second important gastric neurotransmitter is gastrin releasing peptide, or GRP. This neuropeptide is the mammalian homologue of one known as bombesin originally isolated from frog skin. GRP is released by enteric nerves in the vicinity of gastrin-containing G cells in the gastric antrum.

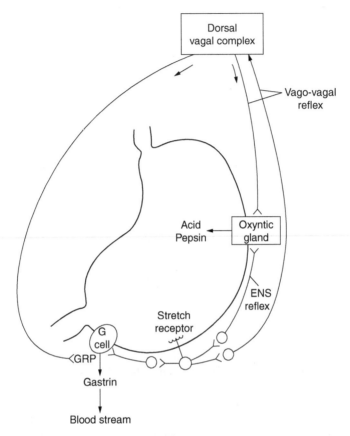

Figure 3–4. Neural regulation of gastric secretion in response to gastric distension. Stretch of the stomach wall increases acid secretion via both intrinsic reflexes and vago-vagal reflexes.

HUMORAL CONTROL

The gastric secretory response is also regulated by soluble factors that originate from endocrine and other regulatory cell types, such as ECL cells (Figure 3–5). The primary endocrine regulator of gastric secretion is gastrin, which actually consists of a family of peptides that are discussed in greater detail in the preceding chapter. Gastrin travels through the bloodstream from its site of release in the antral mucosa to stimulate parietal and ECL cells via their CCK_2 receptors.

Gastric secretion is also modified by paracrine mediators. Histamine is released from ECL cells under the combined influence of gastrin and ACh, and diffuses to neighboring parietal cells to activate acid secretion via histamine H_2 receptors. At one time histamine was thought to be the final common mediator of acid secretion, based in part on the clinical observation that histamine H_2 receptor antagonists can profoundly inhibit acid secretion. However, it is now known that parietal

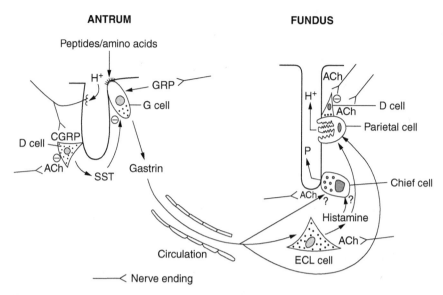

Figure 3-5. Regulation of gastric acid and pepsin secretion by soluble mediators and neural input. Gastrin is released from G cells in the antrum and travels through the circulation to influence the activity of ECL cells and parietal cells. The specific agonists of chief cells are not well understood. Gastrin release is negatively regulated by luminal acidity via the release of somatostatin from antral D cells. Fundic D cells may also exert a tonic negative influence on parietal as well as chief and ECL cells.

cells express receptors for not only histamine, but also ACh (muscarinic m_3) and gastrin (CCK_2) (Figure 3–6). Because histamine H_2 receptors are linked predominantly to signaling pathways that involve cAMP, while ACh and gastrin signal through calcium, when the parietal cell is acted upon simultaneously by all three stimuli, a potentiated, or greater than additive, effect on acid secretion results. The physiological implication of this potentiation, or synergism, is that a greater level of acid secretion can be produced with relatively small increases in each of the three stimuli. The pharmacological significance is that simply interfering with the action of any one of them can significantly inhibit acid secretion. In fact, synergism is a common theme in the control of several different functions throughout the gastrointestinal system.

Acid secretion is also subject to negative regulation by specific mediators. Specifically, somatostatin is released from D cells in response to an axon reflex that releases CGRP in the antral mucosa when luminal pH falls below 3, and inhibits the release of gastrin from G cells. Elsewhere in the stomach, somatostatin can also exert inhibitory influences on ECL, parietal, and chief cells. The SSTR2 somatostatin receptor is responsible for the inhibitory effects of the peptide in the stomach. In fact, there is data to support the idea that gastric secretion under resting conditions is tonically suppressed by somatostatin. When stimulated responses occur, they are due not only to the active stimulatory mechanisms discussed above, but also

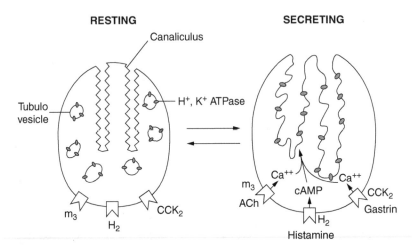

Figure 3–6. Parietal cell receptors and schematic representation of the morphological changes depicted in Figure 3–3. Amplification of the apical surface area is accompanied by an increased density of H⁺, K⁺ ATPase molecules at this site. Note that acetylcholine (ACh) and gastrin signal via calcium, whereas histamine signals via cAMP.

specific suppression of the inhibitory effects of somatostatin, involving the actions of both ACh (via m_2 and m_4 receptors) and histamine (via H_3 receptors) on D cells.

Luminal Regulators

Specific luminal constituents also modulate gastric secretion indirectly. The example of pH is described earlier, but acid output, at least, is also increased by components of the meal. Short peptides and amino acids, derived from dietary protein secondary to the action of pepsin released from chief cells, are capable of activating gastrin release from G cells. Aromatic amino acids are the most potent, and "receptors" for these are assumed to reside on the apical membrane of the open G-type endocrine cells, although their structure remains to be defined. Gastric acid secretion is also activated by alcoholic beverages, coffee, and dietary calcium. The effects of alcoholic beverages may not be due to ethanol itself, but rather the amino acids present in the beverage, particularly in beer and wine. Likewise, the effect of coffee does not appear to be attributable to caffeine, since decaffeinated coffee also increases secretion.

Regulation of Secretion in the Interdigestive Phase

Between meals, the stomach secretes acid and other secretory products at a low level, perhaps to aid in maintaining the sterility of the stomach. However, because no food is present, and thus no buffering capacity of the gastric contents, the low volume of secretions produced nevertheless have a low pH—usually around 3.0. Basal acid output in the healthy human is in the range of 0–11 mEq/h, which can be contrasted with the maximal rates that can be produced by ingestion of a meal, or intravenous administration of gastrin, of 10–63 mEq/h. The basal secretion rate is believed to reflect the combined influences of histamine and ACh, released from ECL cells and nerve endings, respectively, tempered by the influence of somatostatin from fundic D cells. Gastrin secretion during the interdigestive period, on the other hand, is minimal. This is because gastrin release is suppressed by a luminal pH of 3 or below, via the release of somatostatin from antral D cells.

Regulation of Postprandial Secretion

In conjunction with a meal, gastric acid secretion can be considered to occur in three phases—cephalic, gastric, and intestinal. The major portion of secretion occurs during the gastric phase, when the meal is actually present in the stomach. Secretion of other gastric products usually parallels that of the acid.

CEPHALIC PHASE

Even before the meal is ingested, the stomach is readied to receive it by the so-called cephalic (i.e., related to the head) phase of secretion. In fact, during the cephalic phase, the functions of several gastrointestinal systems in addition to the stomach begin to be regulated, including the pancreas and gallbladder. Higher brain centers respond to the sight, smell, taste and even the thought of food, and relay information to the dorsal vagal complex. In turn, vagal outflow initiates both secretory and motor behavior in the stomach and more distal segments. Gastric secretion occurring during the cephalic phase readies the stomach to receive the meal. Vagal outflow activates enteric nerves that in turn release GRP and ACh. Release of GRP in the vicinity of antral G cells releases gastrin that travels through the bloodstream to activate parietal and chief cells in an endocrine fashion. ACh also suppresses ongoing somatostatin release.

The existence of a cephalic phase of secretion was demonstrated by experiments called "sham feeding." Gastric acid output was measured in volunteers who were exposed to the sight and smell of food cooking in the laboratory, and then asked to chew the food, but to spit it out before swallowing. Experiments of this type can also be used to demonstrate the importance of cognitive factors and learned preferences in regulating the extent of the cephalic phase of secretion. Gastric secretory responses are far greater when subjects anticipate, smell, and taste a meal that they themselves have chosen as a favorite, compared to a standard test meal. Conversely, sham feeding with a bland meal elicits little, if any, gastric secretory response above baseline. Likewise, the experiments of Pavlov, where dogs were conditioned to associate the ringing of a bell with a meal, showed that the anticipation of food alone is a powerful trigger for an increase in gastric secretion.

GASTRIC PHASE

The gastric phase of secretion is quantitatively the most important. In addition to vagal influences continuing from the cephalic phase, secretion is now amplified further by mechanical and chemical stimuli that arise from the presence of the meal in the lumen. These include the luminal signals discussed earlier, and signals arising from stretch receptors embedded in the wall of the stomach. Thus, as the stomach distends to accommodate the volume of the meal, these receptors initiate both short and long reflexes to further enhance secretory responses either directly, via the release of ACh in the vicinity of parietal cells, or indirectly, via the release of ACh that activates ECL cells, or GRP that activates G cells to release gastrin. The gastric phase also involves changes in motility, which will be discussed in more detail in Chapter 8. For now, suffice to say that local and vago-vagal reflexes allow the stomach to relax as it distends in the process of receptive relaxation, which is essential for the reservoir function of the stomach. These vago-vagal reflexes also transmit information downstream to ready more distal segments of the intestine to receive the meal. The gastric phase of secretion is also accompanied by a marked increase in gastric blood flow, which supplies the metabolic requirements of the actively secreting cell types.

Due to the combined influence of neurocrine and endocrine signals, further amplified by histamine release from ECL cells, secretory cells of the stomach are highly active during the gastric phase. Moreover, pepsinogen released by chief cells is rapidly cleaved to pepsin in an autocatalytic reaction that occurs optimally at pH 2, and this pepsin then acts on ingested protein to release short peptides and amino acids that further enhance gastrin release. Moreover, many dietary substances, including proteins, are highly effective buffers. Thus, while acid secretory rates remain high, the effective pH in the bulk of the lumen may rise to pH 5. This ensures that the rate of acid secretion during the gastric phase is not attenuated by an inhibition of gastrin release that would otherwise be mediated by somatostatin.

INTESTINAL PHASE

As the meal moves out of the stomach into the duodenum, the buffering capacity of the lumen is reduced and the pH begins to fall. At a threshold of around pH 3, CGRP triggers somatostatin release from D cells in the gastric antrum, which acts on G cells to suppress gastrin release. Somatostatin released from D cells in the oxyntic mucosa, or from nerve endings, likely also acts directly to inhibit secretory function. This acid-sensing response is a neural pathway that involves the activation of chemoreceptors sensitive to pH, which in turn leads to release of CGRP via an axon reflex. Other signals also limit the extent of gastric secretion when the meal has moved into the small intestine. For example, the presence of fat in the small intestine is associated with a reduction in gastric secretion. This feedback response is believed to involve several endocrine and paracrine factors, including GIP and CCK, the latter of which binds to CCK_1 receptors on D cells.

The foregoing discussion of signals that terminate secretion notwithstanding, it is clear that a portion of gastric secretion occurs once the meal is in the intestine. The mediators of this response are largely unknown. The function of the intestinal phase of secretion is likewise not truly understood, but it may serve to sterilize any remaining stomach contents and to ready the stomach for its next meal. Of course, there is also overlap between the gastric and intestinal phases of secretion since only portions of the meal move into the duodenum at any one time while the rest remains in the stomach.

CELLULAR BASIS OF SECRETION
Acid Secretion

The source of gastric acid secretion is the parietal cell, located in the glands of the fundic mucosa. This cell type is remarkably specialized for its function, which is probably the most energetically costly of any electrolyte transport process anywhere in the body. High rates of secretion by the parietal cell are sustained by redundant regulatory inputs. Thus, the basolateral membrane of the cell contains receptors for histamine, gastrin, and ACh, which cause potentiated secretion when all are present simultaneously (Figure 3–6). The downstream targets of the signaling pathways linked to receptor occupancy are emerging, and include cytoskeletal elements, the machinery controlling vesicular trafficking, ion channels, and the receptors themselves; the latter representing a mechanism of negative feedback. Cytoskeletal rearrangements are implied by the dramatic morphological changes that occur as parietal cells transition from rest to secretion. At rest, the cytoplasm is filled with specialized membrane structures known as tubulovesicles, as well as larger blind sacs known as intracellular canaliculi. When the parietal cell is stimulated, the canaliculi fuse with the apical plasma membrane (Figure 3–6). The intracellular tubulovesicles, in turn, fuse to the canaliculi, massively amplifying the surface area of the apical membrane that is in contact with the gland lumen by a factor of approximately five- to 10-fold. These fusion events require the participation of the cytoskeleton to move membrane structures together, as well as the activation of specific signaling proteins that promote membrane fusion.

The morphological change that occurs in parietal cells during the transition from the resting to the secretory state is also accompanied by a biochemical change. At rest, the tubulovesicles are the site for storage of the majority of a membrane-bound transporter, the H^+, K^+ ATPase, or proton pump, where it is therefore sequestered from the lumen. Following fusion of the tubulovesicles and canaliculi, however, their membranes are brought into continuity with the apical membrane, and thus the density of proton pumps in that pole of the cell is massively increased (Figure 3–6). These pumps are the site of active pumping of protons into the gastric lumen.

Protons are generated adjacent to the apical membrane as a result of the activity of the enzyme carbonic anhydrase II (Figure 3–7). This enzyme generates protons and bicarbonate ions from the reaction of water and carbon dioxide. Protons are then pumped out of the cell across the apical membrane in exchange for potassium ions, with the consumption of cellular energy in the form of ATP. The potassium ions are believed to originate also from the cell cytosol, where they are maintained at levels above their chemical equilibrium by the activity of a basolateral transporter, the Na^+, K^+ ATPase, and a sodium/potassium/chloride cotransporter, NKCC1. They can therefore readily exit across the apical membrane through potassium channels that are also localized to the tubulovesicles, and which are opened when the parietal cell is stimulated. Recent evidence from knockout mice suggests that KCNE2/KCNQ1 channels fulfill this role. Chloride channels are also present in this site, and serve to allow the apical exit of chloride

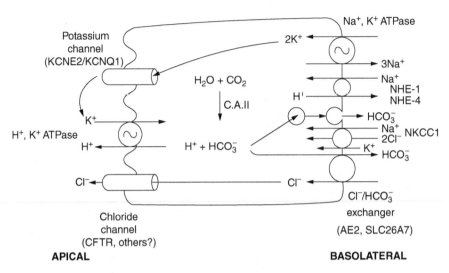

LUMEN   BLOOD STREAM

Figure 3–7. Ion transport proteins of parietal cells. Protons are generated in the cytosol via the action of carbonic anhydrase II (C.A. II). Bicarbonate ions are exported from the basolateral pole of the cell either by vesicular fusion or via a chloride–bicarbonate exchanger.

ions to match the protons pumped from the cell. The molecular identity of these chloride channels remains the subject of debate, although there is some evidence for involvement of CFTR, the protein that is mutated in patients with cystic fibrosis. Chloride derives from the bloodstream, transported by NKCC1 and also in exchange for bicarbonate (see below). The final secretory product is therefore hydrochloric acid, and the process overall is electrically silent due to the complementary charges carried by these two solutes.

The massive rates of secretion conducted by parietal cells represent a considerable challenge to cellular homeostasis. This is because a bicarbonate ion is generated for every proton that is secreted, and if these were allowed to accumulate in the cytosol, deleterious effects on cellular metabolism would result from the resulting increase in pH. Thus, as the protons are secreted apically, the parietal cells also discharge bicarbonate ions across the basolateral membrane to maintain cytosolic pH within narrow limits. At least a portion of this bicarbonate transport occurs in exchange for the chloride ions that are needed for apical secretion, via chloride–bicarbonate exchangers. Some bicarbonate is likely also lost secondary to pumping into intracellular vesicles (distinct from the tubulovesicles) that then move to the basolateral membrane and fuse with it, discharging their contents. The bicarbonate effluxed from the cell by either mechanism is then picked up by the bloodstream, resulting in a measurable increase in circulating pH values when gastric secretory processes are active. The arrangement of the microvasculature in the gastric mucosa also carries a portion of this bicarbonate up to the basolateral pole of surface epithelial cells, which secrete bicarbonates to defend themselves against the potentially injurious effects of acid and pepsin. This movement of bicarbonate into the bloodstream during gastric secretion is referred to as the *alkaline tide.*

The transport mechanisms that exist in parietal cells are depicted in Figure 3–7. In addition to those already mentioned earlier the basolateral membrane contains sodium–hydrogen exchangers (NHE-1 and NHE-4), which expel protons from the cell in exchange for sodium ions, a process driven secondarily by the low intracellular sodium concentration established by the Na^+, K^+ ATPase. At first blush, this may seem counterintuitive, since basolateral fluxes of protons would be predicted to oppose the normal secretion of acid across the apical membrane. However, the role of the exchangers is not to participate in acid secretion, but to fulfill so-called "housekeeping" functions, namely to allow for the efflux of protons generated in resting cells by ongoing metabolic activities. A basolateral potassium channel that has also been identified in parietal cells likely plays a similar homeostatic role. The structure of many of these transport proteins is now understood at the molecular level, which is yielding corresponding insights into potential therapeutic targets. The H^+, K^+ ATPase, in particular, has been shown to consist of two subunits. The transporting α-subunit contains many membrane-spanning regions, and the sites for proton and potassium binding and translocation as well as ATP hydrolysis. The smaller β-subunit, on the other hand, only passes through the membrane a single time, and does not possess any catalytic or transport functions. Instead, the β-subunit appears to be critical for the appropriate targeting of newly synthesized α-subunits to the tubulovesicles, and stabilization of the pump at the apical membrane. Drugs capable of inhibiting the pump, known as proton pump inhibitors, or PPIs, have become the mainstay of treatment for digestive disorders involving inappropriate acid secretion. These PPIs bind either reversibly or irreversibly to a site on the extracellular face of the α-subunit, thereby preventing transport activity.

Other Products

As noted earlier in this chapter, the stomach also secretes a number of additional products that are important in gastrointestinal physiology, including intrinsic factor, pepsinogen, mucus, bicarbonate, and trefoil peptides. Here, we will briefly review how the secretion of these products is controlled at the cellular level, although it should be noted that considerably less information exists on this topic than for the hallmark secretion of gastric acid.

Intrinsic factor is synthesized and released by parietal cells, presumably via a process of exocytosis although the subcellular location of intrinsic factor within parietal cells is not known. Secretion of intrinsic factor is, however, activated by the same secretagogues that activate acid secretion, and therefore presumably involves similar signaling events. However, while intrinsic factor is usually secreted in parallel with acid, these processes are not dependent on each other. Thus, proton pump inhibitors have no inhibitory effect on the secretion of intrinsic factor.

The intrinsic factor is known to be secreted in amounts considerably in excess of physiological requirements for the absorption of cobalamin. This is presumably to account for degradation of a portion of the secreted intrinsic factor by digestive enzymes, although the structure of the peptide is such that it is relatively resistant to degradation, and particularly to digestion by acid and pepsin.

Pepsinogen is secreted by chief cells via a classical process of compound exocytosis, and is thereafter activated to its catalytic form in the presence of a low pH. The active enzyme is particularly effective in degrading collagen, and is inactivated if the pH increases above pH 5 (i.e., soon after the meal has moved into the duodenum, in healthy individuals). As for other cell types that release their products via exocytosis, calcium is a key intracellular mediator effecting the secretory response, and ACh and GRP, both agents which elevate intracellular calcium, are known to be important chief cell secretagogues. The precise roles of gastrin and histamine, on the other hand, remain controversial. One additional secretagogue that may be important, however, is secretin, especially during the intestinal phase of gastric secretion when the presence of the gastric contents in the small intestinal lumen leads to a transient decrease in pH and thus an increase in secretin release.

Surface epithelial cells throughout the stomach secrete mucus and bicarbonate. Mucus is released via exocytosis of granules containing high molecular weight mucins, which are molecules that resemble a bottlebrush with a protein core linked to many long chain oligosaccharides. The oligosaccharide chains are responsible for the unusual physicochemical properties of the mucus. Thus, following the release of mucus, the oligosaccharides expand as they are hydrated, providing a highly viscoelastic substance. The structure of the mucus layer is also stabilized by intramolecular disulfide bonds, as well as by interactions with trefoil peptides. The viscosity of the mucus may limit diffusion of acid through the plane of the gel via a mechanism known as viscous fingering. Thus, acid secreted under hydrostatic pressure from the gastric glands may emerge as a discrete stream through the gel, restricting access of the acid to the gastric surface. Mucus-secreting cells also package phospholipids that are secreted concurrently with mucins, in a manner analogous to the secretion of surfactants in the lung. These phospholipids are believed to confer a hydrophobic nature to the surface of the mucus gel and may thus limit the back-diffusion of apical solutes, such as protons, toward the epithelium, although this attractive hypothesis has yet to be proven. Nevertheless, secretion of the components of the mucus layer is increased by a variety of secretagogues, and is presumed to be under the control of both cholinergic and gastrin-dependent signaling pathways, as well as local reflexes that may involve CGRP and tachykinins. Likewise, prostaglandins are potent mucus secretagogues, providing a partial explanation as to why non-steroidal anti-inflammatory drugs, which prevent prostaglandin synthesis, predispose the gastric mucosa to injury and ulceration. One drug that exploits the protective effect of prostaglandins is misoprostol, which is a synthetic prostaglandin that is often used to counteract the injurious effects of NSAIDs in patients that need to take these chronically.

PATHOPHYSIOLOGY AND CLINICAL CORRELATIONS

An understanding of the physiology underlying gastric secretion allows us in turn to understand how the system can go awry in the setting of disease. Three conditions where dysregulated gastric secretion may occur and/or be important in pathogenesis include ulcer disease, gastrinoma, and atrophic gastritis.

Ulcer Disease

Ulcer disease, more accurately referred to as peptic ulcer disease (which reflects its pathogenesis related to the injurious effects of gastric acid and pepsin), can be subdivided into gastric and duodenal ulcer disease. The names refer to the site in which ulcers, erosions through the lining epithelium that may ultimately lead to bleeding from mucosal blood vessels, are seen, and the two disease states are related but may not share identical pathogenic mechanisms. There is some evidence to suggest that gastric acid secretion may be abnormally high in duodenal ulcer disease patients, both in the interdigestive phase and when maximally stimulated during a meal. Conversely, gastric ulcer disease patients may have lower than normal measured levels of acid secretion following stimulation, thought to be due, in part, to the back-diffusion of secreted acid across the injured gastric mucosa. However, many patients with either gastric or duodenal ulcers demonstrate acid secretory responses that lie entirely within the normal range. For duodenal ulcer disease, at least, it is likely that a failure in mucosal defense mechanisms seems more likely to be the underlying pathogenic defect. Thus, patients with duodenal ulcer disease have abnormally low levels of duodenal mucosal bicarbonate secretion, both resting and after stimulation, and may thus be less capable of neutralizing the gastric acid load that is presented to the small intestine. Gastric ulcers may also arise initially due to a lack of protective factors, such as alterations in blood flow.

There are two major exogenous causes of both gastric and duodenal ulcers; ingestion of nonsteroidal antiinflammatory drugs (NSAIDs) or gastric colonization with a gram-negative, spiral-shaped bacterium known as *Helicobacter pylori*. Ulcer disease associated with the use of NSAIDs likely reflects a loss of protective factors, such as the prostaglandins that normally contribute to the gastric barrier by controlling blood flow, as discussed earlier. The full details of ulcer pathogenesis related to NSAID use are still being worked out, but it is clear that this condition is an increasing problem in developed countries, where aging populations are prescribed more and more NSAIDs to counter degenerative diseases, such as arthritis. NSAIDs thought to be less toxic to the stomach are being developed, but none thus far are completely without the risk of causing ulceration, especially when used chronically.

In the absence of NSAID use, the vast majority of all ulcer patients can be shown to be infected with *H. pylori*, which is specialized to colonize the gastric niche because it secretes large amounts of the enzyme, urease. This product converts urea to ammonium ions in the vicinity of the bacteria, thereby protecting them from the deleterious effects of gastric acidity. In genetically susceptible individuals, infection with *H. pylori* can have profound effects on both gastric and duodenal physiology, including both hyper- and hypo-secretion of acid, alterations in blood flow, and an inhibition of duodenal bicarbonate secretion. These changes may result indirectly from the inflammatory response mounted by the host in a futile attempt to expel the chronic bacterial colonization. Nevertheless, it is clear that acid contributes to ulcer pathogenesis, even if secreted in normal amounts, due to its role in sustaining the activation of pepsin, and, in the case of duodenal ulcers, the direct injurious effects of protons on the epithelial cells at this site which are not designed to withstand prolonged exposure to low pH (contrast with the resilient epithelial cells in the stomach). In fact, a clinical adage: "no acid, no ulcer" also gives clues as to possible treatments.

Patients with ulcer disease are treated typically with drugs that suppress acid secretion, thereby giving the mucosa the opportunity to heal itself. In the past, this was accomplished primarily with H_2 antihistamines, although the protection afforded by such drugs was incomplete because they did not interfere with other important stimuli of acid secretion. More recently, profound acid suppression—essentially total in nature—has been accomplished with PPIs. While there were initially fears that long-term use of these agents would be accompanied by excessive levels of gastrin in the blood, and perhaps by an increased cancer risk given the trophic effects of this hormone, these do not appear to have been borne out by clinical experience and, indeed, one PPI has been transferred to over-the-counter status. The basis of the gastrinemia in patients treated with PPIs is the loss of an inhibitory effect of somatostatin on gastrin release, because luminal pH never falls to levels that would trigger somatostatin release from D cells. Finally, in addition to acid suppression, ulcer patients who can be demonstrated to be infected with *H. pylori* usually receive antibiotics to eradicate the microorganism, a treatment that markedly reduces the risk of any relapse.

Gastrinoma

A rarer disease affecting gastric secretory function is gastrinoma, also known as Zollinger–Ellison or Z-E syndrome. In patients affected by this disorder, a (usually extragastric) endocrine tumor develops whose cells secrete large amounts of gastrin in an unregulated fashion. Such individuals have extremely high rates of gastric acid secretion, both at rest and in response to a meal. Both values may be increased five to ten fold above their normal levels. Moreover, because the tumor cells are unaffected by the normal negative feedback mechanisms that reduce gastrin release from G cells as the luminal pH falls, serum gastrin levels increase yet further.

Patients with gastrinoma often present with symptoms of dyspepsia and even gastric or duodenal ulceration. Duodenal injury, in particular, results because the unremitting load of acid and pepsin from the stomach overwhelms the segment's defensive capacities. This allows pepsin to remain active for longer and to degrade the duodenal epithelial cells, which are not specialized to withstand acid-peptic damage. If the primary tumor can be found in these patients, surgery is usually curative. However, other patients must be managed symptomatically, most often with the use of PPIs.

Atrophic Gastritis

Chronic inflammation of the gastric mucosa, with injury and destruction of epithelial cell lineages, is seen in a number of gastrointestinal infections, especially when microorganisms colonize the stomach. A reaction of this type likely accounts for the fact that a subset of patients infected with *H. pylori* have lower than normal acid output. However, gastric atrophy is also seen in the absence of infection, particularly in the disease of *pernicious anemia*. This latter disease is addressed here because it illuminates several facets of gastrointestinal physiology.

Pernicious anemia is an autoimmune condition where patients develop antibodies to parietal cells and/or intrinsic factor. The immune attack mediated by these antibodies leads to inflammation restricted to the corpus of the stomach, a reduction in parietal cell mass, and destruction of chief cells, likely via a bystander mechanism or secondary to the apparent ability of parietal cells to control the numbers of other cell types present in oxyntic glands. The disease is a progressive one, and clinical manifestations may not occur until parietal cell numbers have been decreased (irreversibly) below a critical number. Acid secretion by the stomach is markedly reduced both at baseline and after meals, and in advanced cases is completely absent. Due to the loss of regulatory feedback, therefore, levels of gastrin in the bloodstream rise sharply, even approaching those seen in some gastrinoma patients in the most serious cases.

The loss of parietal and chief cell function in pernicious anemia significantly reduces the extent to which digestion of the meal can be initiated in the gastric lumen. However, under most circumstances this is not nutritionally significant, since the digestive capacity of the pancreatic enzymes is more than adequate to fully digest dietary macromolecules. On the other hand, the most clinically significant consequence of a reduction in parietal cell function is cobalamin deficiency, which manifests as pernicious anemia and also with neurological disturbances, such as numbness in the extremities and weakness. Some patients may develop iron-deficiency anemia, particularly if their diet is low in heme iron (e.g., in vegetarians). There is also some increased risk of infection via the oral route in patients with pernicious anemia, given the lost ability of the gastric juices to sterilize the ingested meal.

Pernicious anemia is thought to be a relatively rare condition, and often occurs in association with other autoimmune diseases such as Graves disease or thyroiditis. On the other hand, there is a normal decline in parietal cell mass with aging, which may result in cobalamin malabsorption and increased susceptibility to enteric infections in the elderly. The increased susceptibility to infections can also be seen in patients who take PPIs for long periods. However, in this latter group, cobalamin malabsorption does not occur unless present for other reasons, because of the fact that acid and intrinsic factor can be secreted independently by parietal cells.

KEY CONCEPTS

 Gastric secretion plays important roles in digestion, absorption of specific nutrients, and host defense.

 Acid secretion occurs in phases that correspond temporally to the ingestion of a meal.

 Regulation of acid secretion involves neurocrine, paracrine, and endocrine components.

 The stomach secretes other important products such as pepsinogen, intrinsic factor, mucus, and bicarbonate and trefoil peptides.

 Various disease states can result from, or are associated with, abnormal gastric secretory function.

 STUDY QUESTIONS

3–1. *A 40-year-old man comes to his physician complaining of epigastric pain. An upper endoscopy reveals duodenal erosions and a test of gastric secretory function reveals markedly elevated levels of basal acid secretion that are increased only modestly by intravenous infusion of a gastrin analogue. What is the most likely diagnosis?*

A. *Zollinger–Ellison syndrome*

B. *H. pylori infection*

C. *Gastroesophageal reflux disease*

D. *Gastroparesis*

E. *Achalasia*

3–2. In an experiment, rabbits are administered a cholinergic agonist, gastrin, or histamine intravenously, and gastric acid secretion is measured. Which treatment, when coadministered with each of these agents, would be expected to block gastric acid secretion produced by any of the stimuli?

A. Histamine H_2 antagonist

B. Antibodies to gastrin

C. Anticholinergic drug

D. Histamine H_1 antagonist

E. Proton pump inhibitor

3–3. A patient suffering from anemia comes to his physician complaining of frequent bouts of gastroenteritis. A blood test reveals circulating antibodies directed against gastric parietal cells. His anemia is ascribable to hyposecretion of which of the following gastric secretory products?

A. Histamine

B. Gastrin

C. Pepsinogen

D. Hydrochloric acid

E. Intrinsic factor

3–4. Two medical students studying for their physiology final decide to take a break for a lunchtime hamburger. Before reaching the cafeteria, nervous impulses from the dorsal vagal complex will initiate gastric acid secretion by triggering release of which neurotransmitter from the enteric nervous system?

A. Norepinephrine

B. Vasoactive intestinal polypeptide

C. Substance P

D. Gastrin releasing peptide

E. Nitric oxide

3–5. Compared to the cephalic phase, the gastric phase of gastric acid secretion is characterized by which of the following patterns?

	Acid secretion	Gastrin secretion	Somatostatin secretion
A.	Increased	Increased	Increased
B.	Increased	Increased	Decreased
C.	No change	Increased	No change
D.	Decrease	Decreased	Increased
E.	Decreased	Decreased	Decreased
F.	No change	Decreased	No change

SUGGESTED READINGS

Banka S, Tyan K, Thomson W, Newmann WG. Pernicious anemia—genetic insights. *Autoimmun Rev.* 2011;10:455–459.

Gibril F, Jensen RT. Zollinger–Ellison syndrome revisited: diagnosis, biologic markers, associated inherited disorders, and acid hypersecretion. *Curr Gastroenterol Rep.* 2004;6:454–463.

Heitzmann D, Warth R. No potassium, no acid: K⁺ channels and gastric acid secretion. *Physiology.* 2007;22:335–341.

Okamoto C, Karvar S, Forte JG, Yao X. The cell biology of gastric acid secretion. In: Johnson LR, Ghishan FK, Kaunitz JD, Merchant JL, Said HM, Wood JD, eds. *Physiology of the Gastrointestinal Tract.* 5th ed. San Diego: Academic Press; 2012:1251–1279.

Osefo N, Ito T, Jensen RT. Gastric acid hypersecretory states: recent insights and advances. *Curr Gastroenterol Rep.* 2009;11:433–441.

Raufman JP. Gastric chief cells: receptors and signal transduction mechanisms. *Gastroenterology.* 1992;102:699–710.

Samuelson LC, Hinkle KL. Insights into the regulation of gastric acid secretion through analysis of genetically engineered mice. *Annu Rev Physiol.* 2003;65:383–400.

Schubert ML, Peura DA. Control of gastric acid secretion in health and disease. *Gastroenterology.* 2008;134:1842–1860.

Pancreatic and Salivary Secretion

4

OBJECTIVES

- Understand the role played by the pancreas in digestion and absorption of a mixed meal
- Understand the structure of the exocrine pancreas and the cell types that give rise to proteinaceous and fluid components of the pancreatic juice
- Identify key constituents of the pancreatic juice and the enzymes that are secreted in inactive forms
- Describe the factors that regulate the release of secretin and the role of this hormone in stimulating pancreatic ductular secretion
  - Understand the ion transport pathways expressed in pancreatic ducts and their mechanisms of action
- Understand the role of CCK and other factors in regulating pancreatic acinar cells
  - Discuss the relative roles of monitor peptide and CCK-releasing peptide in regulating CCK release
- Identify signaling events activated in pancreatic acinar cells by secretagogues
- Compare and contrast the structure of the salivary glands with that of the exocrine pancreas
- Identify the functions of saliva and the constituents responsible for these
- Define ion transport pathways that produce saliva and modify its composition
- Define regulatory pathways for saliva production
  - Understand conditions where production of saliva may be abnormal

BASIC PRINCIPLES OF PANCREATIC SECRETION

Role and Significance

The pancreas is the source of the majority of enzymes required for digestion of a mixed meal (i.e., carbohydrate, protein, and fat). Pancreatic enzymes are produced in great excess, underscoring their importance in the digestive process. However, unlike the digestive enzymes produced by the stomach and in the saliva, some level of pancreatic function is necessary for adequate digestion and absorption. In general, nutrition is impaired if production of

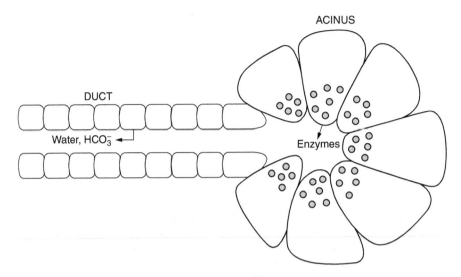

Figure 4–1. Schematic structure of the exocrine pancreas. [Redrawn from the AGA Undergraduate Teaching Project slide set "The Integrated Response to a Meal" (Unit 29, copyright 1995) by S. Pandol and H.E. Raybould, with permission.]

pancreatic enzymes falls below 10% of normal levels, or if outflow of the pancreatic juice into the intestine is physically obstructed.

We should distinguish between the *exocrine* pancreas, responsible for producing secretions that flow out of the body, and the *endocrine* pancreas, the site of synthesis of various important hormones that regulate whole-body homeostasis, the most notable of which is insulin (Figure 4–1). These dual secretory functions of the pancreas are segregated to distinct anatomic locations. The functions and regulation of the exocrine pancreas are the province of gastrointestinal physiology, whereas the endocrine functions are a topic for discussion in a general endocrinology course. Thus, the latter will not be discussed further here.

Pancreatic Secretory Products

The exocrine pancreas is the site of synthesis and secretion predominantly of enzymes. These fall into four main groups—proteases, amylolytic enzymes, lipases, and nucleases—as shown in Table 4–1. In addition, other proteins are produced that modulate the function of pancreatic secretory products, such as colipase and trypsin inhibitors. Finally, the pancreas secretes a peptide known as monitor peptide, which represents an important feedback mechanism linking pancreatic secretory capacity with the requirements of the intestine for digestion at any given moment after the ingestion of a meal; more on that topic later. The quantities of each of the secretory products differ greatly. Almost 80% by weight of the proteins secreted by the exocrine pancreas are proteases, with much lower quantities of the enzymes responsible for breaking down other classes of nutrients. Of the proteases, trypsinogen, the inactive precursor of trypsin, is by far the most

Table 4–1. Pancreatic acinar cell secretory products

Proteases	Amylolytic enzyme	Lipases	Nucleases	Others
Trypsinogen*	Amylase	Lipase	Deoxyribonuclease	Procolipase*
Chymotrypsinogen*		Nonspecific esterase	Ribonuclease	Trypsin inhibitors
Proelastase*		Prophospholipase A_2*		Monitor peptide
Procarboxypeptidase A*				
Procarboxypeptidase B*				

Note: Stored and secreted in inactive forms.

abundant, accounting for approximately 40% by weight of pancreatic secretory products. This likely reflects a central role for trypsin in initiating the digestion of proteins, which will be discussed further in Chapter 15.

As we learned for pepsinogen in the stomach, the proteases synthesized by the pancreas are packaged and stored as inactive precursors. This is also true for at least one lipolytic enzyme, prophospholipase A_2. The need to store these enzymes in their inactive forms relates to the toxicity of the active products toward the pancreas itself. Under normal circumstances, therefore, the pancreas does not digest itself. Only in the setting of disease, particularly if the secretions are retained in the pancreas for a prolonged period, do the enzymes become inappropriately activated resulting in the very painful condition of *pancreatitis*.

ANATOMIC CONSIDERATIONS IN PANCREAS

As alluded to above, the pancreas has both exocrine and endocrine functions. The latter are restricted to endocrine cells located in the islets of Langerhans, which are scattered throughout the bulk of the pancreatic parenchyma. The exocrine functions, on the other hand, are conducted by a series of blind-ended ducts that terminate in structures known as acini. Many such acini, arranged like clusters of grapes, disgorge their products into a branching ductular system that empties into larger and larger collecting ducts, eventually reaching the main pancreatic duct or Wirsung's duct. This duct merges with the common bile duct, coming from the liver, and the mixed bile plus pancreatic juice enters the duodenum a short distance distal to the pylorus, under the control of a sphincter called the sphincter of Oddi. A minor part of the pancreas is drained by an accessory collecting duct, known as the duct of Santorini, which has a separate opening to the duodenum. Both the acinar and ductular cells contribute distinct products to the pancreatic juice and both are regulated during the course of responding to a meal.

Acinar Cells

Pancreatic acinar cells are specialized exocrine secretory cells that are the source of the majority of the proteinaceous components of the pancreatic juice. They are somewhat triangular in shape when viewed in cross-section, with a basolaterally-displaced nucleus. The basolateral membrane faces the bloodstream and contains receptors for a variety of neurohumoral agents responsible for regulating pancreatic secretion. The apical pole of the cell, on the other hand, is packed at rest with large numbers of *zymogen granules* that contain the digestive enzymes and other regulatory factors. These granules are closely apposed to the apical membrane and thus to the lumen of the acinus. When the cell is stimulated by secretagogues, the granules undergo a process of compound exocytosis and fuse with each other and the apical membrane, thereby discharging their contents into the lumen.

Ductular Cells

The cells lining the intercalated ducts of the pancreas also play an important role in modifying the composition of the pancreatic juice. They are classical columnar epithelial cells, comparable to those lining the intestine itself, whose passive permeability is restricted by well-developed intercellular tight junctions. When stimulated, these cells transport bicarbonate ions into the pancreatic juice as it passes along the duct, with water following paracellularly in response to the resulting transepithelial osmotic gradient. Thus, the effect of the duct cells is to dilute the pancreatic juice and to render it alkaline. Quantitatively, the pancreas plays the major role in supplying the bicarbonate necessary to neutralize gastric acid so that appropriate digestion can take place in the small intestine.

The relative roles of acinar and ductular cells in contributing to the pancreatic juice can be demonstrated in animals fed a diet that is deficient in copper while also receiving the drug penicillamine. Among other effects, this treatment leads to atrophy of the pancreatic acini but has no effect on the ducts. Following a meal, such animals are unable to secrete pancreatic enzymes, but remain capable of increasing the volume of pancreatic juice due to the residual duct activity. In fact, the activity of the ductular cells is likely critical to "wash" the pancreatic enzymes out into the small intestine. Later in this chapter, we will consider the effects of cystic fibrosis, a disease state where ductular function is abnormal, on pancreatic secretory function.

REGULATION OF PANCREATIC SECRETION

Phases of Secretion

As we saw for gastric secretion, pancreatic secretory activity related to meal ingestion occurs in phases. In humans, the majority of the secretory response (approximately 60–70%) occurs during the intestinal phase, but there are also significant contributions from the cephalic (20–25%) and gastric (10%) phases. Pancreatic secretion is activated by a combination of neural and hormonal effectors. During the cephalic and gastric phases, secretions are low in volume with high concentrations of digestive enzymes, reflecting stimulation primarily of acinar cells. This stimulation arises from cholinergic vagal input during the cephalic phase, and vago-vagal reflexes activated by gastric distension during the gastric phase. During the intestinal phase, on the other hand, ductular secretion is strongly activated, resulting in the production of high volumes of pancreatic juice with decreased concentrations of protein, although the total quantity of enzymes secreted during this phase is actually also markedly increased. Ductular secretion during this phase is driven primarily by the endocrine action of secretin on receptors localized to the basolateral pole of duct epithelial cells. The inputs to the acinar cells during the intestinal phase include CCK and 5-HT from the intestine as well as neurotransmitters including acetylcholine (ACh) and GRP. The large magnitude of the intestinal phase is also attributable to amplification by so-called enteropancreatic reflexes transmitted via the enteric nervous system. The mechanisms regulating CCK and secretin release during the intestinal phase will be addressed in the following sections.

Role of CCK

CCK can be considered a master regulator of the duodenal cluster unit, of which the pancreas is an important component (Figure 4–2). CCK is a potent stimulus of acinar secretion, acting predominantly via CCK_1 receptor-dependent stimulation of vagal afferents close to its site of release in the duodenum, thereby evoking vago-vagal reflexes that stimulate acinar cell secretion via cholinergic and non-cholinergic neurotransmitters (the latter including both GRP and VIP). There are also CCK_1 receptors on the basolateral pole of acinar cells, but it now seems likely that these are only activated if circulating concentrations of CCK rise to supraphysiologic levels. In addition to its effects on the pancreas, CCK coordinates the

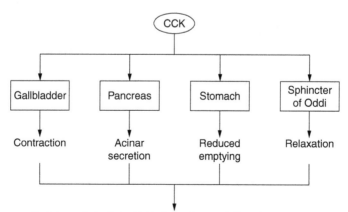

Figure 4–2. Multiple effects of cholecystokinin (CCK) in the duodenal cluster unit. CCK serves to coordinate nutrient delivery to match intestinal capacity.

activity of other GI segments and draining organs, including by contracting the gallbladder (the physiologic function for which this hormone was named), relaxing the sphincter of Oddi, and slowing gastric motility to retard gastric emptying and thereby control the rate of delivery of partially digested nutrients to more distal segments of the gut. The latter activity serves to match luminal nutrient availability to the digestive and absorptive capacity of the small intestine. Finally, CCK can modulate the activity of other neurohumoral regulators in a synergistic fashion. Notably, while CCK is a weak agonist of pancreatic ductular secretion of bicarbonate by itself, it markedly potentiates the effect of secretin on this transport mechanism. During the integrated response to a meal, therefore, it is likely that the ability of secretin to evoke pancreatic bicarbonate secretion is amplified by occurring against the background of a CCK "tone."

Nevertheless, CCK predominantly affects acinar cell secretion. Thus, during the initial response to a meal (i.e., the cephalic and gastric phases), pancreatic secretions are low in volume with a high concentration of enzymes and enzyme precursors. This situation should be contrasted with secretory flows occurring in the intestinal phase, where 5-HT and secretin also play a role. The effects of secretin are mediated predominantly at the level of the ducts. However, 5-HT, released from intestinal enterochromaffin cells in response to nutrients, activates a vago-vagal reflex that mirrors and augments that of CCK itself. It has been calculated that CCK and 5-HT are each responsible for about 50% of pancreatic enzyme secretion during the intestinal phase.

FACTORS CAUSING CCK RELEASE

CCK is synthesized and stored by endocrine cells located predominantly in the duodenum, labeled in some sources as "I" cells (Figure 4–3). Control of CCK release from these cells is carefully regulated to match the body's needs for CCK bioactivity. In part, this is accomplished by the activity of two luminally active CCK releasing factors, which are small peptides. One of these peptides is derived from cells in the duodenum, and called CCK-releasing peptide (CCK-RP). It is likely released into the lumen in response to specific nutrients, including fatty acids and hydrophobic amino acids. The other luminal peptide that controls CCK secretion is monitor peptide, which is a product of pancreatic acinar cells. Release of monitor peptide can be neurally mediated, including by the release of ACh and GRP in the vicinity of pancreatic acinar cells during the cephalic phase, and mediated by subsequent vago-vagal reflexes during the gastric and intestinal phases of the response to a meal. Likewise, once CCK release has been stimulated by CCK-RP, it too can cause monitor peptide release via the mechanisms outlined for acinar cell stimulation discussed earlier.

The significance of having peptide factors that regulate CCK release lies in their ability to match pancreatic secretion of proteolytic enzymes to the need for these enzymes in the small intestinal lumen. When meal proteins and oligopeptides are present in the lumen in large quantities, they compete for the action of trypsin and other proteolytic enzymes, meaning that CCK-RP and monitor peptide are degraded only slowly. Thus, CCK release is sustained, causing further

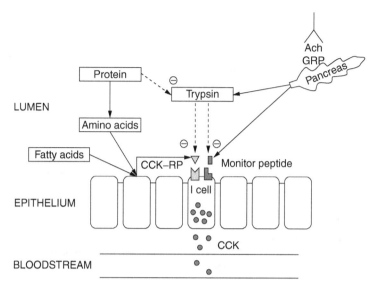

Figure 4–3. Mechanisms responsible for controlling cholecystokinin (CCK) release from duodenal I cells. CCK-RP, CCK releasing peptide; ACh, acetylcholine; GRP, gastrin-releasing peptide. Solid arrows represent stimulatory effects while dashed arrows indicate inhibition.

secretion of proteases and other components of the pancreatic juice. On the other hand, once the meal has been fully digested and absorbed, CCK-RP and monitor peptide will be degraded by the pancreatic proteases. This then leads to the termination of CCK release, and thus a marked reduction in the secretion of pancreatic enzymes. This feedback mechanism for the control of CCK release, and in turn, pancreatic secretion, can be demonstrated in animals in which pancreatic juices have been diverted away from the intestinal lumen. In such experiments, CCK release in response to fatty acids or amino acids is potentiated and prolonged, presumably reflecting the persistence of CCK-RP.

Role of Secretin

The other major regulator of pancreatic secretion is secretin, which is released from S cells in the duodenal mucosa. When the meal enters the small intestine from the stomach, the volume of pancreatic secretions increases rapidly, shifting from a low-volume, protein-rich fluid to a high volume secretion in which enzymes are present at lower concentrations (although in greater absolute amounts, reflecting the effect of CCK and neural effectors on acinar cell secretion). As the secretory rate rises, the pH and bicarbonate concentration in the pancreatic juice rises, with a reciprocal fall in the concentration of chloride ions (Figure 4–4). These latter effects on the composition of the pancreatic juice are mediated predominantly by the endocrine mediator, secretin. The postprandial bicarbonate secretory response can largely be

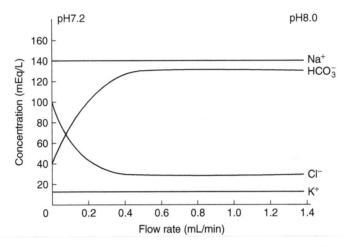

Figure 4–4. Ionic composition of the pancreatic juice as a function of its flow rate. Note that the pancreatic juice becomes alkaline at high rates of secretion.

reproduced by intravenous administration of secretin, particularly if given with a low dose of CCK that potentiates ductular secretion, as discussed earlier.

FACTORS CAUSING SECRETIN RELEASE

The S cells in the duodenal mucosa can be considered to act functionally as pH meters, sensing the acidity of the luminal contents (Figure 4–5). As the pH falls, due to the entry of gastric acid, secretin is released from the S cells and travels through the bloodstream to bind to receptors on pancreatic duct cells, as well as on epithelial cells lining the bile ducts and the duodenum itself. These cells, in turn, are stimulated to secrete bicarbonate into the duodenal lumen, thus causing

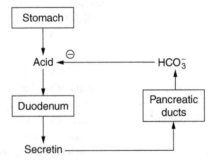

Figure 4–5. Function of secretin. Secretin is released from the duodenum in response to reduced pH, and travels through the bloodstream to evoke bicarbonate secretion from the pancreatic ducts (as well as from the biliary ducts and the duodenal mucosa, not shown), thereby neutralizing gastric acid in the duodenal lumen.

a rise in pH that will eventually shut off secretin release. The pancreas is quantitatively the most important in the bicarbonate secretory response, although the ability of duodenal epithelial cells to secrete bicarbonate may be critically important to protect them from gastric acid, especially in the first part of the duodenum, which is proximal to the site of entry of the pancreatic juice and bile. In fact, patients suffering from duodenal ulcers have abnormally low levels of duodenal bicarbonate secretion both at rest and in response to luminal acidification.

The threshold for secretin release appears to be a luminal pH of less than 4.5. The mechanism by which the S cells sense the change in luminal acidity, and whether secretin release requires a peptide releasing factor and/or the function of mucosal sensory nerve endings is currently unclear. However, while other meal components, such as fatty acids, have been shown in experimental studies to evoke secretin release, the response to acid appears to be the most important physiologically. Subjects who are unable to secrete gastric acid (achlorhydric) secondary to disease or the administration of proton pump inhibitors, or in whom gastric contents have been neutralized by the oral administration of bicarbonate, fail to release secretin postprandially no matter what type of meal is given.

CELLULAR BASIS OF PANCREATIC SECRETION

Acinar Cells

Pancreatic acinar cells are classical secretory cells that synthesize the proteinaceous components of pancreatic juice and package them into zymogen granules that are stored in the apical pole of the cell. The contents of these granules are discharged into the lumen of the acinus via a process of compound exocytosis when the cell receives appropriate neurohumoral inputs. Following the meal, the pancreatic enzymes are then rapidly resynthesized and repackaged into granules, with the process taking less than an hour, leaving the cell ready to respond to the next meal. Evidence exists that the synthetic process is regulated by endocrine effects of CCK and also by other hormones, such as insulin. Pancreatic enzymes are synthesized with a signal peptide at their N-terminus, which directs them to the Golgi apparatus and the secretory pathway, and presumably prevents access of these potentially noxious proteins to the cell cytosol. The various pancreatic proteins are mixed within a given zymogen granule and thus the relative proportions that are released usually reflect the relative rates of initial synthesis. In the long-term, the rate of synthesis of specific classes of enzymes can be regulated in response to changes in the diet. For example, an increase in the proportion of calories supplied by carbohydrates will eventually result in increased expression of amylase as a proportion of the total pancreatic enzymes. This response is mediated by insulin. Corresponding changes occur in the hydrolytic enzymes responsible for digestion of each of the major classes of nutrients (carbohydrates, fat, and proteins) in response to increased or decreased ingestion. Short-term nutrient-related inhibition of pancreatic secretion can also occur in the setting of hyperglycemia, or if free amino acids are infused into the plasma. The mechanism(s) of these latter effects are unknown but their benefit as a feedback mechanism to limit further nutrient digestion and absorption is clear.

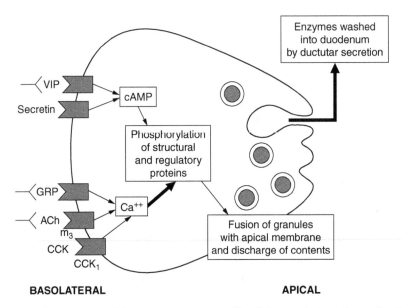

Figure 4–6. Receptors of the pancreatic acinar cell and the regulation of secretion. The block arrow indicates that calcium-dependent signaling pathways play the most prominent role in enzyme secretion. VIP, vasoactive intestinal polypeptide; GRP, gastrin releasing peptide; ACh, acetylcholine; CCK, cholecystokinin.

On their basolateral membranes, acinar cells express receptors for CCK as well as for neural regulators of secretion, including acetylcholine, GRP, and VIP (Figure 4–6). The effects of CCK and ACh are mediated by CCK_1 and m_3 muscarinic receptors, respectively. All of the receptors for the major pancreatic secretagogues are members of the family of G-protein coupled receptors, and link to various downstream effectors such as phospholipase C and adenylyl cyclase. In general, the phospholipase C-dependent pathway, which is utilized by the receptors for CCK, ACh, and GRP and results in increases in cytoplasmic calcium, is the most quantitatively significant for acinar secretion, with cAMP-dependent signaling playing a subsidiary or modifying role.

During activation of pancreatic acinar cells, numerous proteins change their phosphorylation status. These changes are mediated by protein kinases and phosphatases that are activated by either calcium or cAMP, including calmodulin-dependent protein kinase, protein kinase C, protein kinase A and the phosphatase, calcineurin. Altered phosphorylation of structural and regulatory proteins, particularly those of the cytoskeleton, in turn mediates the movement of zymogen granules toward the apical pole of the cell and their eventual fusion with the apical plasma membrane. Effects on the cytoskeleton include dissolution of an actin-rich web at the apical pole of the cell that may function to restrict access of granules to the membrane in the resting state. The fusion events also involve the interaction of specific proteins called SNAREs, which mediate the recognition of vesicles destined to fuse with the apical membrane with their target sites, as well as small G proteins of the Rab family that are expressed on the surface of zymogen granules and regulate exocytosis.

Signaling events that originate at the level of secretagogue receptors are also presumed to regulate the synthesis of pancreatic enzymes as well as acinar cell growth. The precise details of such regulation are still the subject of active investigation, but may involve cross-talk between G-protein coupled secretagogue receptors and those for classical growth factors, which mediate signaling via tyrosine kinases and mitogen-activated protein kinases capable of direct regulation of nuclear transcription factors. Non-secretagogue growth factors, such as epidermal growth factor and insulin, may also have independent effects on growth. Adaptive growth of the pancreas, such as during feeding of a high-protein diet or during the hyperphagia of pregnancy, ensures greater digestive capacity to avert malabsorption.

Ductular Cells

In contrast to acinar cells that secrete their characteristic products via a process of granule exocytosis, the ductular cells that contribute the fluid and bicarbonate components of pancreatic juice are classical polarized epithelial cells that conduct vectorial ion transport via the cooperative activation of membrane transport proteins localized to their apical and basolateral poles. As seen elsewhere in the gastrointestinal tract, while exocytic secretion predominantly involves calcium-dependent signaling with cAMP playing a modulatory role, the membrane transport events that underlie ductular ion secretion are predominantly driven by cAMP, with calcium playing the subsidiary role.

As outlined earlier, the primary stimulus of duct cell secretion is secretin, which binds to a basolateral receptor that links via a G-protein to adenylyl cyclase. The primary target of the cAMP thereby generated is protein kinase A, which phosphorylates the CFTR chloride channel localized to the apical membrane of the cell. This channel allows outflow of chloride ions, which can exchange for bicarbonate across an apical chloride–bicarbonate exchanger (SLC26a6 appears to be the most important isoform) to provide for movement of bicarbonate ions into the duct lumen (Figure 4–7). Water and sodium ions follow paracellularly in response to the electrochemical gradient across the epithelium. The bicarbonate required for the transport mechanism derives from two sources. Some is generated intracellularly, via the activity of carbonic anhydrase, which converts water and carbon dioxide to a bicarbonate ion and a proton; the proton is recycled basolaterally via a sodium–hydrogen exchanger, likely NHE-1 and/or NHE-4, to maintain intracellular pH within the physiological range. Protons may also be recycled by pumping them into vesicles that subsequently fuse with the basolateral membrane, in a process analogous to that used to recycle bicarbonate ions in the actively secreting parietal cell (see Chapter 3). Other bicarbonate ions are taken up from the bloodstream via a basolateral sodium–bicarbonate cotransporter (pNBC1), which takes advantage of the low intracellular sodium concentration established by a

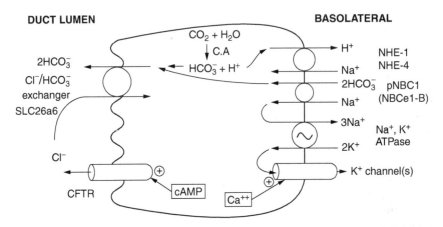

Figure 4–7. Ion transport pathways present in pancreatic duct cells. C.A., carbonic anhydrase; NHE-1(4), sodium/hydrogen exchanger-1(4); pNBC1, sodium-bicarbonate cotransporter; SLC26a6, solute-carrier 26a6 (chloride–bicarbonate exchanger).

basolateral sodium–potassium ATPase. The bicarbonate in the bloodstream, at least in part, is likely derived from the "alkaline tide" that is a by-product of gastric acid secretion. Thus, the gastrointestinal system effectively recycles acid and base equivalents to conduct the processes necessary for digestion and absorption of nutrients without adverse effects on whole body acid–base status. The relative contribution of carbonic anhydrase and pNBC1 to the supply of bicarbonate ions is unknown, but in humans, who are capable of high rates of bicarbonate secretion when the pancreas is maximally stimulated, pNBC1, which takes up two bicarbonate ions for each sodium, may play the primary role. Because this NBC isoform is electrogenic, moreover, its activity will be driven not only by the sodium gradient across the basolateral membrane, but also by the membrane potential. Thus, opening of the CFTR chloride channel, which will act to depolarize the cell, will secondarily drive bicarbonate uptake via pNBC1.

CCK is able to potentiate the bicarbonate secretory response to secretin, without itself serving as a potent independent stimulus of the transport mechanism. Likewise, ACh also potentiates secretion at the level of the ducts, accounting for the fact that bicarbonate secretion is diminished slightly in vagotomized subjects. The intracellular mechanism(s) whereby CCK and ACh synergistically enhance secretin-induced bicarbonate secretion is not well understood, but is presumed to involve increases in cytoplasmic calcium as evoked by these agonists in other cell types. Some studies have suggested the presence of an accessory chloride channel in duct cells that is sensitive to changes in cytoplasmic calcium concentrations, and which may contribute to the chloride needed for bicarbonate exchange. In addition, the ability of calcium to activate basolateral potassium channels may also be involved, by sustaining the electrical gradient needed to drive net bicarbonate efflux across the apical membrane.

The bicarbonate transported by the duct cells, along with the fluid secretion that this transport mechanism drives, is important to wash the proteinaceous components of the gastric juice into the intestinal lumen. Moreover, the alkaline nature of this secretion is critically important in neutralizing gastric acid. Note that the pancreatic digestive enzymes are optimally active at neutral pH, as opposed to the acidic pH optimum of gastric pepsin.

PANCREATIC PATHOPHYSIOLOGY AND CLINICAL CORRELATIONS

The hydrolytic enzymes secreted by the pancreas are produced in quantities that are vastly in excess of those needed to digest a normal intake of nutrients. It has been calculated that pancreatic enzyme output needs to fall below 10% of normal levels before effects on nutrient absorption are seen. Thus, pancreatic insufficiency is relatively rare. However, under specific conditions, it can occur, manifesting as maldigestion and malabsorption. Fat absorption is usually the first affected by alterations in pancreatic output of enzymes and bicarbonate, perhaps due to a relatively limited supply of lipase and because pancreatic lipase is most sensitive to inactivation by low pH. Thus, *steatorrhea*, or fat in the stool, may be an early sign of pancreatic dysfunction.

Cystic Fibrosis

On the basis of our discussion of the mechanisms underlying bicarbonate secretion in the pancreatic ducts, it should not be surprising that pancreatic function is altered in the genetic disorder of cystic fibrosis, where mutations lead to abnormal function of the CFTR chloride channel. Indeed, the disease was named for characteristic histological abnormalities seen in the pancreas in affected patients. Although pancreatic enzyme synthesis and secretion are normal in patients with cystic fibrosis, the relative inability of the ducts to secrete bicarbonate and water means that the enzymes cannot be flushed properly from the organ, and limited quantities reach the intestinal lumen. Moreover, the enzymes that do reach the lumen are inactive because of the failure to neutralize gastric acid. These findings underscore the role of the duct cells in normal pancreatic function. In fact, in patients with severe CFTR mutations causing a marked reduction in channel function, the exocrine pancreas may be largely destroyed during fetal life, due to the action of retained proteolytic enzymes that become inappropriately activated and damage the tissue. Such patients are said to be "pancreatic insufficient" and must receive supplements of pancreatic enzymes, along with antacids, to allow for adequate nutrition. Patients with milder mutations may retain some degree of pancreatic function, at least early in life, but are then at greater risk for the development of inflammation of the pancreas (pancreatitis) with aging.

Pancreatitis

 In addition to patients suffering from cystic fibrosis, others who experience retention of pancreatic enzymes within the organ may experience the painful consequences of autodigestion of the pancreatic tissue. Pancreatic secretions may be retained within the organ due to obstruction (e.g., a gallstone occluding the pancreatic duct, or a malignancy) or inflammation of the tissue, which commonly occurs in patients who abuse alcohol. Alcohol can also be metabolized into products that cause hyperstimulation of acinar cells, resulting in intracellular trypsin activation and cell death. Because of the potential for injurious effects of the pancreatic enzymes, and particularly the proteinases, such as trypsin, the pancreas has several lines of defense to minimize autodigestion under normal circumstances, provided pancreatic enzymes do not linger in the ductular tree. These include the storage of the enzymes with the greatest injurious potential (proteinases, phospholipase A_2) as inactive proforms, which normally cannot be activated until they reach their substrates in the intestinal lumen. Similarly, the pancreas secretes a variety of low molecular weight trypsin inhibitors that can antagonize a small amount of prematurely activated enzyme. Finally, trypsin can degrade itself if it becomes activated prior to reaching the intestine. In one form of hereditary pancreatitis, patients express a trypsin molecule that is mutated such that it is resistant to cleavage by other trypsin molecules. Under these conditions, if the other lines of defense are breached, these patients develop recurrent pancreatic injury due to the effects of trypsin on surrounding tissues.

When the pancreas is injured, malabsorption and maldigestion can occur due to the lack of enzymatic activity in the lumen. These symptoms may occur particularly in obstructive pancreatitis, when the block to enzyme secretion may be total. Moreover, due to injury to the organ, the pancreatic enzymes may spill into the circulation, from which they are normally excluded. Measurement of serum amylase is a sensitive diagnostic marker of pancreatic injury. The loss of luminal enzymes may also result in unopposed stimulation of CCK release, which further stimulates the pancreas causing supraphysiological elevations in acinar cell calcium as well as pain. Some patients with pancreatitis have seen reduced pain as well as benefits with respect to maldigestion following enzyme supplementation.

BASIC PRINCIPLES OF SALIVARY SECRETION

We consider salivary secretion here because of analogies between this process and that of pancreatic secretion (Figure 4–8). Thus, a primary salivary secretion arises in acini, and is modified as it flows through ducts. It is instructive to compare and contrast these two processes, and an understanding of one permits an understanding of the other.

Role and Significance

Saliva plays a number of roles in gastrointestinal physiology (Table 4–2). Its primary function is to lubricate ingested food, and to thereby permit formation of a smooth, rounded portion (known as a *bolus*) that is suitable for swallowing. However, it also performs additional roles. For example, the ability of saliva to solubilize molecules in the meal allows these to diffuse to taste buds on the tongue, affecting appetite and food intake. This has an impact on the function of more distal segments of the gastrointestinal tract. For example, while chewing a bland substance will stimulate some degree of gastric secretion, a much greater response

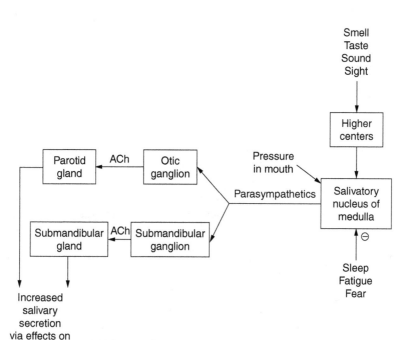

Figure 4–8. Regulation of salivary secretion by the parasympathetic nervous system. ACh, acetylcholine.

is seen when a subject chews a food he or she finds palatable. Salivary secretion can also begin the digestive process.

Saliva also plays important roles in host defense. It contains a variety of antibacterial substances that serve to protect the oral cavity from microbial colonization. Saliva is also slightly alkaline. This property is important in clearing any

Table 4–2. Constituents of saliva and their functions

Constituent	Functions
Water	Facilitates taste and dissolution of nutrients; aids in swallowing and speech
Bicarbonate	Neutralizes refluxed gastric acid
Mucins	Lubrication
Amylase	Starch digestion
Lysozyme, lactoferrin, IgA	Innate and acquired immune protection
Epidermal and nerve growth factors	Assumed to contribute to mucosal growth and protection

refluxed gastric acid from the esophagus, thus acting to prevent esophageal erosions and injury. Finally, saliva clearly aids in speech, as anyone who has had to make a presentation without the aid of a glass of water will know.

Salivary Secretory Products

Saliva contains a number of different solutes. Serous acinar cells largely supply proteinaceous components, whereas mucous acinar cells secrete watery mucus. The protein components of saliva include digestive enzymes. For example, saliva begins the digestion of carbohydrates via the action of salivary amylase. This latter enzyme is not required for adequate digestion of starch in healthy adults, but may assume greater importance in neonates, where there is a normal developmental delay in the expression of pancreatic amylase. Some species also secrete a lipase enzyme into their saliva, although the existence of such a *lingual lipase* is controversial in humans. In any event, the salivary enzymes can be considered as "back-ups" that are only required for digestion if other sources are reduced. In patients with pancreatic insufficiency, for example, salivary enzyme synthesis may be modestly upregulated.

Saliva contains substances that are important for protection of the host. Lysozyme and other antibacterial peptides limit colonization of the oral cavity by microbes. Lactoferrin sequesters iron, thereby inhibiting the growth of bacteria that require this substance. Saliva also contains significant quantities of secretory IgA, which contribute to immune defense. The salivary glands also synthesize a number of growth factors that are presumed to contribute to growth and repair of epithelial and other cell types more distally in the gastrointestinal tract. These include nerve growth factor and epidermal growth factor.

In terms of the lubricating and solubilizing functions of saliva, the most important constituents are mucins and water. Mucin molecules are related to those produced by the stomach, and are large glycoproteins with viscoelastic properties. Water, however, is the main component of saliva and is secreted at very high rates. At maximal rates of secretion, the volumes produced by salivary glands can exceed 1 mL/min/g of gland tissue, necessitating high rates of blood flow to supply this fluid. In an adult, more than 500 mL of saliva are produced daily by the three pairs of major salivary glands (parotid, sublingual, and submandibular) as well as smaller glands located throughout the oral cavity and in the mucosa of the lips, tongue, and palate.

Saliva also contains a variety of inorganic solutes, including calcium and phosphate that are important for tooth formation and maintenance. The primary secretion from the salivary acini has an ionic composition that is comparable to plasma. However, as the secretion moves along the ducts, the composition is modified by active transport processes as will be described later.

SALIVARY GLAND ANATOMY

As for the pancreas, the salivary glands are made up of grape-like clusters of acini that drain into a system of intercalated and intralobular (striated) ducts, and eventually into interlobular ducts that drain into the oral cavity. The individual acini and associated ducts are also surrounded by a sheath of myofibroblasts, which are contractile cells that are presumed to be important in providing a hydrostatic force that expels saliva from the gland, thereby contributing to the very high rates of secretion that are possible from this tissue. The salivary glands also receive extensive sympathetic and parasympathetic innervation. Sympathetic efferents originate in the salivatory center adjacent to the dorsal vagal complex, whereas parasympathetics come from the salivatory nuclei. The salivary glands also have a well-developed blood supply that can sustain blood flows more than 10-fold higher, on a weight basis, than those observed in actively contracting skeletal muscle.

Acinar Cells

Unlike the pancreas, the various salivary glands are somewhat heterogenous in their specific structure and function. The acini of the parotid gland, which drains into the upper part of the mouth via the parotid duct, consist entirely of serous cells, and thus are responsible for providing the protein constituents of saliva. The sublingual gland, under the tongue, has predominantly mucous acini, but also a scattering of serous acini as well. The submandibular gland, below the jaw, has a mixture of serous and mucous acini. In the latter gland, individual acini may contain both serous and mucous cell types.

Ductular Cells

As the saliva makes its way out of the acini, it passes through a ductular system. The intercalated ducts, linked directly to the acini, serve predominantly to convey the saliva out of the acinus and to prevent backflow. Cells of the striated intralobular ducts, on the other hand, are polarized epithelial cells with specialized transport functions that are analogous to those in the renal tubules. The epithelial cells of the intralobular ducts, moreover, have well-developed intercellular tight junctions, which significantly limit the permeability of this segment of the gland relative to the leaky acinus.

REGULATION OF SALIVARY SECRETION

Neural Regulation

The salivary glands are unusual among all components of the gastrointestinal system in that their regulation appears to be essentially exclusively mediated by neurocrine pathways, at least in the short-term. The major gastrointestinal hormones have not been demonstrated to exert any effect on salivary secretion, and likewise there is little evidence available to support a critical role for paracrine mediators. Hormones can, however, have chronic effects on the composition of saliva. The most notable example is that of aldosterone, which, in keeping with its effects on other transporting epithelia, can increase the ability of the salivary ducts to absorb sodium ions. In addition to the reliance on neural regulation, the salivary glands are unusual in that they are positively regulated by both the parasympathetic and sympathetic branches of the autonomic nervous system.

This contrasts with the reciprocal roles of parasympathetic and sympathetic regulation seen in most other locations in the body. However, quantitatively, the predominant regulation of secretory rate and composition is via parasympathetic pathways with sympathetic efferents playing only a modifying role.

PARASYMPATHETIC REGULATION

Nerves that are components of the parasympathetic nervous system are critical to the initiation of salivary secretion and to sustaining secretion at high rates. These nerves originate in the salivatory nucleus of the medulla, and receive input from higher centers that integrate both physiological and pathophysiological requirements. Conditioned reflexes, such as smell and taste, as well as pressure reflexes transmitted from the oral cavity itself markedly stimulate parasympathetic outflow, whereas fatigue, sleep, fear, and dehydration suppress this neurotransmission to the salivary glands. The feeling of nausea, under pathologic conditions, conveys another important stimulus for parasympathetic control of salivary secretion. Nausea strongly stimulates salivation, presumably to protect the oral cavity and esophagus from the injurious effects of vomited gastric acid and other intestinal contents. Parasympathetic input to the salivary glands is mediated by ACh acting at m_3 muscarinic receptors. In addition to effects on the acinar cells and ducts of the glands, parasympathetic innervation causes dilation of the blood vessels supplying the gland, thereby providing both the fluid and metabolic requirements needed to sustain high rates of secretion.

SYMPATHETIC REGULATION

Sympathetic nerves passing through the superior cervical ganglion also terminate at the salivary glands. These nerves are not thought to be capable of initiating or sustaining secretion independently, but can potentiate the effects of parasympathetic regulation via the release of norepinephrine and activation of beta-adrenergic receptors on acinar cells. Sympathetic innervation has a biphasic effect on blood flow to the glands. Initially, alpha-adrenergic receptors on the vasculature produce vasoconstriction. However, as the glands themselves produce vasodilatory substances, including kallikrein, which causes an increase in local levels of bradykinin, blood flow increases over resting levels. The higher inputs to the sympathetic system that bring about effects on salivary secretion via this route are, however, poorly understood, but may include local reflexes originating in the oral cavity. Sympathetic innervation is also believed to stimulate motor responses that help to expel saliva from the gland.

CELLULAR BASIS OF SALIVARY SECRETION

Acinar Cells

Acinar cells release their protein and mucus contents via a process of exocytosis, analogous to our discussion of enzyme release from zymogen granules in the pancreatic acini. These responses involve mobilization of intracellular calcium downstream of the muscarinic receptor for ACh. Acinar cells also actively secrete chloride and potassium ions into the primary salivary secretion. Because the acini

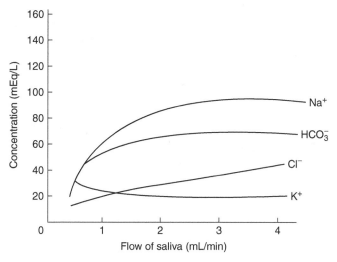

Figure 4–9. Ionic composition of saliva as a function of its flow rate. Note that saliva becomes less hypotonic as flow rates increase.

are relatively leaky, sodium follows paracellularly via the tight junctions. Water may move both paracellularly and transcellularly, the latter pathway being facilitated by apical expression of aquaporin 5. The initial salivary secretion is thus isotonic and has an ionic composition relatively comparable to that of plasma, albeit with a slightly elevated concentration of potassium.

The secretory process in acinar cells is somewhat analogous to that of chloride secretion in the intestine (as discussed in Chapter 5). Driven secondarily by the ability of a basolateral Na^+, K^+ ATPase to maintain low levels of intracellular sodium, a basolateral sodium/potassium/2 chloride cotransporter, NKCC1, accumulates chloride in the acinar cell cytosol above its electrochemical gradient. Chloride can then exit across the apical membrane in response to the elevations in calcium triggered by muscarinic stimulation. The chloride channel involved has recently been identified as TMEM16A, also known as anoctamin. Calcium-dependent potassium channels are also present apically, accounting for net potassium secretion.

Ductular Cells

As we learned for the pancreas, the function of the duct cells in the salivary glands is to modify the composition of the saliva as it passes along their length. The ionic composition of saliva changes as its flow rate increases (Figure 4–9). At low rates of secretion, saliva is hypotonic with respect to plasma and has higher concentrations of potassium than sodium, the opposite of the situation in plasma. The chloride concentration is also much lower than found in plasma. These changes in ionic content are brought about by active transport events taking place in the duct cells (Figure 4–10). Sodium and chloride are reabsorbed across the apical membrane

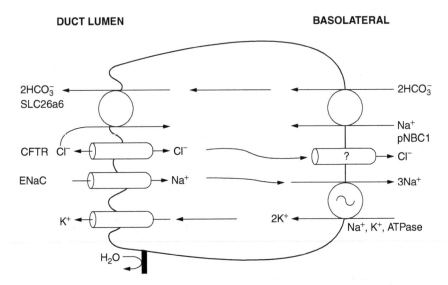

DUCT LUMEN   BASOLATERAL

Tight junctions restrict osmotic reabsorption of water

Figure 4–10. Ion transport pathways in salivary duct epithelial cells. SLC26a6, solute-carrier 26a6 (chloride/bicarbonate exchanger); CFTR, cystic fibrosis transmembrane conductance regulator; ENaC, epithelial sodium carrier; pNBC1, sodium–bicarbonate cotransporter.

via ENaC sodium channels and CFTR chloride channels, respectively, in a coupled mechanism. Chloride can also exit apically via CFTR, to then be recycled via an SLC26A6 anion exchanger, providing for bicarbonate secretion and alkalization of the saliva. The bicarbonate is derived from a basolateral pNBC1 transporter. This process is quite analogous to that providing for bicarbonate secretion in the pancreatic ducts (Figure 4–7), and explains why sodium and chloride are not present in equivalent amounts in the final saliva produced. Potassium is also secreted via apical channels. At the basolateral membrane, the driving force for sodium uptake is provided by a sodium–potassium ATPase, but the pathway for chloride reabsorption across this membrane remains unclear. Because the ductular epithelium has a low passive permeability, water cannot flow across the tight junctions fast enough at moderate rates of salivary secretion to keep pace with the active reabsorption of sodium and chloride, and thus saliva becomes hypotonic. Moreover, due to secretion of bicarbonate into the lumen, the pH of saliva increases progressively along the length of the duct, rising to approximately pH 8 as the saliva enters the mouth under conditions of stimulated flow.

At very high rates of salivary secretion, the concentrations of sodium and potassium more closely resemble those in plasma. The concentration of chloride also increases as the flow rate of saliva increases. These changes in composition are due to the fact that the residence time of the saliva in the ducts is too short for the cells to be able to modify salivary composition significantly, particularly when the saliva is propelled forward by the contractile activity of the surrounding myofibroblasts. Thus, when secretory rates are high, the saliva represents acinar secretion more closely.

SALIVARY PATHOPHYSIOLOGY AND CLINICAL CORRELATIONS

Xerostomia

Xerostomia, literally "dry mouth" is the name given to a variety of conditions where salivary secretion is impaired. While xerostomia may occur congenitally, or as a result of an autoimmune process that targets the salivary glands (Sjögren's syndrome), it is frequently iatrogenic in its etiology, and results as a side effect of several different classes of drugs (antidepressants, psychotropics, and antihypertensives) or secondary to head and neck radiation for malignancies. There are several negative consequences of this condition, which can be predicted from the functions of saliva that we discussed earlier. Thus, patients with impaired salivary secretion have a decrease in oral pH with associated tooth decay and esophageal erosions, difficulty in lubricating and swallowing their food leading to poor nutrition, and opportunistic infections as a result of impaired host defenses. This distressing symptom complex may itself lead to depression.

KEY CONCEPTS

 Pancreatic secretion provides for digestion of the meal.

 Pancreatic acini supply enzymes, whereas ducts supply fluid; major regulators of each cell type are CCK and secretin, respectively.

 Pancreatic secretion is initiated during the cephalic phase, but is most prominent when the meal is in the duodenum.

 The pancreas has several lines of defense to protect against autodigestion. When these lines fail, pancreatitis results.

 Salivary secretion shares several parallels with pancreatic secretion.

 Salivary secretion is predominantly mediated by parasympathetic input arising from higher brain centers. Hormonal regulation is much less important.

STUDY QUESTIONS

4-1. A 4-year-old boy is brought to the pediatrician for an evaluation because of failure to thrive and frequent diarrhea characterized by pale, bulky, foul-smelling stools. Sweat chloride concentrations are measured and found to be elevated. Diminished secretion of which pancreatic product is most likely to be the primary cause of the patient's apparent fat malabsorption?

A. Lipase

B. Procolipase

C. Monitor peptide

D. Cholecystokinin

E. Bicarbonate

4-2. In an experiment, recordings are made of electrical activity in afferent nerves originating in the small intestinal mucosa during sequential luminal perfusion with saline, a solution of hydrolyzed casein, and a solution of intact casein. Rates of neuronal firing were shown to increase markedly during the third period. Firing in these nerves was most likely stimulated by an increase in the mucosal concentration of which of the following?

A. Gastrin

B. Secretin

C. Somatostatin

D. Acetylcholine

E. Cholecystokinin

4-3. A 50-year-old man with a history of alcohol abuse presents at the emergency room with severe, colicky abdominal pain, and a fever. A blood test reveals increased levels of serum amylase and an endoscopic imaging procedure reveals a narrowed pancreatic duct. Pain in this patient is likely predominantly ascribable to premature activation of pancreatic enzymes capable of digesting which of the following nutrients?

A. Triglyceride

B. Phospholipids

C. Protein

D. Starch

E. Nucleic acids

4-4. A researcher conducts a study of the regulation of salivary secretion in a group of normal volunteers under various conditions. Which of the following conditions was associated with the lowest rates of secretion?

A. Chewing gum

B. Undergoing a mock dental exam

C. Sleep

D. Exposure to a nauseating odor

E. Resting control conditions

4–5. *A 50-year-old female patient who has suffered for several years from severe dryness of her eyes due to inadequate tear production is referred to a gastroenterologist for evaluation of chronic heartburn. Endoscopic examination reveals erosions and scarring of the distal esophagus just above the lower esophageal sphincter. Reduced production of which salivary component most likely contributed to the tissue injury.*

A. *Lactoferrin*

B. *Mucus*

C. *IgA*

D. *Bicarbonate*

E. *Amylase*

SUGGESTED READINGS

Argent BE, Gray MA, Steward MC, Case RM. Cell physiology of pancreatic ducts. In: Johnson LR, Ghishan FK, Kaunitz JD, Merchant JL, Said HM, Wood JD, eds. *Physiology of the Gastrointestinal Tract.* 5th ed. San Diego: Academic Press; 2012:1399–1423.

Catalan MA, Ambatipudi KS, Melvin JE. Salivary gland secretion. In: Johnson LR, Ghishan FK, Kaunitz JD, Merchant JL, Said HM, Wood JD, eds. *Physiology of the Gastrointestinal Tract.* 5th ed. San Diego: Academic Press; 2012:1229–1249.

Ebert EC. Gastrointestinal and hepatic manifestations of Sjogren syndrome. *J Clin Gastroenterol.* 2012; 46:25–30.

Lee MG, Ohana E, Park HW, Yang D, Muallem S. Molecular mechanism of pancreatic and salivary gland fluid and HCO_3^- secretion. *Physiol Rev.* 2012;92:39–74.

Liddle RA. Regulation of pancreatic secretion. In: Johnson LR, Ghishan FK, Kaunitz JD, Merchant JL, Said HM, Wood JD, eds. *Physiology of the Gastrointestinal Tract.* 5th ed. San Diego: Academic Press; 2012:1425–1460.

Mossner J. New advances in cell physiology and pathophysiology of the exocrine pancreas. *Dig Dis.* 2010;28:722–728.

Owyang C, Williams JA. Pancreatic secretion. In: Yamada T, Alpers DH, Kalloo AN, Kaplowitz N, Owyang C, Powell DW, eds. *Textbook of Gastroenterology.* 5th ed. Chichester: Wiley-Blackwell; 2009:368–400.

Petersen OH, Tepikin AV, Gerasimenko JV, Gerasimenko OV, Sutton R, Criddle DN. Fatty acids, alcohol and fatty acid ethyl esters: toxic Ca^{2+} signal generation and pancreatitis. *Cell Calcium.* 2009;45:634–642.

Saluja AK, Lerch MM, Phillips PA, Dudeja V. Why does pancreatic overstimulation cause pancreatitis? *Annu Rev Physiol.* 2007;69:249–269.

Williams JA, Yule DI. Stimulus–secretion coupling in pancreatic acinar cells. In: Johnson LR, Ghishan FK, Kaunitz JD, Merchant JL, Said HM, Wood JD, eds. *Physiology of the Gastrointestinal Tract.* 5th ed. San Diego: Academic Press; 2012:1361–1397.

Water and Electrolyte Absorption and Secretion

5

OBJECTIVES

- ▶ *Understand the physiological significance of the regulation of luminal water content and daily fluid balance*
- ▶ *Describe the functional anatomy of the intestinal epithelium that permits it to function as a regulator of fluid movement*
  - ▶ Surface area
- ▶ *Understand how transport function is integrated with intestinal motility*
- ▶ *Define pathways via which electrolytes can be transferred across epithelial barriers*
  - ▶ Passive *versus* active transport
  - ▶ Transcellular *versus* paracellular transport
- ▶ *Describe how a limited collection of membrane transport pathways are arranged to assemble transepithelial transport mechanisms*
- ▶ *Identify the major electrolyte transport pathways of the small and large intestines and their intracellular mechanisms of regulation*
- ▶ *Identify how subepithelial elements and other regulatory systems impact on epithelial transport function*
- ▶ *Define major pathogenic alterations in intestinal electrolyte transport and their consequences*
  - ▶ Heat stable enterotoxin of *E. coli* as an example of molecular mimicry

BASIC PRINCIPLES OF INTESTINAL FLUID TRANSPORT

Role and Significance

The intestinal tract is designed primarily to permit assimilation of nutrients. Because chemical reactions are required to digest nutrients into components that can be absorbed across the intestinal epithelium, a fluid environment is needed to support these. Thus, control of the amount of fluid in the intestinal lumen is critical for normal intestinal function. This fluid environment permits contact of digestive enzymes with food particles, and in turn the diffusion of digested nutrients to their eventual site of absorption. The fluidity of the intestinal contents also provides for their transit along the length of the gastrointestinal tract without damage to the lining of the epithelium.

Thus, control of luminal fluidity is central to gastrointestinal function. In fact, large volumes of fluid are handled by the intestine on a daily basis in the course of digesting and absorbing meals. Although some of this fluid is derived from beverages and from the food itself, the majority is supplied by the intestine and the organs that drain into it. The daily fluid load can vary somewhat depending on the types of food and drink ingested, but in normal adults it approximates 9 liters (Figure 5–1). Obviously, in health, this large volume is not lost to the stool, but instead is reclaimed by the intestine to avoid dehydration. The majority of the fluid is reabsorbed in the small intestine in conjunction with nutrients, although the colon is more efficient in conserving fluid and takes up almost 90% of the fluid presented to it. Moreover, both the small and large intestines have a large reserve capacity for absorption, and it is only when this is exceeded that excessive water loss to the stool occurs, seen clinically as diarrhea. Finally, the intestine is not normally the major determinant of whole body fluid and electrolyte homeostasis, a physiological function that is relegated to the kidneys. However, because large volumes of fluid can move into and out of the intestine, especially in disease states, abnormalities of fluid transport in the intestine have the potential to lead to serious derangements in body-fluid balances.

Electrolytes Involved

The site for control of intestinal fluid movement is the lining epithelium. Epithelial cells express several specialized properties that allow them to control fluid movement. Most important are the intracellular tight junctions, which restrict the passive flow of solutes and back-flow of these once either secreted or absorbed. In fact, despite the large volumes of fluid moved into and out of the intestinal tract, water is transported passively across the intestinal epithelium in response to osmotic gradients established by the active transport of electrolytes and other solutes. Moreover, there is limited evidence to suggest a major role for aquaporin water channels in mediating water movement in the intestinal epithelium, and instead water is believed to move around the epithelial cells, via the so-called *paracellular* route. Nevertheless, emerging evidence suggests that some water that is absorbed by the intestine may "piggy-back" on transport routes through epithelial cells (*transcellular* transport) by being carried along in the transporters that move other solutes, particularly in the absorptive direction. Nevertheless, no matter what the precise pathway for water movement, ultimately the epithelium must establish an appropriate osmotic vector to drive such transport.

Thus, an understanding of water transport in the gut actually rests on an understanding of ion transport, and particularly active ion transport, which takes place transcellulary and is the subject of specific control mechanisms. In common with those in other transporting epithelia, such as the renal system,

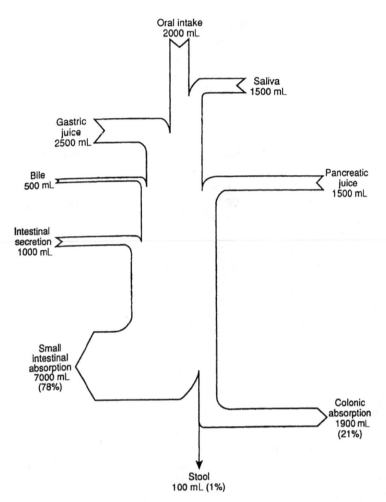

Figure 5-1. Daily water balance in the healthy adult human gastrointestinal tract. The amount of oral intake varies among individuals depending on the types of meals taken. Note that even in health there is a significant secretory flux of fluid from the intestine. (Used with permission from Barrett and Dharmsathaphorn. Transport of water and electrolytes in the gastrointestinal tract: physiological mechanisms, regulation and methods for study. In: Narins RG, ed. *Maxwell and Kleeman's Clinical Disorders of Fluid and Electrolyte Metabolism.* 5th ed. New York; 1994.)

active electrolyte transport pathways share a number of defining characteristics (Table 5–1). These transport pathways move a solute across a single membrane in a polarized epithelial cell. Transepithelial transport mechanisms, in turn, move solutes across the entire epithelium (i.e., two membranes and the cell cytosol), and are made up of a number of transport pathways (typically at least three), arranged asymmetrically in polarized epithelial cells. A distinction is also drawn between transepithelial transport mechanisms that are electrogenic (i.e., associated with

Table 5–1. Characteristics of active membrane transport pathways

Mediates uphill transport against an electrochemical gradient
Effective at low luminal concentrations
Demonstrates saturable kinetics
Requires cellular energy
Demonstrates high ionic specificity

the net movement of charge across the epithelium, thereby establishing a potential difference), or electroneutral. Both types of transport mechanisms can drive the paracellular movement of water, but electrogenic transport pathways will additionally promote the passive movement of a counterion via the tight junctions in an attempt to maintain electrical neutrality. These distinctions also prove important in the ways that these transport mechanisms can be studied experimentally.

The transport pathways that make up the transport mechanisms are of three types. Pumps utilize cellular energy to move ions against a concentration gradient, and are thus defined as active transporters. Channels, on the other hand, are high-capacity "pores" in the plasma membrane through which large numbers of ions can move passively when the channel is open, in response to prevailing electrochemical gradients. Finally, carriers move one or more ions against a concentration gradient by coupling their movement to that of another ion or ions whose transport is favored. Carriers may be either exchangers (the transported species move in opposite directions) or cotransporters (the transported species move in the same direction). Carriers are said to perform "secondary active transport"—while they are not intrinsically active transporters, they take advantage of electrochemical gradients established by other active pumps. Commonly, such secondary active transport pathways in the gut center on sodium ions, taking advantage of the low intracellular sodium concentration established by the basolateral sodium–potassium ATPase that is present in all intestinal epithelial cells.

Another principle that is important to remember about intestinal fluid transport is that both absorption and secretion can occur simultaneously in any given segment of the intestinal tract. This is apparently due, in large part, to the principle that the cells of the villi (or surface cells in the colon) are absorptive whereas crypt epithelial cells are secretory, although there are known to be some exceptions to this general rule. Moreover, the transport mechanisms that are expressed in the small intestine and colon differ, due to the relative paucity of nutrients in the latter segment (Tables 5–2 and 5–3). In general, absorptive mechanisms for fluid center on the active movement of sodium, with or without the coupled transport of chloride, nutrients, or other solutes such as bile acids. On the other hand, most secretory fluxes of the fluid in the intestine are driven by the electrogenic movement of chloride ions, although bicarbonate secretion may assume significance in particular segments of the gut, especially in the stomach and proximal duodenum where it plays an important role in protecting the mucosa from the injurious effects of acid and pepsin. Both secretion and absorption of small amounts of potassium also occur in the intestine, depending on whole-body

Table 5–2. Small intestinal ion transport mechanisms

Bicarbonate secretion
Sodium-coupled nutrient absorption
Proton-coupled nutrient absorption
Electroneutral NaCl absorption
Chloride secretion
Sodium-coupled bile acid absorption
Calcium and iron absorption*

---

*Note: Not major determinants of fluid transport.

potassium status, but these are not quantitatively significant in terms of associated water movement. Similarly, the intestine is a critical portal for absorption of calcium and iron needed for other body systems, but again, the quantities involved play only a very minor role in fluid uptake.

ANATOMICAL CONSIDERATIONS

Amplification of Intestinal Surface Area

The capacity of the intestine for large volumes of water transport is related to its massively amplified surface area. In fact, the surface area of the adult small intestine alone exceeds that of a doubles tennis court. How can this surface area be accommodated within the body? The answer lies in the fact that the intestine is not a simple cylinder, but instead is amplified first by folds in the mucosa, then by the presence of crypts and villi, and finally by the presence of microvilli on the apical poles of individual epithelial cells, which increase the overall surface area by a factor of 20-fold. Overall, the surface area is increased by these physical structures by a factor of 600-fold. This amplification of the surface area not only allows for handling of the large volumes of fluids required for normal functioning of the intestine during digestion and absorption, but also provides a reserve capacity for fluid absorption in disease. However, the surface amplification, particularly in the crypts, also carries a liability in that there is a corresponding reserve capacity for intestinal fluid secretion. Almost all of us have some personal experience of the outcome when secretion is inappropriately stimulated and cannot be balanced by absorption! On a more serious note, if such secretion is extensive and prolonged, it can rapidly lead to serious dehydration if left untreated.

Table 5–3. Colonic ion transport mechanisms

Electrogenic sodium absorption
Electroneutral NaCl absorption
Short chain fatty acid absorption
Chloride secretion
Potassium absorption/secretion*

---

*Note: Not a major determinant of fluid transport.

Innervation and Regulatory Cells

As we learned in earlier chapters, the intestinal epithelium rests on a lamina propria that is a rich source of potential regulatory factors. In addition to endocrine regulators supplied by local blood flow, epithelial functions, including electrolyte transport, are controlled by paracrine mediators supplied by local enteroendocrine cells, immune mediators coming from both resident (in health) and infiltrating (in disease) immune and inflammatory cell types, and neurocrines released from secretomotor efferent nerves originating predominantly in the submucosal plexus of the enteric nervous system. Immunologic effector cells that are known to influence epithelial transport include mast cells, neutrophils, and eosinophils. The epithelial cells themselves may also produce autocrine factors that regulate their transport function, such as growth factors and prostanoids.

The regulatory systems that mediate changes in epithelial transport do not act in isolation. Rather, there is significant cross-talk between the various modes of communication. For example, some immunologic mediators may have both direct effects on epithelial cells, and others that are mediated secondarily via the activation of enteric nerves. Cross-talk between the various regulatory systems also provides for coordinated regulation of transport and motility functions (Figure 5–2).

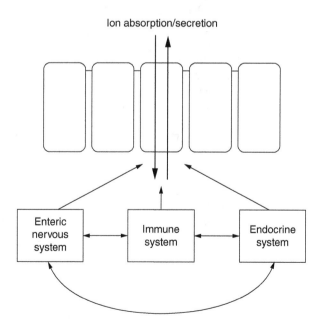

Figure 5–2. Regulation of intestinal ion transport. The balance between fluid and electrolyte absorption and secretion across the intestinal epithelium is regulated by an interplay between endocrine, neurocrine, and immune cell factors.

REGULATION OF WATER AND ELECTROLYTE TRANSPORT
Regulatory Strata

We turn now to a discussion of how transport responses are regulated to sub-serve physiological function. Much of our knowledge surrounding the control of intestinal fluid movement comes from studies of the factors that regulate fluid secretion, which is driven primarily by the secretion of chloride ions. In the post-prandial period when nutrients are present in the small intestinal lumen, fluid absorption has been considered to be more of a passive response that is driven by the presence of these nutrients, and not highly subject to regulation by intra-and inter-cellular mechanisms. On the other hand, when the meal has been fully digested and absorbed, the intestine is still capable of ongoing fluid absorption to balance secretory pathways, and accomplishes this via the absorption solely of sodium and chloride ions, independent of nutrient uptake. Nutrient-independent solute uptake is also an important mechanism in the colon, where there are not usually significant quantities of nutrients, at least in health. The nutrient-independent pathways for fluid absorption are subject to both intra- and intercellular regulation. In general, regulatory pathways that stimulate chloride secretion inhibit electroneutral sodium chloride absorption, and *vice versa*. However, some of the intracellular pathways that stimulate chloride secretion, such as elevations in cAMP, may also stimulate electrogenic sodium absorption in the distal colon. Moreover, reciprocity also does not apply to nutrient-coupled absorption, which can continue unopposed even under circumstances that lead to the stimulation of chloride secretion. This last point underlies the efficacy of so-called *oral rehydration solutions* that are used to treat the dehydration accompanying severe diarrheal diseases, such as cholera, when intravenous fluids are not available. Glucose, or complex carbohydrates such as those in rice water, are added to an electrolyte solution and given orally. This mixture can drive fluid uptake even when chloride secretion is maximally stimulated and electroneutral NaCl absorption is blocked.

As we have seen for control of other parts of the gastrointestinal system, intestinal epithelial transport is regulated by endocrine, neurocrine, paracrine, and immune mediators. However, unlike gastric and pancreatic secretion, for example, endocrine mediators play a relatively limited role in acute regulation of intestinal transport function. Instead, the primary regulation of intestinal epithelial transport appears to occur via neurocrine and paracrine pathways, with regulation by immune mediators also assuming great importance in the setting of disease states such as intestinal inflammation and food allergies.

Short and Long Reflexes

Intestinal epithelial transport is regulated by neurotransmitters originating from nerve endings of the enteric nervous system. The most potent effectors in this regard include acetylcholine (ACh) and vasoactive intestinal polypeptide, (VIP) both of which can directly stimulate epithelial cells to secrete chloride. This should be contrasted with the divergent effects of these neurotransmitters on intestinal motility, as will be discussed in greater detail in Chapters 7–9, where these two neurotransmitters cause smooth muscle contraction versus relaxation, respectively. This may suggest that fluid lubrication is needed at any site along the length of the intestine where motility is occurring, to ease the passage of intestinal contents along the lumen.

Some neural input to the control of intestinal transport almost certainly originates in the central nervous system, and, as we learned in Chapter 2, this input is then interpreted and integrated with local information to impinge ultimately on the activity of secretomotor neurons. In a similar fashion, vago-vagal reflexes likely match intestinal transport function to conditions that result from the physical state of luminal contents, such as via the activation of stretch receptors. In addition to these "long" reflexes, however, there has been an emerging appreciation of the role played by "short" or local reflexes in regulating transport. The most well-studied of such reflexes is initiated by stroking the mucosa, which can be considered to model the local passage of a food bolus. In turn, this releases 5-hydroxytryptamine from local enterochromaffin cells, followed by activation of cholinergic efferents that stimulate a corresponding burst of chloride, and thus fluid, secretion. This reflex may be important in protecting the epithelium from physical damage by the passing meal components.

HUMORAL CONTROL

Although there appears to be a relatively limited role for classical endocrine hormones in mediating changes in intestinal transport function, at least in the short term, other soluble effectors have clear effects and are largely derived from paracrine or immune sources. For example, local production of prostaglandins, likely predominantly by subepithelial elements such as myofibroblasts, plays an important role in stimulating the secretion of both chloride and bicarbonate. Similarly, histamine, released by mast cells residing in the lamina propria, has been shown to be an effective chloride secretagogue, although its effect is transient. Interestingly, rather than activate bicarbonate secretion, histamine is an inhibitor of this process, acting via enteric nerves to stimulate the presumed release of an antisecretory neurotransmitter. Immune effector cells that release substances capable of regulating the epithelium can be considered specialized "sensory" cells that alter transport function in response to specific conditions pertaining in the lumen, such as the presence of food substances to which an individual is allergic. These and other putative humoral regulators of intestinal secretion and/or absorption are listed in Table 5–4.

Table 5–4. Major endogenous regulators of intestinal ion transport

Cyclic nucleotide-dependent	Calcium-dependent
Vasoactive intestinal polypeptide (VIP)	Acetylcholine (ACh)
Prostaglandins	Histamine
Guanylin (cGMP)	5-hydroxytryptamine
5'AMP/adenosine	Bile acids

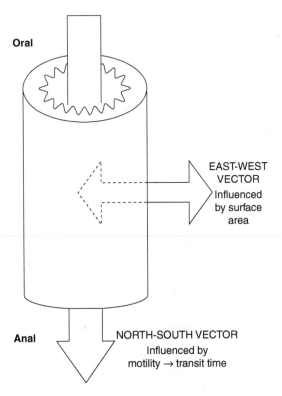

Figure 5–3. Integration of influences on fluid movement in the intestine. Overall fluid fluxes depend on the surface area available for ion transport and residence time in the lumen.

Humoral regulators of intestinal transport typically bind to receptors localized to the basolateral pole of intestinal epithelial cells. It should be emphasized, however, that such effectors may alter epithelial function not only via such direct binding, but also via the secondary activation of other subepithelial elements, such as nerves and the myofibroblastic sheath that lies immediately below the epithelial layer (Figure 5–2). In this way, intestinal secretory and/or absorptive function can be better integrated with other physiological functions of the gut such as motility and blood flow. In turn, agonists that alter these latter functions may have indirect effects on intestinal secretion and absorption. The net rate of movement of any substance across the intestinal epithelium will reflect not only the "east–west" vector of absorption/secretion, but also the "north–south" vector of movement along the length of the gastrointestinal tract (Figure 5–3). Thus, if motility is increased, hastening the transit of substances along the intestine, there will be less time for absorption to take place (or, conversely, for active secretion to add to luminal fluid loads). If transit is slowed, absorption can catch up with the presented fluid volume. This last principle underlies the efficacy of several antidiarrheal medications, and particularly opiate drugs such as Imodium.

Given its location at the interface of the host and the external environment, the epithelium is also positioned to respond to substances present in the intestinal lumen, and indeed, expresses a number of apical receptors for such agents. Guanylin is a novel peptide stimulus of epithelial chloride secretion that is synthesized by enteroendocrine cells and released into the lumen. The physiological role of this substance may be to coordinate salt handling by the small and large intestines with that of the kidneys, since a portion of the peptide enters the bloodstream and can influence salt retention or secretion by renal tubular epithelial cells. Another luminal regulator that may play an important role in modulating epithelial function in the setting of inflammation is 5'-AMP, which is released by activated neutrophils that migrate into the lumen when activated by invading microorganisms or inflammatory cytokines. Finally, bile acids, which are synthesized by the liver to aid in fat digestion and absorption (more on this topic later), are effective as apical stimuli of chloride secretion in the colon. Under normal circumstances, bile acids are reabsorbed in the terminal ileum when they are no longer needed to solubilize the products of fat digestion. However, if this absorptive area is lost to disease or surgery, bile acids can spill over into the colon and cause diarrhea. Whether bile acids are normally functionally significant in driving fluid secretion in the small intestine is the subject of active investigation. Some have suggested that they function as "osmosignals." Thus, when sufficient fluid is present in the small intestinal lumen, their concentration may be below that needed to evoke secretory responses. On the other hand, if the intestinal contents become relatively dessicated, the bile acids may become concentrated to such a degree that they exceed the threshold needed to evoke secretory responses. In keeping with this hypothesis, clinical studies have recently shown that a drug that prevents active reabsorption of bile acids is effective in relieving chronic constipation.

Acute Regulation

Acute regulation of intestinal fluid and electrolyte transport occurs to match needs for luminal fluidity on a minute-to-minute basis, most typically in the context of responding to ingestion of a meal. Altered intestinal transport can also occur independent of the presence of a meal, notably as stimulated by input from the central nervous system at times of threat or stress. In either case, while both secretion and absorption occur simultaneously, in health, the absorptive vector predominates overall and most of the fluid used for digestion and absorption is recycled (Figure 5–4).

Neurotransmitters released from enteric secretomotor neurons, as well as paracrine effectors from local enteroendocrine cells or other subepithelial elements, alter the functional capacity of transporting epithelial cells to conduct transport across their apical and basolateral membranes. For the case of acute regulation, little or none of the change in transport capacity reflects alterations in the synthesis

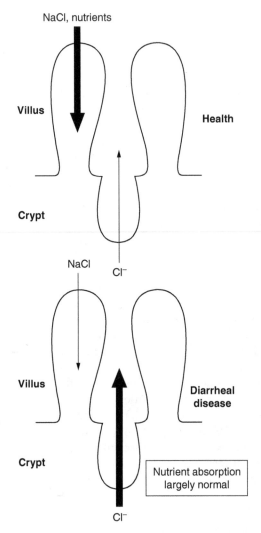

Figure 5–4. Balance between absorption and secretion in health and in secretory diarrheal disease. Note that small intestinal nutrient absorption is usually largely normal in the setting of secretory diarrhea.

of the transporters involved. Rather, second messenger pathways evoked by neurohumoral regulators alter the activation status of the transporters to increase or decrease the corresponding membrane transport event. This can be the result of a direct interaction of an intracellular effector with a transporter, or a posttranslational modification (e.g., phosphorylation) mediated by an intracellular protein (e.g., a protein kinase) activated downstream of the mobilized messenger. Acute regulation of intestinal epithelial transport can also result from redistribution of transporters within the epithelial cells themselves. There is evidence that a number of transporters cycle between sub-membrane vesicles and the plasma membrane, in response to second messenger cascades. Delivery of additional, preformed transporters to the membrane will increase transport capacity whereas endocytic retrieval will reduce it.

Chronic Adaptation

The bowel is also capable of altering its ability to conduct water and electrolyte transport in a chronic fashion, in order to adapt to changes in whole-body electrolyte status. With the cloning of various transport proteins and accompanying molecular insights into their genetic structure, we are beginning to learn how expression of intestinal transporters can be matched to the need to take up or excrete their transported solute. Such chronic regulation of transport takes place over a timescale of days to weeks, in contrast to the acute events discussed earlier.

Aldosterone is an important regulator of sodium transport in the intestine in addition to similar roles in the renal system. When the diet is low in salt, aldosterone is released and increases the expression of transporters required for sodium absorption in the colon, as discussed in more detail later. The net effect is active sodium retention by the colon, with chloride following passively to maintain electrical neutrality. Analogous processes allow for increased or decreased intestinal retention of other important electrolytes. For example, a fall in plasma calcium increases levels of 1,25-dihydroxyvitamin D_3, which stimulates the expression of proteins needed for calcium absorption in the small intestine. Conversely, levels of transporters involved in intestinal iron absorption are decreased in patients suffering from the disease of hemochromatosis, which is associated with overloading of the body's stores of iron.

CELLULAR BASIS OF TRANSPORT

 We will now discuss the distribution of electrolyte transport mechanisms in the various intestinal segments, and how individual transport proteins are arranged to permit electrolyte absorption and secretion in the gut. The transport mechanisms displayed by the major gut segments are designed to subserve their specific physiological functions, while taking advantage of prevailing luminal constituents. Thus, for example, absorptive mechanisms in the small intestine center around nutrients, whereas the colon, which functions critically to conserve fluid and electrolytes, can count on few luminal nutrients to aid in this absorptive process in health.

Absorptive Mechanisms

Absorptive mechanisms expressed in the small intestine and colon are summarized in Tables 5–2 and 5–3. Throughout the length of the small intestine, sodium is taken up in conjunction with a variety of nutrients. These processes are exemplified by that of glucose-coupled sodium absorption, which is depicted diagrammatically in Figure 5–5. This, and related nutrient-coupled transport

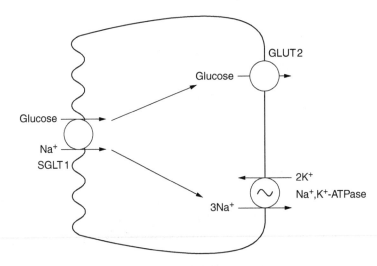

Figure 5–5. Sodium-coupled nutrient absorption exemplified by the uptake of glucose from the intestinal lumen. SGLT1, sodium–glucose cotransporter 1.

mechanisms, such as those driven by specific amino acids, rely on the low intracellular sodium concentration established by the active, basolateral Na, K-ATPase. Apical uptake of sodium and glucose is a coupled process that occurs via a cotransporter, SGLT-1. By tying the movement of glucose to that of sodium, glucose can be moved uphill, even when luminal concentrations of this nutrient are low. Glucose thus absorbed is then utilized by the enterocyte, or is transported to the bloodstream for use elsewhere in the body via a facilitated diffusion pathway called GLUT-2. The overall process is referred to as electrogenic because there is no active transport of a counterion to offset the charge of the actively transported sodium. Instead, anions (largely chloride) and water follow passively via the tight junctions. Notably, glucose-coupled sodium absorption is not inhibited by an increase in intracellular cAMP levels—contrast this with electroneutral sodium chloride absorption discussed later. This fortuitous circumstance permits the use of oral rehydration solutions in cholera. Sodium-coupled transport also allows for the active uptake of conjugated bile acids, although in this case the transport mechanism is restricted to the terminal ileum. In the colon, where luminal glucose is largely absent, a similar mechanism allows for the electrogenic uptake of sodium by replacing SGLT-1 with the epithelial sodium channel, ENaC (Figure 5–6). However, in this case, the absorptive process is stimulated by a rise in cAMP, while it is inhibited by increases in intracellular calcium.

Absorptive mechanisms in the gut can also center around protons. This is the case for the uptake of the short peptides that are the products of digestion of dietary proteins. These are absorbed via an apical transporter known as PepT1, coupled to proton uptake. PepT1 is a remarkable transporter in that it can accommodate a wide range of substrates, including di-, tri-, and perhaps even tetra-peptides

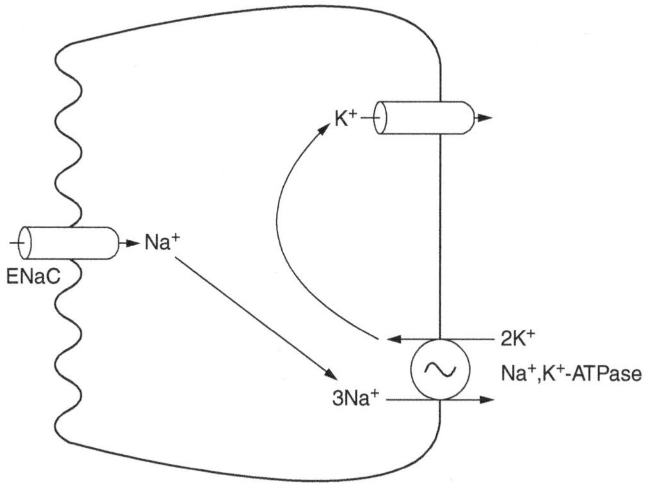

Figure 5-6. Electrogenic sodium absorption in the colon. Sodium enters the epithelial cells via epithelial sodium channels (ENaC).

made up of various combinations of the 20 naturally occurring amino acids. This contrasts markedly with the high degree of specificity usually displayed by membrane transport proteins. The structural basis for the broad specificity of PepT1 is largely unknown. However, it is nutritionally significant, because as we will see in Chapter 15, some amino acids, including essential ones that cannot be synthesized by the body, are only efficiently absorbed in peptide form due to a relative lack of relevant amino acid transporters. PepT1 may also serve as a portal of entry for so-called "peptidomimetic" drugs, including several antibiotics.

Between meals, when nutrients are not available in the lumen, fluid absorption can still continue in the small intestine via an electroneutral mechanism that involves the coupled absorption of both sodium and chloride. This mechanism is diagrammed in Figure 5–7, and also accounts for a variable proportion of fluid absorption in the colon. Coupled ion exchangers on the apical membrane carry sodium and chloride into the cell in exchange for protons and bicarbonate ions, respectively, and both exchange processes require the activity of the other. Notably, the NHE3 sodium–hydrogen exchanger isoform that participates in this transport mechanism is inhibited by cAMP, and thus the overall transport process can likewise be inhibited by this second messenger. This fact has implications for the pathogenesis of cholera and other diarrheal diseases, as will be discussed later.

The small intestine also absorbs iron and calcium in their ionic forms, although as mentioned previously the small quantities of these ions that are handled do not contribute in a major way to fluid handling. Calcium absorption is possible along the length of the small intestine depending on whole-body demands, whereas the majority of iron absorption occurs in the proximal small intestine due to specific expression of the membrane transporters required to facilitate iron movement.

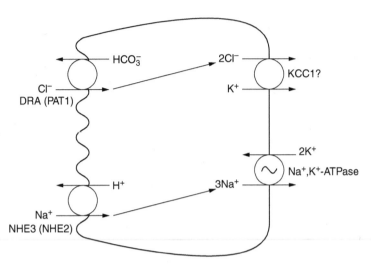

Figure 5–7. Electroneutral NaCl absorption in the small intestine and colon. NaCl enters across the apical membrane via the coupled activity of a sodium/hydrogen exchanger (NHE3, with a minor role for NHE2) and a chloride/bicarbonate exchanger (DRA, down-regulated in adenoma (SLC26a3); PAT1, putative anion transporter 1 (SLC26a6) may play a subsidiary role in some segments). The route of basolateral chloride exit via the potassium/2 chloride cotransporter (KCC1) remains speculative.

Dietary iron is also handled differently depending on whether it is in the form of heme (derived from meat), from which it is released by lysosomal enzymes following uptake of the intact heme molecule, or in its ionized form following release from various food substances, or derived from cast-iron cooking vessels.

The colon also conducts an additional absorptive transport process that reclaims an important by-product of waste metabolism. Dietary fiber and other complex carbohydrates that cannot be digested by mammalian enzymes are degraded in the colon by the resident bacterial flora, and generate short-chain fatty acids such as acetate, propionate, and butyrate. These are taken up by colonic epithelial cells and may contribute to the health of this intestinal segment. Butyrate, in particular, appears to be an important metabolic fuel for the colonocyte.

Secretory Mechanisms

Secretory mechanisms in the gastrointestinal tract center around the active transport of chloride ions. The mechanism for secretion of chloride itself is depicted in Figure 5–8. Chloride is taken up across the basolateral membrane of crypt epithelial cells via a sodium/potassium/2 chloride cotransporter called NKCC1. This transporter conducts secondary active uptake of chloride into the cell cytosol by taking advantage of the favorable gradient for sodium movement established by the basolateral Na, K-ATPase. Potassium that is cotransported is recycled across the basolateral membrane via channels that may be activated by either cAMP or

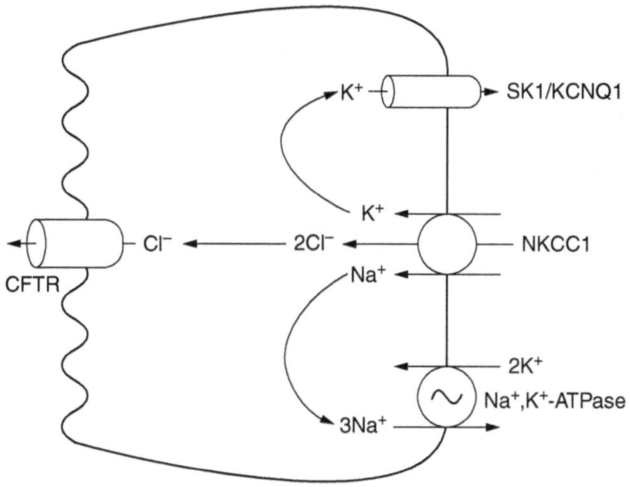

Figure 5–8. Chloride secretion in the small intestine and colon. Chloride uptake occurs via the sodium/potassium/2 chloride cotransporter, NKCC1. Potassium is recycled basolaterally via SK1/KCNQ1 potassium channels. Chloride exit is predominantly via the cystic fibrosis transmembrane conductance regulator (CFTR) chloride channel, as well as via additional chloride channels such as TMEM16A under some circumstances (not shown).

calcium. Chloride thus accumulates in the cytosol, ready to exit the cell across the apical membrane when chloride channels are opened in response to second messenger pathways. The quantitatively most significant pathway for chloride exit is the CFTR channel that we have already encountered in the pancreatic ducts; there is some evidence also to suggest an accessory role played by additional chloride channels such TMEM16A (anoctamin) that are activated by increases in intracellular calcium. The net effect is the electrogenic movement of chloride from the bloodstream to the lumen; water and sodium follow passively via the tight junctions to maintain neutrality.

Due to the combined influence of available model systems and an intense interest in the chloride secretory mechanism spurred by its relationship to cystic fibrosis, we have considerable information as to how secretion actually takes place (Figure 5–9). In response to agonists such as VIP or prostaglandins, cAMP levels are increased in the crypt cell cytosol, which in turn result in activation of PKA. This enzyme can phosphorylate and thereby open the CFTR chloride channel, resulting in an initial burst of chloride secretion. cAMP-dependent agonists of this process are additionally notable for the fact that they evoke sustained, large-magnitude secretory responses until their effect is terminated by agonist degradation. This may be attributable, at least in part, to the fact that cAMP-dependent signaling, perhaps via effects on the cytoskeleton, appears to increase the capacity of the basolateral membrane for chloride uptake via NKCC1, a

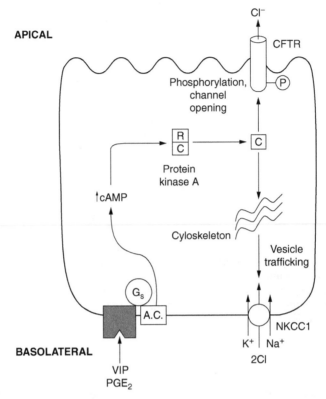

Figure 5-9. Regulation of chloride secretion by cAMP-dependent agonists such as vasoactive intestinal polypeptide (VIP) and prostaglandins. These agonists activate adenylyl cyclase (A.C.) via a stimulatory G protein (G_s) leading to an increase in intracellular cAMP. This in turn activates the cAMP-dependent protein kinase (protein kinase A), causing dissociation of its catalytic (C) subunits from the regulatory (R) subunits. The catalytic subunits are thereby freed to phosphorylate CFTR leading to channel opening, and to stimulate the insertion of additional NKCC1 cotransporter molecules into the basolateral membrane.

response which likely involves vesicular trafficking as discussed earlier. Chloride secretion is also notable for the fact that, unlike many other biological processes, the effects of cAMP and cGMP are comparable rather than opposite. cGMP is an important mediator of a key secretagogue that acts apically, guanylin, and also participates in secretory responses to a specific bacterial toxin that we will discuss later. Finally, agonists such as ACh, histamine and likely bile acids evoke chloride secretion by increasing cytosolic calcium concentrations. In this case, the primary locus for regulation is a basolateral potassium channel. As potassium leaves the cell, the driving force for chloride exit increases, allowing chloride to flow across the apical membrane via the small proportion of CFTR channels that may be open at any given time, and perhaps also via TMEM16A chloride

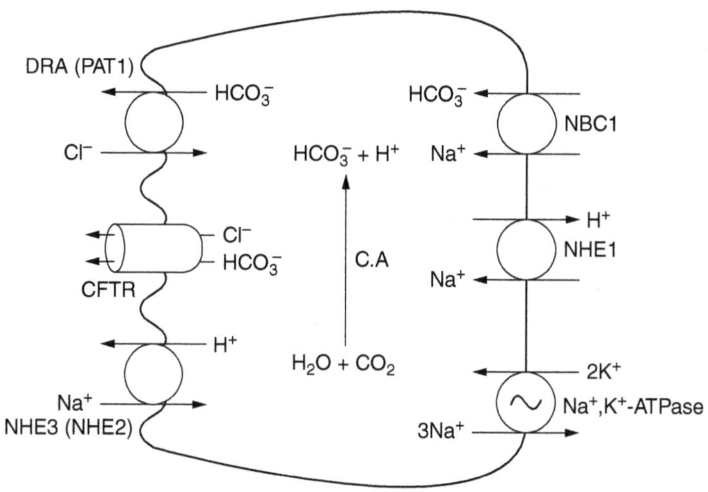

Figure 5–10. Bicarbonate secretion in the duodenum. Bicarbonate exits the apical membrane either in exchange for chloride supplied by CFTR, or via the CFTR channel itself. Bicarbonate is supplied by either intracellular production, or taken up from the bloodstream across the basolateral membrane. CA, carbonic anhydrase; NHE, sodium/hydrogen exchanger; CFTR, cystic fibrosis transmembrane conductance regulator; DRA, down-regulated in adenoma (SLC26a3); PAT1, putative anion transporter 1 (SLC26a6); NBC1, sodium/bicarbonate cotransporter 1.

channels. What is known, however, that the calcium-dependent chloride secretory response is smaller and more transient than those evoked by either cAMP or cGMP elevations. This may imply a physiological need to be able to call upon both brief and sustained secretory responses under specific circumstances during the digestion and absorption of a meal. As we saw for ductular secretion in the pancreas, moreover, when crypt epithelial cells are simultaneously exposed to a combination of agonists acting via cyclic nucleotides and calcium, a synergistic enhancement of secretion results.

The intestine is also capable of active bicarbonate secretion (Figure 5–10). This mechanism is particularly prominent in the proximal duodenum, which must defend itself from the potentially injurious effects of the acidic gastric juices. Bicarbonate is believed to be secreted by both an electroneutral mechanism involving a chloride–bicarbonate exchanger at the apical membrane, or via an electrogenic mechanism, where bicarbonate travels via CFTR. In either case, bicarbonate for secretion can be generated intracellularly via the activity of carbonic anhydrase, or is taken up from the bloodstream by the sodium–bicarbonate cotransporter, NBC1. Like chloride secretion, the overall process of bicarbonate secretion can be stimulated by intracellular increases in cAMP, cGMP, or calcium, with prostaglandins, guanylin, and ACh representing physiologically important secretagogues that utilize each respective second messenger. The primary physiological stimulus for duodenal bicarbonate secretion appears to be the presence of an acidic pH in the lumen, which presumably is sensed by enteric afferents as well as, perhaps, enterochromaffin cells that release 5-hydroxytryptamine, which activates secretion via both direct and indirect (cholinergic) pathways.

Pathophysiology and Clinical Correlations

Given the importance of maintaining an appropriate amount of fluid in the intestinal lumen, it is not surprising that disease results when the underlying transport mechanisms are dysregulated.

Secretory Diarrhea

Diarrhea can result when intestinal chloride secretion is stimulated excessively, and the resulting luminal fluid load exceeds the absorptive capacity of the small and large intestines (Figure 5–4). The prototypic disease state in which this occurs is cholera, in which *Vibrio cholerae* bacteria, present in the intestinal lumen, secrete a toxin that can bind to and enter intestinal epithelial cells. The active subunit of this toxin translocates to the basolateral membrane where it irreversibly activates the stimulatory G_s G-protein, resulting in a massive accumulation of cAMP and stimulation of downstream signaling pathways. In turn, this produces uncontrolled and sustained chloride secretion and an outpouring of fluid into the lumen. Stool volumes of up to 20 liters per day are not uncommon in this disorder, which can rapidly lead to death due to the complications of dehydration if left untreated. The severity of fluid loss in cholera is likely amplified by a simultaneous inhibition of electroneutral NaCl absorption (although importantly, not of sodium-coupled nutrient absorption) and by activation of enteric reflexes that further potentiate secretion.

Active intestinal secretion may also underlie diarrhea caused by a number of other enteric pathogens, including rotavirus that expresses a protein capable of elevating intracellular calcium. *Clostridium difficile* is a pathogen that is often acquired in hospital settings, particularly in patients whose normal enteric flora has been disrupted by the administration of antibiotics, and secretes toxins that provoke chloride secretion via calcium-dependent pathways in addition to damaging the barrier function of the epithelium. Finally, the endogenous peptide regulator of chloride secretion, guanylin, was actually discovered on the basis of knowledge of a heat-stable toxin produced by certain strains of pathogenic *E. coli*, which is the major cause of traveler's diarrhea. This toxin was known to bind to an apical receptor in epithelial cells and to evoke chloride secretion via increases in cGMP. It was hypothesized, and subsequently proven, that there must also be a natural ligand for this receptor, and in fact, the bacterial toxin displays structural homology to guanylin and thus represents an example of "molecular mimicry."

"Secretory" (watery) diarrhea can also occur in settings where the underlying mechanism appears to be a reduction in electrolyte absorptive capacity in the absence of elevated chloride secretion, or indeed in settings where chloride secretion may actually be suppressed. In particular, when the epithelium is exposed to a barrage of immune and inflammatory mediators, such as in the inflammatory bowel diseases of Crohn's disease and ulcerative colitis, there is an inhibition of sodium and chloride absorption (both electroneutral and electrogenic), seen clinically as diarrhea, which is the most frequent symptom of these conditions. Similar mechanisms may account for the diarrhea produced by invasive bacterial pathogens, as opposed to that seen in infections by bacteria that produce toxins, discussed above.

Two rare genetic conditions further illustrate the importance of a balance between secretion and absorption in intestinal fluid homeostasis. Patients with congenital chloride diarrhea have a mutation in the *DRA* gene that encodes the chloride–bicarbonate exchanger that participates in the electroneutral sodium chloride absorptive mechanism. The disease presents neonatally as a severe, chloride-rich, acidic diarrhea that can rapidly result in dehydration and death if left untreated. Similarly, congenital sodium diarrhea results from a defect in epithelial apical sodium–hydrogen exchange, and results in a sodium-rich, alkaline stool. While extremely rare in clinical practice, these "experiments of nature" are important because they provide insights into the molecular basis of intestinal transport mechanisms.

Diarrheal diseases continue to be major public health problems, particularly in developing countries where sanitation is inadequate and enteric infections are common. Diarrheal illnesses represent an important cause of infant mortality in such countries, second only to respiratory infections. Diarrheal diseases also have a major impact in developed countries, though more frequently in terms of discomfort, inconvenience, and lost productivity than mortality. Nevertheless, thousands of deaths from diarrheal diseases occur each year even in the United States, and many of these take place even after the patient has reached a health facility due to an under-appreciation of how rapidly diarrhea can cause dehydration and metabolic disturbances.

Malabsorption

Because water is absorbed passively in the gastrointestinal tract, its uptake is dependent on adequate absorption of luminal substances. If nutritional products remain in the lumen due to defects in digestion and/or absorption, then an "osmotic" diarrhea can result. In this case, there is no excessive stimulation of chloride secretion as seen in cholera and other disease states discussed earlier. Rather, the absorptive vector for fluid is impaired and not all of the large volume of fluid used daily for the digestive process can be reclaimed. A common example of osmotic diarrhea occurs in the disease of lactose intolerance, which will be discussed in more detail in Chapter 15. For now, suffice to say that individuals suffering from this condition cannot fully digest the dietary disaccharide, lactose, which is found in milk and other dairy products. Thus, when dairy products are ingested, the lactose can remain in the lumen in quantities sufficient to pull water from the bloodstream by osmosis.

Cystic Fibrosis

There is an exquisite balance among transport mechanisms in the intestine in health, and both under- or over-expression of a given mechanism can lead to disease (Figure 5–4). We have already learned the result of over-expression of chloride secretion, but under-expression of this process may be at least as deleterious. By now, you should be able to predict the effect of a failure of the gut to secrete adequate amounts of chloride, as occurs in the genetic disorder of cystic fibrosis. In fact, patients with this condition suffer from intestinal obstructions with thick, inspissated plugs of intestinal contents that are inadequately hydrated. When this occurs in newborns, it is called *meconium ileus*, and it is often the first sign of the disorder, but similar obstructions may occur throughout the lifespan of a patient with cystic fibrosis. Presumably, if other chloride channels participate in intestinal chloride secretion in addition to the CFTR chloride channel that is mutated and dysfunctional in cystic fibrosis, their activity is insufficient to drive secretion of the amount of fluid that is needed for normal intestinal function.

KEY CONCEPTS

1 *The intestine handles large volumes of fluid in fulfilling its physiological functions.*

2 *Dysfunction can rapidly impact whole-body electrolyte homeostasis.*

3 *Water is moved passively in response to active electrolyte transport.*

4 *Transport mechanisms are heterogenous along the length of the intestine and between crypt and villus cells.*

5 *Transport mechanisms consist of the asymmetrical arrangement of a limited number of electrolyte transport pathways.*

6 *Certain pathogens can cause diarrheal disease by hijacking normal cellular signaling pathways.*

7 *Diarrheal disease remains a major health problem in both developed and developing countries.*

STUDY QUESTIONS

5–1. Individuals being housed in a camp in South-East Asia following a natural disaster develop wide-spread watery diarrhea. Increased activity of which of the following transport proteins might be exploited therapeutically to reduce fluid losses?

   A. SGLT-1

   B. CFTR

   C. NHE3

   D. Na,K-ATPase

   E. NKCC1

5–2. A 50-year old man on a business trip to a developing county develops severe diarrhea and begins taking Imodium in an attempt to lessen his symptoms. Any relief he obtains can most likely be ascribed to an increase in which of the following?

   A. Intestinal transit time

   B. Mucosal blood flow

   C. Chloride secretion

   D. Peristalsis

   E. Epithelial proliferation

5–3. A 30-year old woman with Crohn's disease undergoes a surgical resection of her terminal ileum. After recovering from the surgery, she develops chronic diarrhea, with a daily stool output of approximately 2 liters (10x normal). Which of the following substances is/are most likely primarily responsible for her symptoms?

   A. Prostaglandins

   B. Inflammatory cytokines

   C. Vasoactive intestinal polypeptide

   D. Bile acids

   E. Short chain fatty acids

5–4. An infant develops chronic diarrhea and failure to thrive. Tests reveal glucosuria. Further studies show that urinary excretion of lactulose given orally, as well as uptake of oral alanine, are comparable to that seen in a normal child, whereas oral galactose absorption is markedly impaired. Diarrhea in this child is most likely due to a mutation in which of the following proteins?

   A. CFTR

   B. ENaC

   C. NHE3

   D. PepT1

   E. SGLT-1

5-5. *In a healthy adult, the volume of fluid presented to the intestine on a daily basis is approximately 8 liters. Assuming a normal diet, reabsorption of the bulk of this fluid in the small intestine is driven primarily by which of the following?*

A. *Nutrient-coupled electrogenic sodium absorption*

B. *Electroneutral NaCl absorption*

C. *Nutrient-coupled proton absorption*

D. *Potassium absorption*

E. *Electrogenic sodium absorption via ENaC channels*

SUGGESTED READINGS

Barrett KE, Keely SJ. Chloride secretion by the intestinal epithelium: molecular basis and regulatory aspects. *Annu Rev Physiol.* 2000;62:535–572.

Cooke HJ. Neurotransmitters in neuronal reflexes regulating intestinal secretion. *Ann NY Acad Sci.* 2000;91:77–80.

Donowitz M, Alpers DH, Binder HJ, Brewer T, Carrington J, Grey MJ. Translational approaches for pharmacotherapy development for acute diarrhea. *Gastroenterology.* 2012;142:e1–e9.

Eggemont E. Gastrointestinal manifestations in cystic fibrosis. *Eur J Gastroenterol Hepatol.* 1996;8: 731–738.

Field M. Intestinal ion transport and the pathophysiology of diarrhea. *J Clin Invest.* 2003;111:931–943.

Harris JB, LaRocque RC, Qadri F, Ryan ET, Calderwood SB. Cholera. *Lancet.* 2012;379:2466–2476.

Keely SJ, Montrose MH, Barrett KE. Electrolyte secretion and absorption: small intestine and colon. In: Yamada T, Alpers DH, Kalloo AN, Kaplowitz N, Owyang C, Powell DW, eds. *Textbook of Gastroenterology.* 5th ed. Chichester: Wiley-Blackwell; 2009:330–367.

Kopic S, Geibel JP. Toxin-mediated diarrhea in the 21st century: the pathophysiology of intestinal ion transport in the course of ETEC, *V. cholera* and rotavirus infection. *Toxins.* 2010;2:2132–2157.

Zachos NC, Tse M, Donowitz M. Molecular physiology of intestinal Na$^+$/H$^+$ exchange. *Annu Rev Physiol.* 2005;67:411–443.

Intestinal Mucosal Immunology and Ecology

6

OBJECTIVES

▶ *Understand the role played by the mucosal immune system in protecting the host from infections acquired via the oral route while failing to respond to innocuous antigens*
  ▶ Define the mechanisms and relative roles of innate versus adaptive immunity
  ▶ Understand the specialized features of the mucosal immune system compared with immunity expressed in the periphery
▶ *Identify the cell populations that contribute to immunity in the gut and their locations*
  ▶ Describe mechanisms that result in cellular homing to the gut and other mucosal sites
  ▶ Describe the characteristics of IgA that make it especially suited to function in the gut
▶ *Describe the immune responses that occur to antigens encountered in the gut*
  ▶ Understand the concept of oral tolerance
▶ *Understand the origins, make-up and physiological importance of microbial populations that exist in the normal intestine*
▶ *Define the consequences of abnormal immune responses in the intestine*

BASIC PRINCIPLES OF MUCOSAL IMMUNOLOGY

Concept of a Mucosal Immune System

As we have learned in previous chapters, the surface of the gastrointestinal tract represents a vast frontier that can potentially serve as a portal of entry into the body. Moreover, by the very nature of the physiological function of the gut, its lumen is frequently filled with a complex mixture of nutrients that constitute an attractive "culture medium" for a variety of microbes. Indeed, the intestine is challenged to distinguish between potentially harmful microorganisms, against which it must defend itself, versus the innocuous antigens that occur in food. The intestine also has a special need for immune surveillance against malignancy. Thus, the rapid rate of proliferation of intestinal epithelial cells, coupled with exposure of these cells to potential toxins in the intestinal lumen, renders the epithelium uniquely sensitive to cell transformation. It is likely that the immune system is important in detecting many transformed cells before they have the opportunity to develop into a tumor, although clearly this line of defense is not perfect. Finally, over millennia, humans and other animals have been exposed to a barrage of intestinal pathogens via contaminated food and water; inadequate sanitation still persists in many underdeveloped areas of the world. This constant exposure has driven the development of a highly specialized branch of the immune system, referred to as the mucosal immune system, which encompasses the mucosa-associated lymphoid tissues, or MALT.

In fact, the intestine represents the largest immunological compartment of the body, and has also evolved nonimmunologic barriers to invasion by pathogens. The nonimmune barriers include secretion of the acid by the stomach, the potential antimicrobial actions of other components of the digestive juices such as enzymes and bile acids, the mucus layer, which overlies much of the epithelium, that limits microbial attachment to the epithelial surface, specific antibacterial products secreted by specialized epithelial cells or by the salivary glands, and the epithelium itself, which, when intact, represents a physical barrier to the uncontrolled flux of microbes into the body. The immune barriers include both the so-called innate immune system, and adaptive, or acquired immunity. Innate immunity consists of a series of mechanisms to respond to molecular structures that are broadly specific for classes of microbes, but are not expressed by host cells. These structures are referred to as pathogen-associated molecular patterns, and are recognized by pattern-recognition receptors. This event sets in motion a number of rapid responses that are designed to repel invading pathogens. In contrast, adaptive immunity develops more slowly, but is exquisitely specific, potentially more effective, and generates a "memory" in the host that permits an amplified response if the same pathogen is encountered again. Adaptive immunity is mediated by lymphoid cells, notably T and B lymphocytes, and soluble antibodies. Overall, the combined activity of the more primitive, or ancient, innate system, and adaptive immunity, is remarkably effective in protecting us from the potential perils of intestinal infections.

The intestinal immune system, particularly with respect to the adaptive limb, is also part of a broader immune system that protects other mucosal surfaces in the body, including the airways, eyes, urogenital tracts, and the mammary glands. Lymphocytes specific for antigens encountered via any of these mucosal routes undergo regulated trafficking that allows them to engage in homing back not only to the site where their expansion was stimulated, but also to all of the other mucosal sites listed. This provides a common system of mucosal protection. The concept of the common mucosal immune system is also relevant to immune protection of neonates by maternal antibodies. The majority of antibodies secreted in breast milk are specific for antigens that the mother has encountered via the gut, and provide similar protection to the baby, whose immune system is not mature at birth.

Special Features of the Immune System of the Intestine

The immune system in the intestine is specialized to subserve the specific functions discussed earlier. First, in conditions of health, the lymphocytes that traffic to mucosal sites encounter antigens in a controlled fashion. This is accomplished by limiting the uptake of significant quantities of particulate antigens only to specific sites within the epithelial monolayer, via specialized epithelial cells known as M cells. M cells overlie organized lymphoid aggregates known as Peyer's patches. The lymphocytes in these structures are immunologically naive and represent the afferent arm of the mucosal immune system; after they have been stimulated by their cognate antigen, they traffic back to the lamina propria via draining lymph nodes, the thoracic ducts, and the bloodstream, from where they reenter the mucosa. During this migration the lymphocytes mature and differentiate, and then represent an efferent arm of the system, capable of effector functions in the mucosa. Second, unlike the peripheral immune system, where the primary immunoglobulin is IgG, the humoral aspects of mucosal immunity are predominantly served by secretory IgA molecules, which will be discussed in more detail later. Third, the intestinal mucosa can be considered to be constantly in a state of "physiological" inflammation, even in health. Presumably this reflects the constant stimulation the system receives from the intestinal microflora, and renders the intestine armed and ready to respond rapidly at times of threat by pathogens. Finally, the specific lymphocyte subsets present in the intestine can promote a particular type of immune response called oral tolerance, where a local antibody response to a specific antigen can be mounted at mucosal sites in the absence of a response in the periphery.

FUNCTIONAL ANATOMY OF THE MUCOSAL IMMUNE SYSTEM

Cellular Mediators of Innate Immunity

As discussed earlier, the innate arm of the mucosal immune system is designed to mount rapid responses to pathogens, and does so by expressing pattern-recognition receptors that recognize molecules that are important to broad classes of pathogenic microbes, such as lipopolysaccharides and peptidoglycans. Macrophages represent one important class of effectors of such innate immune responses, but in fact pattern-recognition receptors may be more widely distributed, including on cells not classically considered to be immune effector cells, such as the epithelium. Pattern-recognition receptors include the Toll-like receptors, so-called because of their homology to the *Drosophila* defense molecule, Toll, and other proteins that may respond to pathogen molecules presented intracellularly, such as Nod 1 and Nod 2. In general, activation of the innate immune response generates chemotactic molecules that stimulate the influx and activation of further inflammatory cells, including additional monocytes that can differentiate into tissue macrophages, as well as, importantly, neutrophils. Collectively, these cells can effect microbial killing by releasing a variety of toxic products, including reactive oxygen species, which have the unfortunate side effect that they may also cause bystander damage to adjacent, uninfected tissues. Activation of the innate immune response may also generate cytokines that facilitate the later, and more specific, adaptive immune response.

Cellular Mediators of Adaptive Immunity

Unlike the limited selection of pathogen factors recognized by innate immunity, adaptive immunity involves the exquisitely specific recognition of literally millions of discrete antigenic sequences that are found in microorganisms as well as in abnormal host cells, such as those that have undergone malignant transformation or which are virally infected. Such recognition is mediated by specific receptors expressed on two classes of lymphoid cells, T and B cells. T cells recognize peptides derived from antigenic sequences via a heterodimeric, variable cell surface T-cell receptor that originates from recombination of various distinct gene segments as well as subsequent editing to provide for additional diversity. The peptides are presented bound to major histocompatibility complex (MHC) molecules on antigen-presenting cells, which include dendritic cells and likely intestinal epithelial cells. A positive response also requires costimulation of the T cell via accessory molecules and ligands. The binding of antigen to a specific T-cell receptor then drives the expansion of a clone of cells expressing that receptor; some of these differentiate into effector T cells capable of secreting cytokines that regulate additional immune responses, others remain as memory cells to jump-start an adaptive immune response if the same antigen is encountered again. T cells in the mucosal immune system can be subdivided into those expressing the differentiation marker CD4, and those expressing CD8. The former cell population recognizes antigens, derived from the extracellular environment via endocytosis, that are displayed on the surface of antigen-presenting cells in the context of MHC class II molecules. Such antigens likely include components of pathogenic microorganisms. In general, CD4-positive T cells help to regulate immune responses, and also further differentiate into specific subsets that secrete characteristic products depending on the specific threat to the system, under the influence of specific cytokine messages. CD4-positive cells can further be subdivided into effector and regulatory subsets. The effector cells are so-called "helper" cells (Th) that promote the development of B cells and thereby "help" them to produce antibodies. Regulatory T cells, on the other hand, suppress the activity of other T cells at sites of inflammation or in response to the commensal microbiota. There is evidence that some inflammatory diseases of the intestine may arise, in part, from the failure to develop sufficient numbers of regulatory T cells. CD8 positive T cells, on the other hand, recognize abnormal intracellular proteins in the context of MHC class I molecules. Like CD4 cells, CD8 cells may generate cytokines that regulate the network of immune responses, but CD8 cells may also be directly cytotoxic. Thus, CD8 T cells provide important protection against potentially harmful intracellular events, such as viral infection or malignant transformation. MHC class I molecules are expressed on essentially all cell types in the gut, underscoring the significance of this protective pathway.

Adaptive immunity is also mediated by B cells, which differentiate into plasma cells and begin to secrete antibodies specific for a given antigen under the influence of antigen-specific T cells and the cytokines they produce, especially transforming growth factor-β, interleukin (IL)-4, IL-5, and IL-6. This exemplifies a central principle in intestinal adaptive immunity, which is that an effective immune response typically requires the cooperation of several different cell types as well as soluble mediators. Antibodies produced by B cells may additionally mediate activity of another class of effector cells known as natural killer or NK cells. These cells represent a link between the adaptive and innate branches of the immune response. NK cells can destroy particles (e.g., microbes) that have been *opsonized*, i.e., coated with antibodies specific for cell surface components. However, NK cells also exert cytotoxic effects that are independent of any aspects of the adaptive response. Thus, they recognize cells that have downregulated MHC class I molecules, which is a strategy commonly employed by virally infected or tumor cells in an attempt to evade the immune attack that would otherwise be mounted by CD8-positive T cells. In either case, however, NK cells lyse their targets via the release of cytotoxic products that include an enzyme, granzyme, and a substance capable of forming pores in target cell membranes, called perforin.

Organization of Lymphoid Tissues

It is also important to appreciate how lymphoid tissues are organized in the intestine. As mentioned earlier, in the small intestine, the afferent arm of the adaptive system (i.e., the arm that responds initially to a threat) occurs in structures known as Peyer's patches, as shown diagrammatically in Figure 6–1. In the colon, these

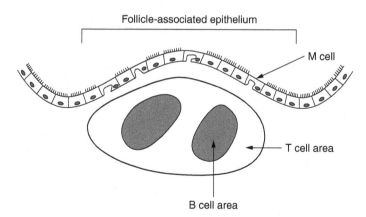

Figure 6–1. Structure of a Peyer's patch in the small intestinal mucosa. The follicle-associated epithelium contains M, or microfold cells, that have a subapical pocket in which antigens can be presented to immune cells. Lymphocytes are aggregated underneath the epithelium with T and B lymphocytes restricted to distinct areas. Peyer's patchers also contain dendritic cells (not shown), which can present antigens to lymphocytes.

aggregates of lymphocytes are more loosely organized, but analogous in function. Naive T and B cells from the bloodstream are targeted to migrate into Peyer's patches because they recognize a specific type of endothelial cell that is found in the blood supply to these lymphoid structures. The other important components of the Peyer's patch include the M cell, which replaces normal enterocytes as an epithelial covering for the lymphoid follicle, and is important in initial uptake of luminal particulates, and dendritic cells and macrophages, which serve to process and present antigens to the T and B cells. Once stimulated, activated T and B cells migrate out of the lymphoid follicle and, via the pathways discussed earlier, eventually back to the lamina propria.

Dendritic cells are also more widely distributed in the intestinal mucosa beyond the Peyer's patches. They are thought to be important in additional sensing/sampling of luminal antigens, because they can project their dendrites between the tight junctions of adjacent epithelial cells. The antigens thus taken up are presented to lymphocytes in the lamina propria (Figure 6–2).

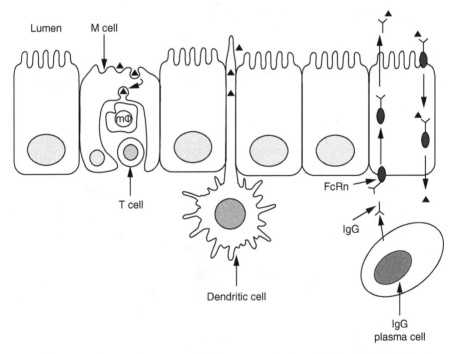

Figure 6–2. Pathways for antigen uptake across the intestinal epithelium. Proteins (small triangles) are taken up by M cells or the processes of dendritic cells, or after binding to specific IgG molecules that are subsequently trafficked in a retrograde fashion by the neonatal Fc receptor (FcRn) expressed on intestinal epithelial cells. mΦ, macrophage.

A final class of organized lymphoid cells in the intestine consists of a subset of lymphocytes that are anchored immediately adjacent to the epithelial layer via specific adhesion molecules. These are called intraepithelial lymphocytes, and appear predominantly to consist of memory T cells capable of responding to only a subset of luminal antigens. They likely function primarily to secrete cytokines involved in the regulation of the epithelium, and may also participate in immune surveillance for emerging malignancies.

SECRETORY IgA SYSTEM

Effector B cells in the lamina propria are capable of synthesizing a range of immunoglobulins. Following maturation into a plasma cell, a given B cell retains the ability to synthesize only one specific antibody type. However, the distribution of immunoglobulin subtypes in the mucosal immune system is quite different from that seen in the peripheral immune system, as represented by circulating B cells. Thus, while IgG is the major antibody in the bloodstream, in the intestine, 70–90% of the B cells in the lamina propria secrete IgA, with the remainder largely making IgM, and a few cells making IgE. Very few cells in the lamina propria make IgG in healthy individuals. In fact, given the large numbers of lymphocytes that normally reside in the gut, the daily synthesis of IgA exceeds that of all other immunoglobulins.

Structural Aspects of IgA

There are two subclasses of IgA, coded by separate genes in the immunoglobulin locus. IgA_1 is the predominant form of this antibody found in the circulation, and the majority of serum IgA is also in the form of monomers. On the other hand, the IgA plasma cells that localize to the intestinal lamina propria show a greater predominance of IgA_2, and essentially all of the IgA is in the form of dimers.

The two IgA molecules in dimeric IgA are bound together by a short polypeptide sequence known as the J (or joining) chain. J chain is also a component of other polymeric immunoglobulins, such as IgM. The other critical component of secretory IgA that is found in the lumen of the intestine derives from intestinal epithelial cells (Figure 6–3). Thus, dimers of IgA plus J chain are taken up at the basolateral surface of the epithelium by binding to a structure known as the polymeric immunoglobulin receptor, or pIgR. The complex of IgA plus pIgR is internalized and translocated across the epithelial cell. At the apical membrane, the IgA dimer is released into the lumen bound to a cleaved portion of pIgR, known as secretory component. Secretory component stabilizes the IgA dimer against proteolytic cleavage by either the digestive juices or bacterial proteases.

It should be noted that the small quantities of IgG produced in the gut can also be translocated across the epithelium. However, rather than utilizing pIgR, monomeric IgG is instead trafficked across the epithelium following

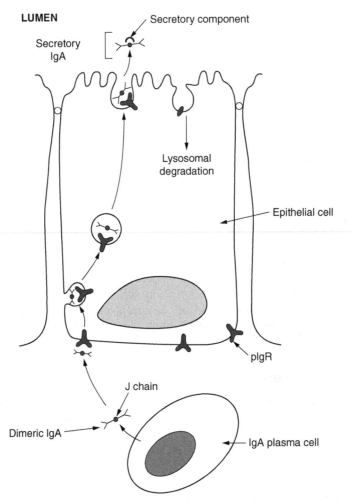

Figure 6–3. Secretion of IgA across the intestinal epithelium. IgA is secreted by plasma cells in the lamina propria as a dimer, with two IgA molecules linked by a J, or joining, chain. J chain is recognized by the polymeric immunoglobulin receptor (pIgR) expressed on the basolateral membrane of epithelial cells, and once bound, the complex is internalized and trafficked across the cytosol to the apical membrane. Apical proteases cleave the extracellular portion of pIgR, which remains associated with the IgA dimer as secretory component. The remnant of the pIgR is internalized and degraded.

binding to the so-called neonatal Fc receptor (FcRn). Another important difference from IgA transport is that FcRn-mediated transport can be bidirectional. Thus, IgG transport can contribute another mechanism for antigen uptake from the lumen, particularly in disease states when mucosal IgG synthesis may be upregulated (Figure 6–2).

Mechanisms of Protective Effects

Secretory IgA exerts protection in the intestine via several mechanisms. IgA released into the lumen of the gut can bind microbial antigens, food antigens, and viruses to prevent their interaction with, and uptake by, intestinal epithelial cells. Thus, secretory IgA exerts at least part of its function via a process of immune exclusion. There is also evidence for a second line of defense that takes place within epithelial cells themselves. Thus, if any antigens are internalized by these cells, they can encounter vesicles bearing IgA bound to pIgR that are destined for the apical membrane. The IgA in these vesicles can bind the foreign antigen and traffic it back to the apical membrane, thus resulting in its elimination. Finally, some IgA molecules doubtless function to sequester antigens that are able to penetrate to the lamina propria.

IgA has an additional specialization relative to other antibody classes that particularly suits it to function in the gut. Thus, the antibody is not capable of fixing complement via the classical pathway, rendering it relatively noninflammatory upon antigen binding. This is likely an important consideration given the vast antigenic load that is presented to the intestine, representing the combined influences of potentially antigenic food proteins along with microbial products.

Physiological Functions

The secretory IgA response that is predominant in the intestine serves to protect the body from potentially injurious substances that might otherwise stimulate a more generalized immune/inflammatory reaction in the periphery. Note that the IgA system is not well-developed in newborns. In the breast-fed infant, protection can be obtained via IgA antibodies secreted into the mother's milk. This is one benefit of the common mucosal immune system, discussed earlier, where lymphocytes activated by antigens encountered in the intestine also traffic to other mucosal sites, including the mammary glands. The IgA system becomes mature in the child by the age of 5–6 months, in part driven by the gradual acquisition of the microbiota.

IMMUNE RESPONSE TO ENTERIC ANTIGENS

There are three potential outcomes when the adaptive immune system encounters an antigen in the intestine, depending, in part, on the type of antigen that is encountered and its quantity. A localized response can occur, such as the stimulation of antigen-specific IgA production. The antigen can also, at least theoretically, drive a systemic immune response with the production of circulating antibodies plus expansion of antigen-specific T cells. However, it is clear that this would be an undesirable outcome under normal circumstances, given the number of antigens encountered by the intestine on a daily basis and the deleterious consequences of systemic reactions to these, particularly if they stimulate a generalized inflammatory reaction. Thus, an additional response to orally delivered antigens has also evolved in the mucosal immune system, which limits these adverse consequences in the systemic immune system. This specialized response is referred to as "oral tolerance."

Oral Tolerance

Oral tolerance refers to a mucosal immune response where local IgA is produced, yet there is no detectable immune response in the periphery. Oral tolerance is the most frequent outcome for antigens that are presumably innocuous, such as food antigens and antigens derived from commensal microorganisms that normally inhabit the gut. The determination as to whether oral tolerance will occur depends on the type of antigen, the amount given, the frequency of exposure, and host factors, including the age of the recipient.

The lack of response in the periphery requires active suppressive mechanisms that are mediated by the regulatory T cells discussed above and are highly specific, because they extend only to the substance that is fed and not to other antigens. The phenomenon of oral tolerance is being exploited for the treatment of some systemic autoimmune diseases. Thus, feeding patients with a self-antigen that is capable of driving a systemic disease, such as collagen in the case of arthritis or myelin basic protein in the case of multiple sclerosis has resulted in some diminution of disease symptoms, associated with a reduction in circulating autoantibodies. While such treatments remain experimental at present, they are likely to represent a powerful alternative to other, more toxic antiinflammatory therapies if they can be optimized.

Immune Responsiveness

Under different circumstances, it may be appropriate for the intestine to respond to an antigen and additionally for this response to spread to the periphery. This is particularly the case for immune responses to pathogens, where the mucosal immune system responds to the large amounts of antigens produced by these rapidly replicating microbes, some of which are capable of physically invading across the epithelium. Generalized immune responses to otherwise innocuous antigens can also be driven by administering these in the presence of an adjuvant. This latter approach might ultimately prove useful in exploiting the oral route to vaccinate people against disease-related antigens, such as by expressing these along with an adjuvant in transgenic plants. However, we do not currently have enough understanding of the mechanisms that determine whether an immune response versus tolerance occurs for such approaches yet to be reliable.

Generalized immune responses can also be deleterious to the host under specific circumstances. For example, if the barrier function of the epithelium is compromised, it is possible to generate both local and systemic immune responses to the normal commensal flora of the gut, which in turn can lead to tissue injury.

Autoimmunity

During the development of immunity, clones of T and B cells capable of reacting to self-antigens are mostly actively deleted. However, even in healthy individuals, a few such lymphocytes are thought to remain in the mucosal immune system, and may be needed to respond to microbes that engage in "molecular mimicry," i.e., expressing antigens that resemble proteins of the host, in an attempt to evade immunity. Under normal circumstances, these autoreactive clones are likely held in check by regulatory T cells and inhibitory cytokines. Likewise, self-antigens may be presented in the absence of appropriate costimulatory molecules, which results in anergy rather than an immune response. On the other hand, under pathologic conditions, this regulation may be lost with the resulting emergence of autoreactivity and tissue inflammation and injury. These mechanisms may be important in contributing to disease in conditions such as inflammatory bowel diseases, celiac disease, and atrophic gastritis.

INTESTINAL MICROECOLOGY

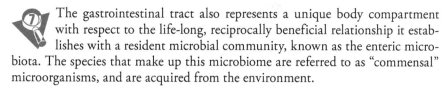 The gastrointestinal tract also represents a unique body compartment with respect to the life-long, reciprocally beneficial relationship it establishes with a resident microbial community, known as the enteric microbiota. The species that make up this microbiome are referred to as "commensal" microorganisms, and are acquired from the environment.

Development of Intestinal Microbiota

At birth, the intestinal tract is sterile. However, by the age of 1 month, the infant begins to become richly colonized with organisms derived from the environment in an oral-to-anal direction. The microbiota then matures to an "adult" phenotype by about 3 years of age, which is shared among family members and across generations. Over the long-term, diet also influences the microbiota, with systematic changes in the diet resulting in society-level changes in the microbiome.

INDIGENOUS POPULATIONS

The entire gastrointestinal tract can be shown to be colonized with bacteria, but the types of bacteria and their numbers vary along the gastrointestinal tract. The stomach and the majority of the small intestine contain relatively few bacteria, and lack anaerobes. On the other hand, beginning in the distal small intestine, the numbers of bacteria rise sharply, and anaerobes also appear. The largest numbers of bacteria, by far, occur in the colon, where anaerobes vastly outnumber aerobic bacteria (Table 6–1).

Table 6–1. Enteric bacterial populations

	Stomach	Jejunum	Ileum	Cecum/Colon
Total bacteria/g	$0–10^3$	$0–10^4$	$10^4–10^8$	$10^{10}–10^{12}$
Aerobes and facultative anaerobes/g	$0–10^3$	$0–10^4$	$10^4–10^5$	$10^2–10^9$
Anaerobes/g	0	0	$10^3–10^8$	$10^{10}–10^{12}$
pH	3	6–7	7.5	6.8–7.3

The flora in the colon is complex, likely containing at least 1500 different bacterial species. However, the precise proportions of each species tend to differ between individuals, while remaining relatively constant in a given individual over time in the absence of disruptive events (see later). This has led to the concept that the bacterial flora of a given subject is essentially equivalent to a "fingerprint," representing the interplay between the host and bacterial factors that determine the relative ability of each individual commensal species to colonize the colonic lumen. We are also learning that the indigenous microbiota likely exists predominantly in loose communities known as "biofilms" that associate with colonic mucus on the surface of the epithelium. This may account for the relative stability of the flora over time. Finally, while we are far from being able to generate a complete catalogue of all of the species that colonize the colon, we do know that the major anaerobic species include bacteroides, bifidobacteria, clostridia, eubacteria, and anaerobic streptococci. Likewise, important aerobes include enterobacteria such as *E. coli*, streptococci, and staphylococci.

FACTORS CONTROLLING MICROBIOTA

The bacterial colonization of the upper gastrointestinal tract is kept in check by a number of physical and humoral factors. Gastric acid, for example, significantly limits the initial inoculum of bacteria that enters the system with food or drink. Many gastrointestinal secretions, such as saliva and bile, also contain substances that are toxic to bacteria, including bile acids, small antimicrobial peptides known as defensins, and lysozyme. In the small intestine, moreover, the overall bacterial burden is kept in check by the combined influences of motility (especially peristalsis) and the ability of the mucosa to secrete fluids and electrolytes that can wash bacteria out of the lumen before they have the opportunity to organize into loosely adherent biofilms. Secretion of IgA may also limit the growth of some commensals, although under normal circumstances, the mucosal immune system does not mount a significant immune response to the indigenous microbiota.

In the colon, on the other hand, the relatively slow motility permits the growth of large numbers of bacteria. These are largely retained in the large intestine by the action of the ileocecal valve. Upwards of 10^{12} bacteria can be found per gram of colonic luminal contents, and the majority of the formed mass of the stool, after water, consists of dead bacteria. Indeed, the number of intestinal bacteria in the average person is greater than the total number of cells in the human body. This raises the question of who is the host, and who are the commensals! In the short-term, the make-up of the colonic microbiota is relatively insensitive to diet, although a diet rich in fiber, which constitutes a fuel for anaerobic bacteria (as discussed later), may result in an increase in overall bacterial numbers. Conversely, intestinal colonization can be dramatically reduced in patients taking broad-spectrum antibiotics, which may result in alterations in bowel function, at least temporarily.

Physiological Functions of the Microbiota

Experiments in animals reveal that the intestinal microbiota is not essential to life. Thus, animals that are raised in a totally sterile environment from birth are apparently healthy and reproduce normally. Nevertheless, the microbiota clearly has measurable effects on the host. First, in germ-free animals, the mucosal immune system is poorly developed, illustrating the critical role of luminal stimuli in driving the development and maturation of intestinal lymphoid populations. Second, epithelial proliferation and differentiation is also slowed in the absence of luminal bacteria, although the mechanisms underlying this and its significance for the host are not currently understood.

Colonic bacteria, in particular, also supply metabolic functions that cannot be performed by mammalian enzymes. Indeed, the overall human metabolic phenotype can be considered to represent the combination of capacities encoded by both the host and microbial genomes. The metabolic activity of the microbiota can be divided into effects on endogenous substances and those on substances that originate outside the body. Colonic bacteria utilize reductases to convert bilirubin, a product of heme metabolism that is secreted in the bile, into urobilinogen. Bacterial dehydroxylases also act on primary bile acids to generate secondary bile acids that enter the enterohepatic circulation (more about this in Chapter 11) and bacterial enzymes are also responsible for deconjugating any conjugated bile acids that escape active reabsorption in the terminal ileum, to then permit their passive reuptake across the colonic mucosa (Table 6–2).

Table 6–2. Metabolic effects of enteric bacteria

Substrate	Enzymes	Products	Disposition
Endogenous substrates			
Urea	Urease	Ammonia	Passive absorption or excretion as NH_4^+
Bilirubin	Reductases	Urobilinogen stercobilins	Passive reabsorption Excreted
Primary bile acids	Dehydroxylases	Secondary bile acids	Passive reabsorption
Conjugated bile acids	Deconjugases	Unconjugated bile acids	Passive reabsorption
Exogenous substrates			
Carbohydrates (fiber)	Glycosidases	SCFAs* H_2, CO_2, CH_4	Active absorption Expired in breath or excreted in flatus
Amino acids	Decarboxylases and deaminases	Ammonia, HCO_3^-	Reabsorbed or excreted (for ammonia) as NH_4^+
Cysteine, methionine	Sulfatases	Hydrogen sulfide	Excreted in flatus

*SCFA: short chain fatty acid.

(8) Bacterial enzymes also salvage nutrients that cannot be degraded by pancreatic or other digestive enzymes (Table 6–2). This is particularly important for dietary fiber, a form of carbohydrate that is resistant to breakdown by amylase. Breakdown of fiber occurs via a metabolic process known as fermentation, and requires a strict anaerobic environment. Fermentation can also break down any carbohydrates that escape digestion and absorption in the small intestine, such as lactose in patients who are intolerant of this sugar. There is evidence that obesity is associated with a biasing of the microbiota towards bacterial species that are more efficient at nutrient salvage. The products of fermentation are the short-chain fatty acids acetate, propionate, and butyrate, which can be absorbed by colonic epithelial cells and used as fuel. Short-chain fatty acids can reach millimolar concentrations in the colonic lumen, depending on the diet, and account in part for the fact that the colonic lumen is mildly acidic. In addition to short-chain fatty acids, fermentation also yields energy for the bacteria and the gases hydrogen, carbon dioxide, and methane. Bacteria can also act on other dietary components to yield by-products, although these are usually quantitatively less significant than the products of carbohydrate fermentation. Nevertheless, bacterial peptidases, decarboxylases, and deaminases can sequentially degrade luminal proteins into amino acids, carbon dioxide, and ammonia. Bacterial sulfatases can yield hydrogen sulfide by acting on amino acids carrying sulfhydral groups, and bacterial oxidases can act on unabsorbed fatty acids.

Bacterial metabolism may also be exploited for pharmacological purposes. Thus, to target a drug to be released in the colon, it can be given as a prodrug form where the active component is linked to an inactive moiety via a bond that is resistant to host intestinal enzymes. Bacterial enzymes may also detoxify some carcinogens, but equally, they may be responsible for the generation of carcinogens from compounds in the lumen that would otherwise be innocuous. This liability of the microbiota may be another reason why colon cancer is a relatively common malignancy.

(9) A final, and likely critical, role of the microflora is to increase the resistance of the intestinal mucosa to colonization with pathogenic microorganisms. Germ-free animals are exquisitely sensitive to enteric pathogens, succumbing to infection with only a few pathogenic bacteria presented orally compared to the millions needed to cause disease in a normal animal. Likewise, the enteric flora protects the host from overgrowth of bacteria that are innocuous when present in low numbers, but can cause disease if allowed to dominate the flora. The best example of this is found with the bacteria *C. difficile*, which synthesizes a toxin that damages the colonic epithelium causing diarrhea and colitis. *C. difficile* often proliferates markedly when the normal flora has been disrupted secondary to antibiotic treatment, and is the most commonly identified causative agent of antibiotic-associated diarrhea.

Generation of Gas in the Intestine

The intestinal microbiota is also the source of the majority of the gas that originates in the gastrointestinal tract. While large volumes of air may be swallowed with meals, most of this is expelled from the stomach by belching. That which remains is supplemented by carbon dioxide that is generated when gastric acid is neutralized by bicarbonate; the majority of the carbon dioxide can diffuse across the wall of the bowel and is excreted via the lungs. The gas which remains in the intestine is moved back and forth by motility patterns, resulting in bowel sounds, or borborygmi, that can be heard through a stethoscope and sometimes even by the naked ear as a "rumbling stomach." The absence of such bowel sounds is a reliable indicator that bowel motility has been inhibited, which happens commonly (and usually reversibly) after abdominal surgery. More distally, fermentation and other metabolic pathways promoted by bacterial enzymes in the colon results in the formation of large volumes of gas on a daily basis, even in normal individuals who do not complain of any problem with flatulence. Reliable estimates of the amount of gas produced are difficult to come by, but the volume of gas produced by a healthy individual is likely to average 1 liter per day. However, there is considerable variation among individuals, and the amount of gas also depends on the quantity of fermentable residues which depends, in turn, on the diet.

Most of the gases present in flatus are nonodorous, with the majority consisting of nitrogen and hydrogen (Figure 6–4). The amount of methane produced varies considerably among individuals, accounting for that fact that some people,

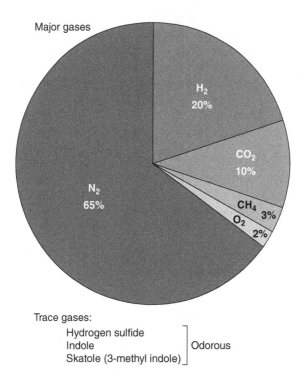

Figure 6–4. Composition of normal intestinal flatus.

but not all, are able to "light" their flatus, which results from the explosive mixture of methane and hydrogen. On the other hand, the gases that are responsible for the odor of flatus are present in very small, or trace, amounts. These include hydrogen sulfide, indole, and skatole.

PATHOPHYSIOLOGY AND CLINICAL CORRELATIONS

Small Bowel Bacterial Overgrowth

While there are small numbers of bacteria present in the normal small intestine, their numbers are low compared to the immense flora in the colon and anaerobic bacteria are either rare or completely absent as one moves more proximally. However, under certain conditions, usually associated with abnormal motility or obstructions, overgrowth of bacteria in the small bowel can occur. This is also referred to as the "stagnant loop system," indicating that the problem arises from stasis of intestinal contents. The abnormal presence of large numbers of bacteria, and particularly anaerobes, in the small bowel has a number of physiological consequences. First, the large load of carbohydrate seen by these bacteria results in brisk fermentation, which can be experienced by the patient as gas and bloating. Second, bacteria can compete with the host to take up vitamin B_{12}, and if overgrowth becomes severe, the patient may develop anemia due to a systemic lack of this vitamin even in the face of adequate intake. Third, the bacteria can cause deconjugation of bile acids, permitting their passive reabsorption before fat digestion and absorption has been completed, and thus potentially resulting in malabsorption and steatorrhea (or fat in the stool). Finally, if the overgrowth is severe, the bacteria may evoke immune and inflammatory reactions in the affected loop, again resulting in intestinal dysfunction and a reduction in absorptive capacity.

Small bowel bacterial overgrowth can be diagnosed by orally administering a disaccharide that is not normally broken down by mammalian enzymes and monitoring the excretion of hydrogen in the breath. Lactulose is commonly used for this purpose. In a normal individual, the appearance of hydrogen in the breath will be delayed until the lactulose has entered the colon; this can also be used to estimate "transit time," or the time needed for the meal to move from the mouth to the end of the small intestine (around 2 hours, on average). In contrast, if there is overgrowth of anaerobic bacteria in the small intestine, hydrogen will be detected in the breath much earlier.

Inflammatory Bowel Diseases

The inflammatory bowel diseases, comprising Crohn's disease and ulcerative colitis, involve chronic inflammation of the bowel. Crohn's disease can occur in any segment of the gut from the mouth to the anus, whereas ulcerative colitis is confined to the colon. Current views of pathogenesis hold that the inflammatory reaction reflects an inappropriate immune response to the normally innocuous intestinal microbiota, likely as a result of genetically determined host defects in immune regulation. A vicious cycle then ensues, as damage to the epithelial barrier permits additional access of bacterial products into the lamina propria, further driving immunologic injury. In various animal models of colitis, inflammation does not occur if animals are raised under germ-free conditions, emphasizing the role of the normal flora in triggering and/or sustaining disease activity.

Inflammatory bowel diseases can have a number of physiologic consequences. Damage to the small intestinal epithelium in Crohn's disease can lead to maldigestion and malabsorption. If the disease process is localized to the terminal ileum, bile acid reabsorption will be impaired which can lead, in turn, to fat malabsorption and diarrhea resulting from the effect of bile acids on colonic electrolyte transport and patients with either Crohn's disease or ulcerative colitis commonly experience diarrhea as a result of the effect of immune and inflammatory mediators on intestinal transport, as well as defects in barrier function.

Current therapies for inflammatory bowel diseases target the excessive immune response, in the absence of a more definitive understanding of the cause of these diseases. Some treatments, as a consequence, have undesirable side effects due to their relative lack of specificity. This is particularly true for the use of systemic corticosteroids, which remain important in the treatment of very severe disease.

Food Allergy

In certain individuals, likely as a result of a genetic predisposition, the intestinal immune system inappropriately generates IgE antibodies to food proteins or other components of the diet, such as nucleic acids. These antibodies bind to mast cells that reside in the lamina propria, which are then said to be "sensitized." The sensitization process also results in upregulation of pathways that permit transfer of the offending protein across intestinal epithelial cells. The net result is that the next time the person eats the protein in question, it is transferred rapidly across the epithelium and cross-links IgE antibodies on the surface of mast cells causing cell activation and release of a host of potent chemical mediators. These mediators can increase intestinal chloride secretion and alter motility, which can be observed clinically as diarrhea. Stimulation of enteric nerve endings by mast cell mediators may further amplify these responses. In the seriously allergic subject, the antigen may also gain access to the circulation from which it can trigger reactions in extraintestinal sites, such as the skin and airways, or cause the generalized allergic reaction throughout the body known as systemic anaphylaxis. Food allergies can be life-threatening if they lead to responses such as laryngeal edema or severe hypotension.

Certain foods are more commonly seen as triggers of allergic responses, perhaps reflecting the relative stability of component proteins during the digestive process. Such foods include peanuts, eggs, certain fruits, and shellfish. Unless an individual is allergic to multiple foods, the best treatment for food allergy is to avoid the food in question, especially if very severe allergic reactions occur. However, it may not always be a simple matter to avoid a given food, particularly outside the home, and for this reason, those who are seriously affected by food allergies are usually advised to carry a self-injector containing epinephrine, which can counter serious symptoms, including bronchospasm. Studies are underway to determine whether seriously-allergic individuals can be desensitized to the offending antigen by specific regimens of oral immunotherapy.

Intestinal Infections

Despite the exquisitely specialized mucosal immune system, and the protection afforded by our resident microbiota, the large surface area of the gastrointestinal tract and its inherent need to allow selective uptake of substances from the lumen means that the gut remains vulnerable as a portal of entry for pathogenic microbes. In fact, diarrheal diseases caused by intestinal infections are second only to respiratory infections as a cause of infant mortality in developing countries.

Infectious agents use a variety of strategies to establish themselves in the intestine and cause disease. Some dwell strictly in the lumen, but may secrete products that alter the physiology of the intestine (e.g., cholera, as discussed in greater detail in the previous chapter). Others may invade the wall of the intestine, and may subsequently evoke intestinal transport, barrier, and motility dysfunction by virtue of the fact that they attract large numbers of inflammatory cells to the site of infection, as well as having direct effects on the epithelium and smooth muscle. Some of the most important infectious pathogens that lead to intestinal disease in humans are listed in Table 6–3. Overall, the most common symptoms evoked by gastrointestinal infections include diarrhea and associated pain, cramping, and bloating. The diarrheal response can in fact be considered a primitive host response, designed to flush the offending microorganism out of the lumen, and indeed many infectious diarrheal illnesses are acute and self-limited. However, particularly in vulnerable individuals, such as the very young, the elderly, and those who are immunocompromised, this "host defense" may come at the cost of severe dehydration and derangements in whole-body electrolyte status.

Given the role of the commensal microbiota in normally protecting the epithelium from colonization with pathogens, in recent years, the use of so-called "probiotics" to restore a healthy balance of the intestinal ecosystem has gained in popularity. Probiotics are preparations of live bacteria, some of which may exist normally as commensals, and these have been shown to have some efficacy not

Table 6–3. Selected important intestinal pathogens and their pathophysiologic mechanisms

Luminal (toxigenic) pathogens	Adherent pathogens	Invasive pathogens	Viral pathogens
V. cholerae	Giardia	Salmonella spp.	Rotavirus
Enterotoxigenic E. coli	Enteropathogenic E. coli	Shigella	Norwalk virus
	H. pylori	Campylobacter	
		Listeria	

only in reducing the symptoms of intestinal infections, but also in some inflammatory conditions of the intestine, such as the inflammatory bowel diseases discussed earlier. A related approach is to consume "prebiotics," foodstuffs that are believed to promote colonic colonization with beneficial bacteria by providing additional substrates for fermentation. We are far from a clear understanding of the mechanism of action of either probiotics or prebiotics, but their apparent efficacy in various digestive disorders does underscore the important role played by the intestinal ecosystem in promoting intestinal health and homeostasis.

KEY CONCEPTS

 The mucosal immune system is uniquely specialized to protect the vast interface between the host and environment represented by the GI tract.

 Mucosal immune responses are shared among several mucosal sites beyond the intestine.

 The intestine can be considered to be "physiologically inflamed," even in health, priming it to respond promptly to invaders.

 Secretory IgA provides important humoral protection against infections in the gut.

 Presentation of antigens via the oral route often leads to a response known as oral tolerance, where a local immune response exists in the face of systemic unresponsiveness.

 Oral tolerance may protect us from inappropriate reactions to food antigens. This response may also be exploited for therapeutic benefit in autoimmune diseases.

 The intestine maintains a life-long, reciprocally beneficial relationship with a complex microbiota that is predominantly contained in the colon.

 Colonic bacteria supply metabolic functions, especially fermentation, and contribute to intestinal gas production.

 Commensal bacteria may provide important protection against colonization by pathogens.

 Derangements in intestinal physiology occur when immune responses are inappropriately stimulated in the intestine, or when defenses fail to protect us from infection with pathogens.

6-1.   A scientist interested in gut ecology studies intestinal responses in germ-free mice. Compared with normally housed animals, what combination of findings would be expected in the colonic lumen?

	sIgA	Secondary bile acids	Short chain fatty acids
A.	Increased	Increased	Decreased
B.	Decreased	Decreased	Decreased
C.	Increased	Decreased	Increased
D.	Decreased	Increased	Increased
E.	Increased	Increased	Increased

6-2.   A biotechnology company attempts to develop an oral vaccine for use in developing countries by expressing a viral protein in transgenic bananas. However, clinical trials reveal that consumption of the bananas fails to confer protective immunity against the viral infection. What immune response likely accounts for this failure?

A. IgA secretion

B. Phagocytic uptake

C. Oral tolerance

D. T-cell sensitization

E. Toll-like receptor activation

6-3.   In a diagnostic test conducted in a patient with suspected Giardia infection, fecal samples are screened for the presence of antibodies reactive with giardial antigens. Assuming such antibodies are found, what is their likely class?

A. Monomeric IgG

B. Monomeric IgA

C. Dimeric IgA

D. Monomeric IgM

E. Pentameric IgM

6-4.   A patient with a severe chest infection is treated with a broad-spectrum antibiotic. Shortly after beginning this treatment, she develops severe diarrhea. Stool samples are most likely to reveal evidence of overgrowth with which of the following organisms?

A. Shigella dysenteriae

B. Vibrio cholerae

C. Lactobacillus acidophilus

D. Campylobacter jejuni

E. Clostridium difficile

6-5.   A scientist working to develop a new diagnostic test administers a solution of lactulose orally to a group of volunteers as well as to a patient with symptoms of malabsorption. She then measures the concentration of hydrogen in expired breath from each group. Hydrogen is present in negligible amounts in both groups prior to lactulose administration, and increases in the control group only after a 1–2 hour lag period. However, in the patient, breath hydrogen levels begin to rise almost immediately. What is the most likely cause of this more rapid appearance?

A.   Celiac disease

B.   Cystic fibrosis

C.   Crohn's disease

D.   Small bowel bacterial overgrowth

E.   H. pylori infection

SUGGESTED READINGS

Cominelli F, Arseneau KO, Blumberg RS, Stenson WF, Pizarro TT. The mucosal immune system and gastrointestinal inflammation. In: Yamada T, Alpers DH, Kalloo AN, Kaplowitz N, Owyang C, Powell DW, eds. *Textbook of Gastroenterology*. 5th ed. Chichester: Wiley-Blackwell; 2009:133–168.

Kau AL, Ahern PP, Griffin NW, Goodman AL, Gordon JI. Human nutrition, the gut microbiome and the immune system. *Nature*. 2011;474:327–336.

MacDonald TT, Monteleone G. Immunity, inflammation and allergy in the gut. *Science*. 2005;307: 1920–1925.

Pabst O, Mowat AM. Oral tolerance to food protein. *Mucosal Immunol*. 2012;5:232–239.

Sampson HA. Food allergy: when mucosal immunity goes wrong. *J Allergy Clin Immunol*. 2005;115: 139–141.

Suarez FL, Springfield J, Levitt MD. Identification of gases responsible for the odor of human flatus and evaluation of a device purported to reduce this odor. *Gut*. 1998;43:100–104.

Tarr PI, Bass DM, Hecht G. Bacterial, viral, and toxic causes of diarrhea, gastroenteritis, and anorectal infections. In: Yamada T. Alpers DH, Kalloo AN, Kaplowitz N, Owyang C, Powell DW, eds. *Textbook of Gastroenterology*. 5th ed. Chichester: Wiley Blackwell; 2009:1157–1224.

Esophageal Motility

7

OBJECTIVES

- ▶ *Describe the functional anatomy of the esophagus and related structures, and their innervation*
- ▶ *Understand the roles played by the oral cavity, pharyngeal structures, and esophagus in transferring food from the mouth to the stomach during swallowing*
  - ▶ Discuss how the contents of the respiratory and digestive systems are kept separate
  - ▶ Define the mechanisms and functions of primary and secondary esophageal peristalsis
- ▶ *Describe the roles played by the upper and lower esophageal sphincters in esophageal motility*
  - ▶ Understand how the relaxation of these structures is coordinated with the swallow
  - ▶ Describe how the lower esophageal sphincter protects against reflux of gastric contents
  - ▶ Understand how belching occurs
- ▶ *Discuss disease states in which esophageal motility and/or swallowing are abnormal*

BASIC PRINCIPLES OF ESOPHAGEAL MOTILITY

Role and Significance

The esophagus is a muscular tube that serves to transfer food from the mouth to the stomach. Under normal circumstances, food resides in the esophagus for only a few seconds and thus there is no time for it to be acted upon by any esophageal secretions. Thus, an understanding of the physiology of the esophagus relates primarily to its motility functions. In addition to moving the food along its length in the process of swallowing, the movements of the esophagus and related oral and pharyngeal structures must be carefully regulated to avoid misdirection of the food into the respiratory tract, or respired air into the digestive system. At rest, the esophagus is a relaxed structure that is closed off at both ends by sphincters—the upper and lower esophageal sphincters, respectively. These sphincters not only cooperate in the act of swallowing, or *deglutition*, but also prevent backflow of gastric contents into the esophageal lumen or oral cavity. However, under specific circumstances, the esophagus does allow for retrograde movement. This occurs normally for air swallowed with the meal, in the process of belching, or abnormally during vomiting. During retrograde movement in humans and most mammals, the esophagus itself is a passive conduit; that is, there are no specific motility functions that propel vomitus or air along the length of the tube. Note that the process of vomiting will be discussed in detail in Chapter 8.

The process of swallowing, as well as other esophageal motility functions, is under close regulatory control. Swallowing can be initiated voluntarily, but thereafter reflects an automatic reflex that involves, sequentially, impulses from the brainstem, processing of this information through vagal centers in the central nervous system, direct effects of parasympathetic vagal efferents on esophageal muscle layers, and relay of information via the enteric nervous system (Figure 7–1). Movement of materials along the length of the esophagus is aided by gravity, but predominantly depends on a coordinated series of muscle contractions and relaxations that make up the propulsive motility pattern known as *peristalsis*.

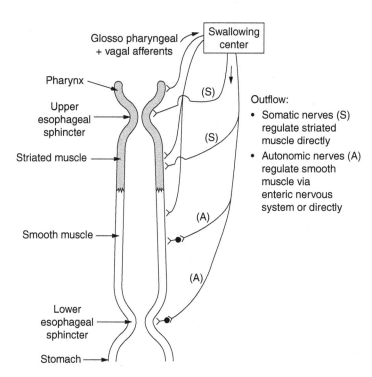

Figure 7–1. Functional anatomy and innervation of the esophagus. Note that the mode of innervation differs between the portions of the esophagus made up of smooth versus striated muscle.

FUNCTIONAL ANATOMY OF THE ESOPHAGEAL MUSCULATURE

Muscle Layers

The esophagus is a muscular tube, 18–25 cm long in adult humans, with its length varying with the total body height. Like the remainder of the gastrointestinal tract, it is surrounded by two muscle layers; the innermost (i.e., closest to the lumen) oriented in a circular fashion and the outer oriented longitudinally. However, unlike the exclusive occurrence of smooth muscle in all more distal segments of the gastrointestinal tract, the esophagus contains striated (or skeletal) muscle in its upper third, both striated and smooth muscle in its middle third, and exclusively smooth muscle in its most distal third. The distinction between muscle types also corresponds approximately to different types of neural control, as discussed later.

Other structures associated with the esophagus are important in swallowing and normal esophageal function. We have already mentioned the upper and lower esophageal sphincters, which are areas of specialized muscle that occlude both ends of the esophagus at rest. The esophagus is situated within the low-pressure thorax, and thus the presence of these sphincters is important to prevent the entry of air and gastric contents. The pharynx, which connects the nose and mouth to both the esophagus and trachea, is also critically involved in swallowing. The pharynx is traditionally divided into three regions—nasopharynx, oropharynx, and hypopharynx. The nasopharynx is not a part of the alimentary tract, but muscles in this structure contribute to swallowing by preventing the movement of the food bolus into the nasal passages. The oropharynx is responsible for propulsion of the food bolus backward into the esophagus. The hypopharynx, extending from the base of the tongue to the cricoid cartilage, contains the upper esophageal sphincter. In total, the pharynx is critically involved in segregating food and air as they pass through this region.

Innervation

The function of the pharynx is controlled by the central nervous system, via outflow from a region known as the central swallowing center (Figure 7–1). The pharynx thereby permits complex coordination of voluntary swallowing with other higher functions, such as respiration and speech. Central input also controls the contractile function of the upper one third of the esophagus, corresponding to the segment of the esophagus that consists of striated muscle. The somatic nerves that innervate these structures have motor end plates that terminate directly on the striated muscle fibers. They originate in brain regions known as the nucleus retrofacialis and the nucleus ambiguus. They release acetylcholine (ACh), which acts on the striated muscle cells via nicotinic receptors.

The smooth muscle of the esophagus is innervated predominantly by the vagus nerve. The vagal efferents synapse with myenteric neurons via ACh and with the smooth muscle directly via ACh and substance P (the former acting via muscarinic receptors). Sensory afferents located in the esophagus likewise project via the vagus to a brain region known as the nucleus tractus solitarius in the dorsal vagal complex. Cell bodies in this region also project to the motor neurons in the nucleus ambiguus, which control a pattern generator for the oral and pharyngeal components of swallowing. This neural circuitry ensures that control of the muscle groups involved in deglutition is linked to the function of more distal regions of the esophagus, as well as to the regulation of opening of the lower esophageal sphincter.

The esophagus is also richly supplied with enteric neurons. These clearly contribute to both sensing the presence and nature of esophageal contents, and coordinating local reflexes that supplement central control of swallowing and esophageal peristalsis. This network of enteric neurons can produce secondary peristalsis of the smooth muscle portion of the esophagus even in the absence of vagal input.

FEATURES OF ESOPHAGEAL MOTILITY

The motility functions consist sequentially of the movement of food from the mouth into the esophagus itself, propulsion along the length of the esophagus via the process of peristalsis, and relaxation of the lower esophageal sphincter to permit entry of the food bolus into the stomach. In health, these components of deglutition are tightly integrated, but for simplicity we will consider each in turn here.

Swallowing

Although the term swallowing can refer to the entire process required to move food from the mouth to stomach, here we will consider it to include only those motility events that move the bolus beyond the upper esophageal sphincter, as well as their regulatory controls. As noted earlier, swallowing is initiated when we sense that food particles in the mouth have been reduced in size sufficiently to permit their passage into the esophagus. While we consider this to be a voluntary response, during its course it in fact becomes an involuntary reflex involving significant input from a pattern-recognition center in the brainstem. This recognizes a food bolus as suitable for swallowing and generates the required neuromuscular response. However, it is possible to override this recognition system voluntarily, such as in the case of swallowing a pill or capsule. But in either case, the subsequent events that contribute to swallowing are entirely involuntary.

First, the tongue shapes and lubricates the bolus and moves it backward in the mouth. Subsequently, a rapid series of pharyngeal effects occur, initiated by mucosal mechanoreceptors in the pharynx that activate afferent nerves traveling through the glossopharyngeal nerve to the swallowing center. In turn, efferent motor nerves run through the vagi to control the contractile state of the pharyngeal muscles. The sequence of contractions that ensues has been observed in experimental subjects by fluoroscopic (X-ray image) analysis. Such studies have shown the events to occur almost simultaneously, which contrasts to the slower motility changes that occur more distally in the esophagus, as will be discussed later. First, the larynx and soft palate move upwards, closing off the airway and nasopharynx, respectively. Next, contraction of several muscles in the anterior portion of the pharynx causes forward displacement of the larynx and pharynx as well as helping to open the upper esophageal sphincter. Sphincter opening also depends on relaxation of the encircling cricopharyngeal muscle.

This is accomplished by a suppression of impulses normally occurring to this region, coordinated by the swallowing center via the nucleus ambiguus. Longitudinal contractions of the pharynx also bring the upper esophageal sphincter close to the base of the tongue, whereupon a pressure gradient developed by the tongue and pharyngeal muscles serve to force the bolus through the sphincter. Finally, the posterior wall of the pharynx contracts in a transverse fashion to clear the area of any remaining food residues. These transverse contractions are propagated aborally (i.e., in the direction away from the mouth) and can be considered the harbinger of the peristaltic wave that later will carry the bolus through the esophagus and down into the stomach. The sequence of events involved in normal swallowing is shown diagrammatically in Figure 7–2.

The nerves that innervate the muscular structures of the pharynx and upper esophageal sphincter release ACh, which causes muscle contraction via binding

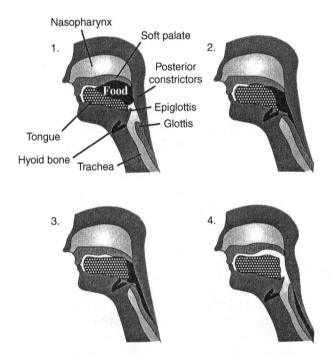

Figure 7–2. Stages involved in swallowing. 1. The tongue moves the bolus backward and the soft palate moves upwards to close off the nasopharynx. 2. The posterior tongue continues to move the bolus backward. 3. The upper pharyngeal muscle contracts at the posterior wall of the pharynx, forcing the bolus down into the pharyngeal channel away from the nasopharynx. The distal pharynx relaxes to receive the bolus, the upper esophageal sphincter relaxes, and the trachea is closed off by movement of the glottis. 4. As the bolus moves into the esophagus, the various structures return to their resting positions. (From Chang EB, Sitrin MD, Black DD. *Gastrointestinal, Hepatobiliary and Nutritional Physiology*. Philadelphia: Lippincott-Raven; 1996:37.)

to nicotinic receptors. Although these nerves accompany the vagus anatomically, functionally they are somatic motor nerves that terminate directly at motor end plates on the striated muscle of this region. This should be contrasted with the autonomic nerves that control the function of the smooth muscle in the more distal segment of the esophagus.

Peristalsis

Once the bolus has moved through the upper esophageal sphincter into the esophageal lumen, it is moved along the length of the tube via a series of coordinated muscular contractions and relaxations known as peristalsis (Figure 7–3). The sequencing and thus the direction of this propulsive

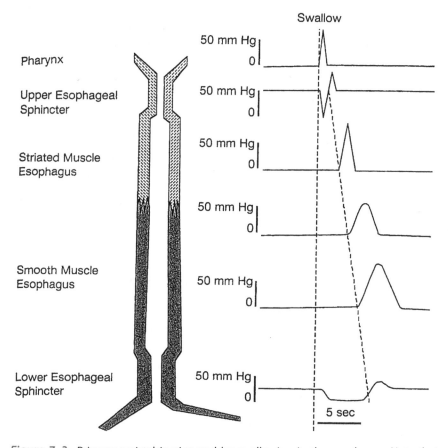

Figure 7–3. Primary peristalsis triggered by swallowing in the esophagus. Note that the pressure wave that moves down the esophagus is coordinated with opening of the lower esophageal sphincter. (Reprinted with permission from Biancani et al. Esophageal motor function. In: Yamada T, Alpers DH, Kaplowitz N, Laine L, Owyang C, Powell DW, eds. *Textbook of Gastroenterology.* 4th ed. Philadelphia: Lippincott Williams and Wilkins; 2003.)

process appears to be hardwired, with contraction of more distal segments occurring at longer latencies following the swallow than in those close to the pharynx. The striated muscle region contracts within 1–2 seconds after the swallow, the middle third of the esophagus within 3–5 seconds, and the lower third within 5–8 seconds. This means that the ability of the body to transfer food from the mouth to stomach is largely independent of body orientation—one can swallow food while hanging upside down, if one is so inspired! Nevertheless, gravity can be an important determinant of transit rate, particularly when liquids are ingested. Indeed, liquids may reach the lower esophageal sphincter before the peristaltic wave has reached this site, which is normally coordinated with its relaxation. The peristaltic wave requires up to 10 seconds, on an average, to sweep solid esophageal contents along its length. Peristalsis in the esophagus is stimulated by its distension. Mechanoreceptors on sensory afferents transmit impulses to the dorsal vagal complex, which in turn activates somatic and vagal efferents that terminate either directly on the striated muscle in the upper third of the esophagus, or onto nerves of the enteric nervous system, respectively. The latter activate enteric nerves capable of releasing ACh (to induce contraction) above the location of bolus-induced distension, or nitric oxide (to induce relaxation) below the bolus (Figure 7–4). The net effect of the sequential contractions and relaxations is to move the bolus aborally. The nature of the bolus also influences the intensity of the motility pattern. Thus, larger or more viscous boluses are propelled with greater force, but more slowly. Conversely, warm boluses are moved more rapidly than cold ones.

The primary wave of peristalsis along the length of the esophagus may also be followed by a secondary wave that is restricted to the smooth muscle portion (Figure 7–5). Secondary peristalsis is likely to be important in clearing a bolus that was not wholly expelled from the esophagus during the

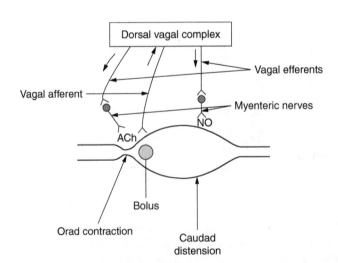

Figure 7–4. Control of peristalsis by vago-vagal reflexes in the lower esophagus. ACh, acetylcholine; NO, nitric oxide.

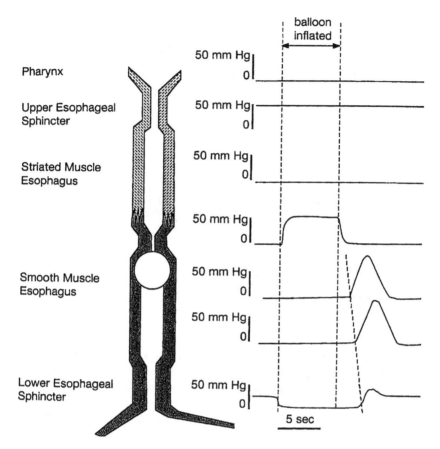

Pharynx

Upper Esophageal
Sphincter

Striated Muscle
Esophagus

Smooth Muscle
Esophagus

Lower Esophageal
Sphincter

Figure 7–5. Secondary peristalsis triggered by distention in the smooth muscle portion of the esophagus. Contraction orad to the bolus is followed by a descending pressure wave that is coordinated with lower esophageal sphincter opening. (From Biancani et al. Esophageal motor function. In: Yamada T, Alpers DH, Kaplowitz N, Laine L, Owyang C, Powell DW, eds. *Textbook of Gastroenterology.* 4th ed. Philadelphia: Lippincott Williams and Wilkins; 2003.)

primary wave, or in removing any gastric contents that reflux back into the lower esophagus. The peristaltic response is triggered by distension, and involves both local reflexes within the enteric nervous system as well as vago-vagal reflexes (Figure 7–6). Studies suggest that the presence of acid alone within the distal esophagus, in the absence of significant distension, may also be sufficient to generate a secondary peristaltic response, implying perhaps that chemosensitive afferents may also contribute.

 Movement of a bolus along the length of the intestine is also regulated by the rate of swallowing events occurring more proximally. In particular, if a second swallow occurs within about 5 seconds of the first, peristalsis is

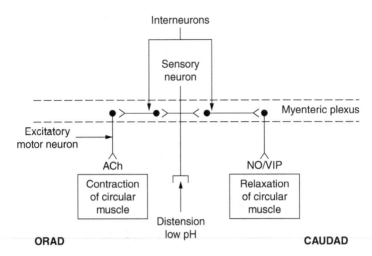

Figure 7–6. Control of peristalsis by the enteric nervous system. Peristalsis can be triggered when a sensory nerve detects distension or luminal acidity. Interneurons convey the signal to excitatory and inhibitory nerves above and below the site of stimulation, respectively. ACh, acetylcholine; NO, nitric oxide; VIP, vasoactive intestinal polypeptide.

inhibited such that both boluses can move in tandem. If a series of rapid swallows is taken, referred to as guzzling, peristalsis is inhibited until after the last swallow is taken. This avoids having the contraction that would normally occur above a bolus from interfering with the movement of the bolus immediately following. This response, known as deglutitive inhibition, is critical to the prowess of those who are successful in drinking competitions!

The esophagus also transmits information about its contents back to more proximal segments. Thus the presence of water, or more potently, acid in the esophagus can be shown to increase the pressure of the upper esophageal sphincter. The intensity of this stimulation increases as one moves closer to the upper part of the esophagus, and the reflex presumably represents a protective mechanism to restrict esophageal (or refluxed gastric) contents from returning to the pharynx from where they might otherwise be aspirated. This response depends, at least in part, on vago-vagal signaling. On the other hand, if air is present in the esophagus, it induces opening of the upper esophageal sphincter, which is critical to belching, or the retrograde movement of air that is swallowed along with food. Although both reflexes presumably involve activation of sensory afferents by distension, the mechanisms that allow for discrimination between air and liquid are unknown.

LES Relaxation

The final component of esophageal motility is relaxation of the lower esophageal sphincter, allowing the bolus to move into the stomach. Under resting conditions, the lower esophageal sphincter is tonically contracted. This tonic contraction involves, in part, a mechanism described as *myogenic*—that is to say, the contractile state of the muscle is independent of neural input, and increases intrinsically as it is stretched, apparently secondary to sustained increases in intracellular calcium. Moreover, the tone of the sphincter can also be increased by neurohumoral agents released in concert with ingestion of a meal, including ACh and gastrin. The extent of this effect is dependent on the composition of the meal, with proteins increasing sphincter tone to a greater extent than fat. This may relate, in turn, to differing extents of release of neurohumoral agents from more distal segments of the gastrointestinal tract in response to these two nutrients, or products of their digestion. Finally, LES pressure is substantially augmented by the crural diaphragm, which wraps around the esophagus. This also accounts for the increase in LES pressure during inspiration and coughing. Overall, the basal tone of the sphincter is critical in light of the positive pressure gradient from the abdomen to the thorax. It protects the lower portion of the esophagus from the corrosive effect of the gastric contents, especially those mediated by acid and pepsin, and particularly after gastric secretion is stimulated. The squamous epithelium lining the esophagus is much less able than the gastric epithelium to defend itself from these injurious substances.

When a food bolus is swallowed, relaxation of the lower esophageal sphincter is closely coordinated with the preceding motility events, such that it occurs just as the peristaltic wave reaches the end of the esophagus (Figures 7–3 and 7–5). The careful integration of peristalsis and sphincter relaxation is brought about by the combined activity of the vagus nerve and enteric nervous system, and is mediated by the release of nitric oxide from inhibitory nerves whose cell bodies lie in the myenteric plexus. There is evidence to suggest that vasoactive intestinal polypeptide (VIP) is also contained within these nerves, and that this peptidergic neurotransmitter also contributes to LES relaxation. In general, the contractile state of the lower esophageal sphincter at any given moment can be considered to reflect a summation of both positive and negative inputs. The movement of the food bolus through the sphincter is also facilitated by a pressure gradient. The peristaltic wave pushes the bolus distally whereas negative pressure in the gastric cavity also contributes to rapid movement through the sphincter.

Even in healthy individuals, the lower esophageal sphincter relaxes transiently from time to time in a manner that is independent of either swallowing or secondary peristalsis. These responses are triggered by gastric distension, which in turn activates vago-vagal pathways that reduce the tone of both the LES and the crural diaphragm via NO and CCK. Such relaxations facilitate belching of swallowed air, occur only during waking, and are more common when we are upright (which presumably protects against acid reflux to some extent). However, in individuals with reflux disease, these transient relaxations are more frequently associated with reflux of the gastric contents into the distal esophagus (see later).

PATHOPHYSIOLOGY AND CLINICAL CORRELATIONS

Dysphagia

Dysphagia refers to difficulty in swallowing, which can result from abnormalities in any of the components of the swallowing reflex or the anatomical structures involved. For example, abnormalities of the tongue can result in dysphagia because the bolus cannot be propelled backward toward the pharynx with sufficient force. In general, dysphagia can be considered as arising from either the oropharynx and striated muscle region of the esophagus, or the smooth muscle portion of the esophagus, corresponding to the different innervation and mechanisms of sensation and control in these two areas. Likewise, dysphagia can result from either structural or functional causes. Dysphagia is a common medical problem that is especially frequent in the elderly, and associated with much distress, as well as the risk of aspiration, choking, and malnutrition. It is estimated that up to 13% of hospitalized patients and as many as 60% of nursing-home residents have feeding problems, most of which are the result of oropharyngeal dysphagia. All patients with dysphagia will experience problems with solid food, and may have varying degrees of difficulty swallowing liquids as well, depending on the severity of the underlying cause.

Structural causes of dysphagia extend to diverticula (outpouchings of the pharyngeal or esophageal wall in which food can become trapped) or to various forms of obstruction. The latter include mucosal or muscular rings that circumferentially occlude a portion of the esophageal lumen. These are seen frequently in patients with a hiatal hernia, a condition where a portion of the stomach protrudes above the diaphragm. Ring-like strictures can also occur in response to long-standing tissue injury secondary to reflux disease (see below); the inflammation eventually leads to scarring and fibrosis that may occlude the lumen. Finally, esophageal tumors can also impede passage of esophageal contents.

Functional causes of dysphagia relate to either neurological control of the oropharyngeal phase of swallowing, peristalsis, and esophageal sphincter relaxation, or defects in the muscle layers themselves. Dysphagia is seen frequently after stroke, which may disrupt the exquisite coordination of contraction and relaxation of the pharyngeal structures needed to swallow without aspirating food particles. Other neurological disorders, including amyotrophic lateral sclerosis and Parkinson's disease may likewise alter the control of the pharyngeal region such that difficulties with swallowing ensue. Disorders at the level of the striated muscle of the pharynx and upper third of the esophagus have also been described, including myasthenia gravis, an autoimmune disease that attacks nicotinic ACh receptors at the neuromuscular junction.

Treatment of dysphagia depends on the underlying cause. When there are structural abnormalities, surgery to repair diverticula, cut overly tight muscles, or remove an obstructing tumor can often bring some relief. Mechanical dilatation of a strictured segment is also attempted, with varying degrees of success. In the case of functional disorders, on the other hand, effective therapy usually depends on whether treatment is available for the underlying disorder, and surgery is much less helpful.

A final cause of dysphagia relates not to esophageal motility function, but rather to a lack of salivary secretion in the mouth. The subjective feeling of mouth dryness is called *xerostomia*, and is covered in more detail in Chapter 4. This condition can lead to dysphagia because of a lack of the normal lubricating properties of saliva.

ACHALASIA

A special form of dysphagia is known as achalasia, which means "failure to relax." This condition occurs when the lower esophageal sphincter does not open fully in concert with the peristaltic wave that sweeps the bolus along the length of the esophagus, and thus food becomes retained at the level of the LES. The disorder has been recognized for more than 300 years, and is now known to reflect a chronic disorder in the functional innervation of the sphincter region. Histologic studies have revealed degeneration of nerve ganglion cells within the myenteric plexus of the enteric nervous system. The cause of this degeneration in most patients apparently results from an autoimmune attack, triggered after an initial insult in genetically-susceptible individuals. In regions where the disease is endemic, Chagas disease can also result in achalasia during its chronic phase, again as a result of selective destruction of the myenteric ganglia. However, in this latter case, other body systems are also affected, such as the heart, urinary, and respiratory tracts, and other segments of the gut itself.

A decrease in postganglionic neurotransmission in the sphincter region, secondary to ganglion destruction, could theoretically affect both contraction and relaxation of the lower esophageal sphincter. Recall that the tone of the LES is the net reflection of stimulatory and inhibitory neural inputs. Evidence for altered stimulatory input comes from studies where muscle strips obtained from patients with achalasia are examined in the laboratory. These can be shown to contract in response to ACh, but not in response to nicotine, underscoring the deficiency in postganglionic excitation. In fact, the lower esophageal sphincter of patients with achalasia may be hypersensitive to ACh at the level of the muscle itself, particularly if the disease is long-standing, which is an example of postdenervation supersensitivity. This heightened excitatory response forms the basis of a diagnostic test, where an ACh analogue is injected directly into the sphincter via an endoscope, resulting in a profound contraction. However, many patients retain at least some degree of postganglionic excitatory signaling, because LES pressure decreases on administration of atropine.

Considering deficiencies in inhibitory input to the LES, it is clear that impairment of the inhibitory ganglia occurs early in the disease process. These nerves are crucial for coordinating relaxation of the LES after the swallow, as well as the propagation of the esophageal peristaltic wave by producing a caudad relaxation ahead of the bolus. As we have discussed, these nerves use nitric oxide to produce their inhibitory effects. Patients with achalasia lack nitric oxide synthase, the enzyme responsible for production of nitric oxide, at the gastroesophageal junction, along with a decrease in the other inhibitory neurotransmitter, VIP.

The underlying cause of achalasia is a "wiring defect" and thus cannot be corrected. Therapy for this condition therefore focuses on symptomatic relief. Specifically, the goal is to reduce LES pressure, thereby allowing gravity to clear the esophagus. Forceful dilatation of the sphincter using balloons, or surgical myotomy, offers relief to many patients, but sometimes only at the cost of reflux disease. However, since reflux can usually be managed medically, this is a reasonable trade-off. Recently, endoscopic injection of botulinum toxin into the sphincter region has also gained favor as a treatment for achalasia. This toxin irreversibly inhibits the release of ACh from presynaptic terminals, effectively removing the major stimulus involved in sphincter tone. However, this effect will eventually be reversed by the growth of new axons, and so the effectiveness of the treatment wanes over time unless repeated toxin injections are administered.

Gastroesophageal Reflux Disease

One of the most frequent complaints that brings people to consult a gastroenterologist is the occurrence of heartburn, which is usually a symptomatic reflection of reflux of gastric contents into the distal esophagus. One needs only to watch television advertisements to gain an appreciation of the massive market for pharmaceutical and over-the-counter preparations for this disease. Gastroesophageal reflux disease, or GERD, is one of the commonest human ailments, and has a huge economic impact, although the majority of sufferers will never seek care from a physician. Likewise, it has been estimated that untreated GERD has a greater impact on a patient's quality of life than many other chronic diseases, including hypertension, mild heart failure, and angina. Finally, in addition to the distress of disease symptoms, chronic injury of the esophageal mucosa may ultimately cause a phenotypic change in the lining epithelial cells, known as Barrett's esophagus, which is recognized as a precancerous lesion.

It should be stressed that gastroesophageal reflux, *per se*, is not a disease, but a normal physiological process. Small volumes of gastric contents reflux into the esophagus many times per day, especially after large meals, but do not cause symptoms. Refluxed materials are rapidly cleared under normal circumstances by secondary esophageal peristalsis, and the acidity of the contents can also be neutralized by bicarbonate contained in swallowed saliva. In patients suffering from GERD, on the other hand, contact of the gastric contents with the esophageal mucosa is presumably prolonged, or they may regurgitate into the pharynx; in some individuals, the aggressive effects of the refluxed materials can lead to actual injury of the esophagus and perhaps later to more serious complications.

GERD results in intermittent symptoms in many patients, and may or may not result in inflammation of the esophagus (*esophagitis*) regardless of the severity of symptoms. This underscores the delicate balance that exists between aggressive and defensive factors in the distal esophagus. The aggressive factors include the aforementioned gastric contents, with acid and pepsin, or occasionally even effects of duodenal contents that include bile acids. Defensive factors include the anatomic barriers to reflux inherent in the lower esophageal sphincter and its surrounding (and supporting) muscles such as the diaphragm. Other defensive factors are mechanisms that promote acid clearance, and resistance of the tissue itself to the passage of protons and degradation by pepsin. GERD results when the balance between the aggressive and defensive factors is disrupted.

As we discussed earlier, the lower esophageal sphincter transiently relaxes at frequent intervals to permit belching, but in patients with GERD these relaxations apparently allow acid as well as gas to move in a retrograde fashion. The pressure developed in the LES may also be impaired by disease or inflammation affecting the cholinergic neurotransmission pathways that are responsible for LES tone. Under these conditions, pressure within the LES falls, and the sphincter may be "blown open" if there is an abrupt increase in intraabdominal pressure, such as may occur during bending or straining.

Some patients may also have defective esophageal clearance of refluxed materials. If peristalsis is sluggish, the refluxate may stay in contact with the esophageal mucosa for prolonged periods, and resulting inflammation can cause further injury to esophageal innervation, resulting in a vicious cycle. The failure to clear refluxed material also accounts for the fact that many patients report a worsening of reflux symptoms at night. When the patient is supine, gravity can no longer aid in bolus clearance. Compromised salivation, or the normal physiological decrease in salivation that occurs during sleep, can likewise reduce the ability to neutralize the refluxate.

Finally, GERD may be due to alterations in the resistance of the esophageal mucosa itself to injury. Normal individuals can withstand exposure to acid in the esophagus, sometimes for lengthy aggregate times during the day. However, the mucosa is protected by the combined effects of the squamous epithelium, which is 25–30 cells thick, local bicarbonate and mucus secretion, the ability of the epithelial cells to buffer and extrude protons, and subepithelial blood flow which can carry away protons and carbon dioxide to sustain tissue pH homeostasis. It is unclear at present whether defects in tissue resistance can be primary causes of GERD, but they certainly can contribute once injury has begun due to the other causes listed. GERD also reflects the impact of gastric factors, which will be discussed in more detail in the succeeding chapter.

The extent of reflux can be documented by ambulatory pH monitoring, usually over a 24 h period; a small pH probe is passed through the nose into the esophagus and relays pH information to a battery-powered data recorder worn by the patient. Therapy for patients with GERD centers mainly on the control of gastric secretion. Lifestyle modifications, such as eating smaller meals, avoiding evening snacks and alcohol, weight loss, and elevating the head of the bed are all helpful in mild disease. If symptoms are more severe, medical therapy is usually attempted. With new and potent acid-suppressive, proton pump inhibitors, patients can often become completely asymptomatic and the lack of acid secretion also provides time for the esophageal mucosa to heal. However, in some patients, GERD will be so severe that a surgical procedure known as a fundoplication is undertaken. This procedure has the goal of reinforcing the lower esophageal sphincter by folding a portion of the gastric fundus around the LES.

KEY CONCEPTS

 Together with the structures of the mouth and pharynx, the esophagus serves to move food from the oral cavity to the stomach.

 Regulation of swallowing involves somatic neurotransmission in the upper third of the esophagus, comprised of striated muscle, and autonomic regulation via the vagus and enteric nervous system in the lower two thirds, composed of smooth muscle. Swallowing is initiated voluntarily, but thereafter reflects a complex integration of regulatory influences coordinated by the swallowing center in the brain.

 Precise control of swallowing is important to segregate food and air in the pharynx.

 Two sphincters, normally closed, regulate the movement of the bolus into and out of the esophagus. The upper esophageal sphincter is opened in concert with pharyngeal motility. The lower esophageal sphincter opens to allow the bolus to enter the stomach, coordinated with esophageal motility.

 Solids are primarily moved along the esophagus by peristalsis; liquid movement is additionally assisted by gravity. Primary peristalsis sweeps the bolus along the length of the esophagus.

 Secondary peristalsis, initiated by distension, clears any remaining food or material refluxed from the stomach.

 Peristalsis is inhibited by a second swallow that rapidly follows the first.

 Upper esophageal sphincter tone is increased by the presence of liquid in the proximal esophagus.

 Distressing diseases states occur when swallowing and other aspects of esophageal motility are deranged. Dysphagia and achalasia result in an inability to swallow properly and/or to move food into the stomach.

GERD is a common disorder that relates to abnormal function of the lower esophageal sphincter.

STUDY QUESTIONS

7-1. A 30-year-old woman comes to the doctor's office complaining of progressively worsening difficulties with swallowing. A manometric study is conducted to examine pressure generation along the length of her esophagus. This test reveals that contractions in response to a swallow are poorly synchronized and pressure in the lower esophageal sphincter remains elevated. Production of which of the following neurotransmitters is likely to be reduced at the level of the lower esophageal sphincter?

A. Acetylcholine

B. Substance P

C. Norepinephrine

D. Nitric oxide

E. Gastrin releasing peptide

7-2. In the patient described in question 1, what is the most likely diagnosis?

A. Gastroesophageal reflux disease

B. Hiatal hernia

C. Achalasia

D. Esophageal cancer

E. Barrett's esophagus

7-3. In a study of the control of esophageal motility, a scientist instills a small amount of dilute hydrochloric acid into the upper third of the esophagus of a human volunteer, using an endoscope. This treatment is most likely to produce which of the following responses?

A. Peristalsis

B. Retroperistalsis

C. Esophageal spasm

D. Relaxation of the upper esophageal sphincter

E. No response

7-4. A bed-ridden, 90-year-old man in a nursing home is referred for endoscopy because of difficulty in swallowing that developed rapidly after he took his pain medication for arthritis the night before, when he was supine. The endoscopy reveals that the pill is lodged in the esophagus and has triggered an inflammatory response. Compared to the upright position, the reduction in which of the following influences on esophageal transit most likely contributed to the adverse outcome in this patient?

A. Primary peristalsis

B. Secondary peristalsis

C. Nucleus ambiguus activity

D. Pharyngeal contraction

E. Gravity

7–5.   A 50-year-old man who is markedly overweight comes to his primary care physician complaining that he suffers nightly from a burning sensation in his chest after retiring, which is made worse if he has had a snack close to bedtime. Which of the following would be the most appropriate treatment for this patient if his symptoms are not resolved by weight loss and eliminating night time meals?

A.   Cholinergic agonist

B.   Smooth muscle relaxant

C.   Nitric oxide donor

D.   Nicotinic agonist

E.   Proton pump inhibitor

SUGGESTED READINGS

Castell DO, Murray JA, Tutuian R, Orlando RC, Arnold R. Review article: the pathophysiology of gastroesophageal efflux disease—oesophageal manifestations. *Aliment Pharmacol Ther.* 2004; 20(suppl 9):14–25.

Gockel HR, Schumacher J, Gockel I, Lang H, Haaf T, Nothen MM. Achalasia: will genetic studies provide insights? *Hum Genet.* 2010;128:353–364.

Kahrilas P, Pandolfino JE. Esophageal motor function. In: Yamada T, Alpers DH, Kalloo AN, Kaplowitz N, Owyang C, Powell DW, eds. *Textbook of Gastroenterology.* 5th ed. Chichester: Wiley-Blackwell; 2009:187–206.

Mittal RK. Motor function of the pharynx, the esophagus, and its sphincters. In: Johnson LR, Ghishan FK, Kaunitz JD, Merchant JL, Said HM, Wood JD, eds. *Physiology of the Gastrointestinal Tract.* 5th ed. San Diego: Academic Press; 2012:919–950.

Mittal RK, Bhalla V. Oesophageal motor function and its disorders. *Gut.* 2004;53:1536–1542.

Gastric Motility

BASIC PRINCIPLES OF GASTRIC MOTILITY

Role and Significance

As we have learned from previous chapters, the stomach is a segment of the gastrointestinal tract in which important aspects of digestion and secretory function are initiated. However, in addition to these functions, which are largely dependent on gastric secretory function, the stomach also plays critical roles that depend on its motility properties.

First, the stomach can be considered as a homogenizer, mechanically breaking down ingested food into an emulsion of small particles with a vastly increased total surface area, thereby amplifying the effects of digestion. Second, the stomach is a critical contributor to the matching of food delivery to the digestive and absorptive capacity of more distal segments of the gut. Under normal circumstances, the stomach allows the delivery of approximately 200 kcal/h into the small intestine, although this may vary somewhat depending on the physical form of the meal (solid vs. liquids) and the nutrient(s) of which it is comprised, as will be described further. The stomach thus serves as a reservoir, allowing food particles to move only slowly into the duodenum to maximize their chances for assimilation. To accomplish this function, the stomach exhibits remarkable pressure/volume characteristics, which are vital in accommodating the volume of the meal without allowing significant reflux of the gastric contents back into the esophagus, or forcing them prematurely into the duodenum. Distention of the stomach also delivers important information to downstream segments of the gastrointestinal tract, as well as contributing to the signaling of satiety. These latter features likely underlie the effectiveness of gastric-reduction surgery for the treatment of morbid obesity, since the small remaining stomach reservoir only allows the patient to take small meals comfortably.

Finally, the stomach possesses distinct motility functions during the fasted state. Most importantly, it has developed mechanisms whereby ingested solids that cannot be digested or mechanically dispersed can be expelled from the stomach under normal conditions. This can be considered a "housekeeping" function, which sweeps undigested materials or ingested foreign objects along the length of the entire gastrointestinal tract, beginning at the stomach. This housekeeping function, mediated by a specific motility pattern known as the *migrating motor complex* or *MMC*, accounts for the fact that coins or similar objects that are swallowed by small children will eventually be passed in the feces.

FUNCTIONAL ANATOMY OF THE GASTRIC MUSCULATURE

From a motility standpoint, the stomach is a muscular sac with the largest caliber of any intestinal segment. It is a particularly distensible organ, and its ability to increase its volume is also enhanced by the fact that its distension is not highly constrained by adjacent organs, which can be contrasted with the more densely packed organs surrounding more distal segments of the gastrointestinal system. The stomach can also be divided into two functional regions for considerations of motility (Figure 8–1). The proximal stomach, consisting of the cardia, fundus,

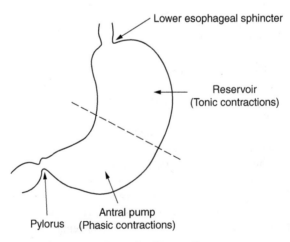

Figure 8–1. Regions of the stomach involved in motility responses.

and proximal portion of the body (corpus) of the stomach, serves primarily as a reservoir and to move gastric contents to the distal stomach. Tonic contractions of the proximal stomach are additionally important in gastric emptying. The distal stomach, on the other hand, consisting of the distal portion of the body and the antrum, serves predominantly to grind and triturate the meal. Finally, the *pylorus* acts as a sphincter that controls the amount and size of food particles that can exit the stomach in the fed state. Conversely, full relaxation of the pylorus is critical during the housekeeping MMC.

Muscle Layers

As elsewhere in the gastrointestinal tract, the muscle layers of the stomach consist of a circular layer of smooth muscle arranged circumferentially, and closer to the lumen, and a longitudinal layer that is oriented along the length of the organ. However, because the stomach is shaped as a sac rather than a simple tube, these different muscle layers may assume greater or lesser importance in the different functional regions of the stomach, likely also important for specific motility patterns. Thus, circular muscle is prominent throughout the stomach, although it is notable that it is largely electrically isolated from the circular muscle in the small intestine because of the presence of a connective tissue septum at the level of the pylorus. On the other hand, longitudinal muscle is more prominent in the distal stomach, and these muscle fibers are mostly continuous with those of the duodenum. There is also a small region of obliquely oriented muscle fibers in the lesser curvature of the stomach that is continuous with the gastroesophageal junction, and restricted to the cardia. Finally, the pylorus represents a specialized region of circular muscle at the point where the caliber of the gastric lumen is sharply reduced prior to entry into the duodenum; it serves as a mechanical barrier to food exit that is also enhanced by a folded, redundant mucosa.

The smooth muscle cells of the different functional regions of the stomach also display distinctive contractile properties, which are intrinsic to these cells (myogenic properties) and independent of either neural or humoral input. Most important for our discussion is the distinction between phasic and tonic contractions. Some smooth muscles contract and then relax in a matter of seconds, known as phasic contractions, which are prominent in the distal stomach. Tonic contractions, on the other hand, are sustained contractions that are prominent in the proximal stomach, and may persist for many minutes. Each type of contraction is important in mediating the specific motility properties that are needed for the function of each region of the stomach.

Innervation

The stomach is richly endowed with both intrinsic and extrinsic neural inputs. The major extrinsic pathways for regulation of gastric motility are parasympathetic in nature, and are contained within the vagus nerve. Most vagal efferents that terminate in the stomach are stimulatory, cholinergic nerves although a few nerves with high thresholds for activation are inhibitory, releasing vasoactive intestinal polypeptide (VIP) and nitric oxide as their major neurotransmitters. Vagal afferents are also critical for the control of motility functions. These are of both mechano- and chemosensitive types, and activate sites in the nucleus tractus solitarius of the dorsal motor nucleus in the brain. In a more limited fashion, sympathetic innervation arrives at the stomach by way of the splanchnic nerve, and these nerves release noradrenaline as a postganglionic inhibitory neurotransmitter at the level of enteric ganglia. The physiological role of sympathetic innervation to the stomach in producing the motility patterns that characterize the response to a meal is minor compared to vagal influences. On the other hand, sympathetic influences may contribute importantly to a decrease in gastric motility during times of threat.

Intrinsic innervation via the enteric nervous system is also critically important to the full expression of gastric motility responses. Indeed, many of the stereotypical motility responses of the stomach are largely, if not wholly, independent of central input. Myenteric neurons of the stomach also provide for coordination of gastric motility functions with those of the more distal segments of the gut, particularly during fasting periods. These nerves also communicate with the pacemaker cells of the intestine, known as *interstitial cells of Cajal*, located within the circular muscle layers of the stomach and proximal gut. This communication establishes the rate at which contractions of the tissue can maximally occur if an additional excitatory signal is also received, which is known as the *basal electrical rhythm*, or *BER*.

FEATURES OF GASTRIC MOTILITY

Basal Electric Rhythm

The BER refers to waves of rhythmic depolarization of intestinal smooth muscle cells, which originate at a specific point and then are propagated along the length of the gastrointestinal tract. The pacemaker potentials originating at this point determine the contractile parameters of the stomach as a whole—namely the maximal frequency of contractions, their propagation velocity, and the direction in which they propagate. For the stomach specifically, the waves appear to begin at a point in the body along the greater curvature of the stomach, and then sweep across the stomach toward the pylorus (Figure 8–2). It should also be emphasized that the BER represents only the maximal rate of contraction of the stomach or indeed of any other segment of the gastrointestinal tract. The waves of depolarization that occur in response to the pacemaker activity of the network of interstitial cells of Cajal are not of sufficient magnitude to initiate action potentials in the smooth muscle. Rather, it is only when the release of stimulatory neurotransmitters from enteric nerve endings is superimposed on these waves of depolarization that the threshold for contraction of the smooth muscle will be reached (Figure 8–3). The BER differs in the various intestinal segments. For example, in the stomach the BER is approximately 3 cycles per minute (cpm), whereas the duodenum has a BER of 12 cpm. This presumably reflects the presence of dominant and separate pacemakers in each distinct segment, which then relay electrical

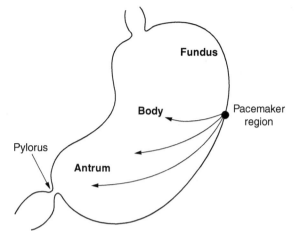

Figure 8–2. Location of the gastric pacemaker.

information throughout the segment that they control via the corresponding network of interstitial cells of Cajal.

Receptive Relaxation

The ability of the stomach to relax as its volume increases is essential to its reservoir function. The process by which this occurs is referred to as *receptive relaxation*, and results in a drop in gastric pressure immediately after eating that persists until all solids have been emptied from the stomach. Some further divide this response into two phases—true receptive relaxation, which is a response that occurs coincident with swallowing, and *accommodation*, a relaxation of the stomach that is mediated by gastric mechanoreceptors that are

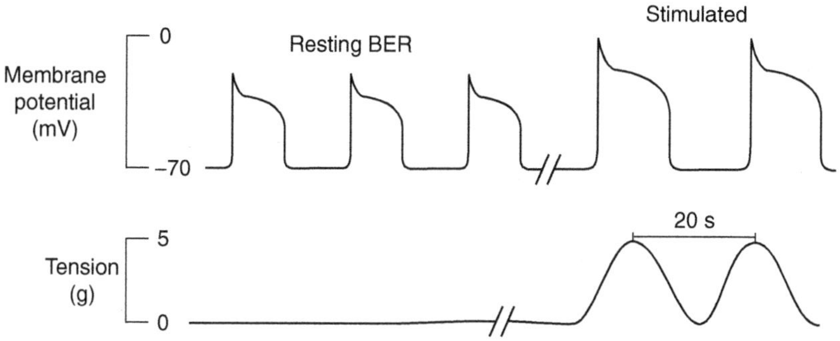

Figure 8–3. Basal electrical rhythm established by the gastric pacemaker. Note that waves of depolarization initiated by the pacemaker are insufficient to trigger contractions unless these are superimposed with a contractile stimulus.

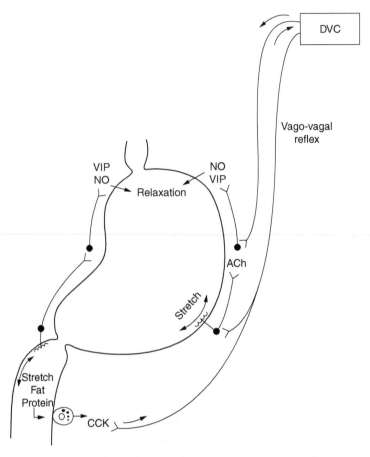

Figure 8–4. Intrinsic and vago-vagal reflexes involved in receptive relaxation of the stomach. The figure indicates that signals triggered by nutrients in the duodenal lumen, or duodenal distension, also result in relaxation of the gastric fundus. ACh, acetylcholine; NO, nitric oxide; VIP, vasoactive intestinal polypeptide; CCK, cholecystokinin; DVC, dorsal vagal complex.

activated as the wall of the stomach is stretched by the entry of the meal. For our purposes, however, the overall process can be considered as a single, integrated response, which involves vagal input coincident with food intake, vago-vagal reflexes, and intrinsic reflexes mediated wholly within the wall of the stomach (Figure 8–4). Vago-vagal and intrinsic reflexes are triggered by the activation of mechanosensitive nerve endings within the stomach wall. In turn, acetylcholine (ACh) released by vagal pathways acts presynaptically to release additional neurotransmitters that actively relax the gastric smooth muscle layers, particularly in the proximal part of the stomach. Both VIP and nitric oxide have been implicated in this response, although other mediators may also be involved.

Gastric tone may also be affected by feedback signals coming from more distal segments of the gastrointestinal tract. For example, distension of the duodenum results in a decrease in the tone of the gastric fundus. Similar reflexes are triggered if the concentration of acid, fat, or protein rises in the duodenal lumen. In this way, gastric emptying is retarded until the duodenum is able to process additional nutrients. Colonic distension also causes relaxation of the stomach as does perfusion of glucose or fat into the ileum. This latter response has been referred to as the "ileal brake," and serves a physiologic function in that it reports that the absorptive capacity of the proximal small intestine has been exceeded, to which an appropriate response again is to retard the release of nutrients from the stomach. In addition to reflexes mediated by the enteric nervous system to produce these gastric motility patterns, retrograde signaling of the type described has also been attributed to CCK. As we have seen previously, CCK is a major hormonal mediator during the intestinal phase of the response to a meal. In altering gastric motility, this hormone most likely acts by binding to CCK_1 receptors expressed on vagal sensory afferents.

Gastric distension, conversely, signals forward to more distal segments to ready them for the arrival of the meal. Probably the best known of these reflexes is the gastrocolic reflex, which may induce the need to defecate shortly after ingesting a meal. In a similar fashion, the gastroileal reflex allows the ileocecal valve to relax in response to gastric distension. Simultaneously, peristalsis is stimulated in the ileum. This reflex therefore allows the ileum to empty any remaining contents into the colon to prepare it to receive the incoming meal. The relative contribution of neurotransmission via the enteric nervous system and humoral factors in producing these reflexes is still a matter of some debate among investigators of intestinal motility.

Mixing and Grinding

The primary motility pattern of the distal portion of the stomach during the fed state consists of rapid phasic contractions that occur circumferentially, and which can even occlude the lumen (Figure 8–5). The rate of these contractions depends on the gastric basal electrical rhythm, and they occur when the release of contractile agonists is superimposed on this rhythm, thereby increasing the magnitude and duration of individual contractions. The contractions proceed from the gastric pacemaker region and move toward the pylorus in a peristaltic pattern. As these waves of contraction begin, they force the gastric contents toward the outlet of the stomach. However, as the velocity of the peristaltic wave increases, it overtakes all but the smallest particles in the gastric lumen, and thus the majority of the meal is forced back toward the body of the stomach. The net result of this backward movement, which has been called *retropulsion*, is to mix the gastric contents thoroughly with the gastric juices and to mechanically reduce the size of the food particles. Mechanical dispersion of the meal is also promoted by impelling the smaller particles against a largely closed pylorus, causing them to be acted on by shear forces. In effect, the stomach acts as a sieve as

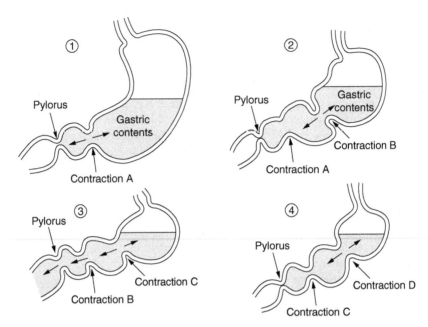

Figure 8–5. Gastric motility patterns contributing to mixing, grinding, and sieving of gastric contents. 1. A circumferential contraction, A, sweeps toward the pylorus resulting in anterograde and retrograde propulsion of material. 2. As contraction A subsides, a second contraction, B, mixes contents further. 3. Contraction B is sufficient to cause transient and partial opening of the pylorus, allowing particles smaller than 1 mm to exit the stomach. Larger particles are propelled back into the stomach to be further dispersed by contraction C. 4. Further cycles of contraction against a closed pylorus continue mixing and grinding until all of the meal is emptied from the stomach.

well as a homogenizer, gradually moving small particles of food closest to the stomach outlet while retaining those that need to be reduced further.

The neurohumoral mediators of the fed pattern of motility in the distal stomach are not fully understood. A vagal component is apparent, in that vagotomy decreases phasic contractions in this region whereas stimulation of the vagal nerve increases them. Distension of the proximal stomach may trigger intramural reflexes that increase motility, such as a fundoantral reflex. A circulating mediator that contributes to the regulation of distal gastric motility has also been suggested, but its identity is not yet known.

Gastric Emptying and the Role of the Pylorus

 When the stomach is filled with a meal, the pylorus remains closed for prolonged periods with only intermittent openings that allow small food particles to enter the duodenum. During the fed state, the pylorus never relaxes completely, and thus exhibits enhanced sieving properties. While the meal is in the stomach, particles larger than 1–2 mm are held within the stomach, which has implications for the delivery of medications in the form of enteric coated pills, which are designed not to dissolve at the acidic pH of the gastric lumen. The pylorus is regulated by both inhibitory and excitatory vagal pathways as well as ascending and descending intrinsic reflexes, and its function is clearly regulated independently of contractions of the gut segments on either side. Nitric oxide has been identified as a key mediator of pyloric relaxation, arising from both vagal and intrinsic pathways, whereas opioids released from vagal efferents have been implicated in contractions. CCK may also increase contractile function of the pylorus in the postprandial period. Feedback reflexes from the duodenum also contribute to pyloric closure. Specifically, the presence of nutrients, hypertonicity or acid in the duodenum causes the pylorus to close, with acetylcholine and 5-hydroxytryptamine identified as mediators.

Actual emptying of the stomach involves both the primary contribution of tonic contractions of the proximal region and phasic distal contractions, which serve as a pump. Extrinsic innervation, working together with the enteric nervous system, is vital for normal emptying, with 5-hydroxytryptamine being identified as a key mediator. $5HT_1$ receptors have been implicated in delaying gastric emptying while $5HT_3$ receptors increase it. Evidence also exists for humoral control. Specifically, a physiological role for CCK in delaying gastric emptying has been proposed on the basis of observations that emptying of mixed meals is accelerated by antagonists of this hormone. Overall, knowledge related to the control of gastric emptying may lead to therapeutic approaches when this process is abnormal, as discussed later. The rate of gastric emptying also depends on both the physical state of the contents as well as their chemical characteristics (Figure 8–6). Inert liquids empty most rapidly from the stomach, according to first-order

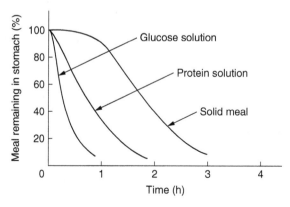

Figure 8–6. Gastric emptying depends on the nature of the gastric contents. Note that emptying of a solid meal does not begin immediately, but only after a lag of approximately 1 hour.

kinetics. However, this pattern is altered if the liquid contains nutrients. A rapid initial phase is then followed by slowed exit, apparently reflecting feedback from the small intestine. Overall, the rate of emptying depends on caloric density of the contents. Their osmolarity also acts independently to slow emptying, via a reflex involving intestinal osmoreceptors as well as vagal input.

Emptying of solids from the stomach is slower yet, with a half time of approximately 1–2 hours. Moreover, emptying of solids from the stomach does not begin immediately, but occurs only after a lag phase of up to 1 hour during which retropulsion and mixing take place. This lag phase is increased in duration if large particles are swallowed whole. After the lag phase, a linear phase of emptying of a particulate suspension occurs at a relatively constant rate, with the size exclusions discussed earlier. The ability of the stomach to deliver only small particles to the small intestine is nutritionally significant. If this size discrimination is lost, it takes longer to digest and absorb the meal constituents in the small intestine, and the anatomic reserve may need to be called into play to fully assimilate such nutrients. The motility functions associated with gastric emptying are also notable in that the organ can distinguish between the liquid and solid phases of the meal, and empty the former more rapidly.

Fatty meals are handled somewhat differently than the mixed meals discussed earlier. While dietary fats are converted to liquid form at body temperature, these are emptied more slowly than would be the case for aqueous solutions. Retention of lipids in the stomach for a prolonged period likely improves their emulsification due to the mixing properties of the stomach, and thus their ultimate digestion and absorption. The slowed emptying of lipids likely results from several factors. First, fats float on top of the other stomach contents due to their lower density, and can coalesce in large globules or adsorb to solid particles due to their poor aqueous solubility. Second, lipids potently activate enterogastric reflexes to diminish propulsive motility, such that any lipid that does manage to leave the stomach will markedly decrease emptying of the remainder, via the release of CCK and activation of the enteric nervous system. For these reasons, patients who have diminished gastric emptying due to disease are advised to avoid very fatty meals (more details of this later).

Gastric Motility During Fasting

In the period in between meals, the stomach, in common with more distal segments of the gastrointestinal tract, undergoes the stereotypical pattern of motility known as the migrating motor complex (MMC). In the absence of feeding, cycles of motility lasting approximately 100 minutes, and consisting of three phases, begin in the stomach and are propagated aborally (Figure 8–7). Phase I comprises 40–60% of the cycle, and is characterized by quiescence. During phase II, contractile activity increases, but the contractions are irregular and fail to propel luminal contents. This phase comprises 20–30% of the overall cycle. Finally, phase III involves a 5–10 minute period of intense, luminally occlusive contractions that sweep from the body of the stomach to

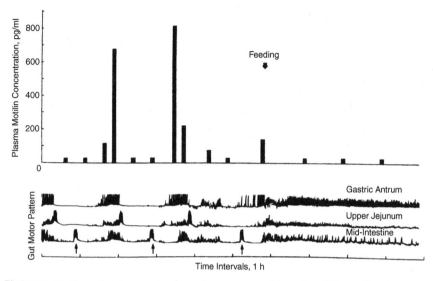

Figure 8–7. The migrating motor complex as assessed in a dog, followed by the motility pattern in the fed state. Each antral phase III complex is accompanied by an increase in plasma motilin, whereas motilin release is suppressed after feeding. (From Hasler WL. Physiology of gastric motility and gastric emptying. In: Yamada T, Alpers DH, Kaplowitz N, Laine L, Owyang C, Powell DW, eds. *Textbook of Gastroenterology*. 4th ed. Philadelphia: Lippincott Williams and Wilkins; 2003.)

the pylorus, and from there move into the duodenum. During this time, the pylorus opens fully in normal subjects, allowing any indigestible residues that remain in the stomach to be cleared from the lumen. This housekeeping function is important for intestinal health, since in its absence, large quantities of indigestible materials may accumulate and even obstruct the lumen, particularly in the stomach. Such aggregations are known as *bezoars*. Following phase III, the stomach and intestine return to quiescence, and continue to cycle until a meal is taken.

Neurohumoral control of the MMC is incompletely understood, but some aspects are known. For example, a phase III activity persists following transection of both the vagal and splanchnic nerves, indicating that it is independent of either parasympathetic or sympathetic input. Instead, the onset of phase III activity is correlated with levels of plasma motilin (Figure 8–7). However, the trigger for cyclical release of this hormone into the bloodstream from its site of production in the duodenal mucosa is not known, other than the fact that release is suppressed by feeding. Nevertheless, it enhances propulsive motility via both direct and indirect actions, the latter involving the release of ACh, 5-hydroxytryptamine, and nitric oxide. Moreover, while phase III can occur in the absence of vagal input, impulses from the vagus can amplify the response. Similarly, phase II of the MMC is abolished by vagotomy. Central input to the regulation of the MMC is more generally apparent from the fact that its intensity is subject to diurnal variation, with reduced activity during sleep, and also by the fact that stress slows MMC cycling via the release of CRF centrally and associated activation of a cholinergic vagal pathway.

PATHOPHYSIOLOGY AND CLINICAL CORRELATES

 Several disease states result in alterations in gastric motility and/or emptying. Gastric function may also be altered iatrogenically, via the undesired actions of a variety of medications.

Pyloric Stenosis

Hypertrophic pyloric stenosis is a congenital condition usually presenting in infancy. It is more common in boys than girls, with one in 150 births of boys resulting in an infant with the disease. The pylorus fails to relax appropriately after a meal, leading to regurgitation and nonbilious projectile vomiting. Infants also develop malnutrition and dehydration due to inadequate delivery of nutrients and fluids to the absorptive small intestine, and, in severe cases, oliguria and electrolyte imbalances. Constipation is also seen. The definitive therapy for this condition is surgical myotomy, making a longitudinal incision into the muscles surrounding the pyloric region. In fact, surgical treatment of pyloric stenosis is the most common cause of surgery in the first 6 months of life. The condition can be compared with achalasia, the failure of the lower esophageal sphincter to relax, which we discussed in the previous chapter. Likewise, the pathogenesis of pyloric stenosis may also relate to the absence of inhibitory influences to the pylorus, and perhaps to inadequate generation of nitric oxide at this site. Indeed, genetic contributors to disease pathogenesis, such as mutations in nitric oxide synthase and mechanosensitive ion channels, are beginning to be understood. Occasionally, adults may present with symptoms of pyloric stenosis. Sometimes this reflects recurrence of congenital disease first suffered in infancy. However, pyloric dysfunction may also be a complication of inflammation and scarring due to gastric ulcer disease, or secondary to a gastric tumor.

Gastroparesis

Gastroparesis refers to a collection of disorders of varied etiologies in which gastric emptying is impaired or delayed, yet without evidence of obstruction. The symptoms of the disorder include early satiety, nausea, vomiting, bloating, and upper abdominal discomfort. A typical pattern is for patients to exhibit late postprandial vomiting of undigested or only partially digested food. Usually, there is a more profound effect on the emptying of solid meals and patients can tolerate liquid feeding quite well.

Gastroparesis may arise for several different reasons. While idiopathic gastroparesis is more common, the disorder may also result from a systemic disease resulting in abnormalities of neuromuscular function, such as diabetes or scleroderma.

It may also occur as a result of either surgical or medical treatments. For example, surgery that injures the vagus will impair gastric emptying since extrinsic input to the stomach is needed to mediate the full expression of this response. Likewise, several medications (typically anticholinergics and opiates) are known to impair gastric emptying.

Clinically, perhaps the most challenging form of gastroparesis is that experienced by patients with long-standing diabetes mellitus. The gastric dysfunction is usually a reflection of a more generalized neuropathy in these patients, but may aggravate their underlying disease. For example, because the delivery of nutrients to the duodenum is unpredictable, this has implications for the ability of the subject to maintain glycemic control. Hyperglycemia *per se* may also exert effects on gastric motility, either directly or via effects on the vagus nerve. Indeed, gastric emptying can be reduced by infusion of glucose, fatty acids, or amino acids parenterally.

The management of gastroparesis rests on an understanding of the physiology of gastric emptying. Patients are encouraged to take small meals, and to increase the proportion of their nutrients supplied by liquids, which can empty rapidly from the stomach. Low fat diets are also recommended, to avoid a large increase in CCK that would feedback to inhibit emptying still further. Some prokinetic medications that increase the motility of the stomach are also available.

Vomiting

Vomiting, while not a disorder of gastric motility *per se*, is nevertheless considered here because it results primarily in evacuation of the gastric contents. Vomiting reflects the coordinated interaction of neural, humoral, and muscular phenomena. Vomiting may be prompted by both central and peripheral triggers (Figure 8–8), but pivotally requires the involvement of central brain regions to coordinate the responses required. A chemoreceptor trigger zone, located in the area postrema of the medulla, receives input from cortical, oral, vestibular, and peripheral afferents. In addition, the blood–brain barrier in this region is relatively leaky. This means that the chemoreceptor trigger zone can sample chemical constituents of both the blood and cerebrospinal fluid. Various stimuli can lead to both nausea (the sensation that vomiting is imminent) and actual vomiting. Thus nausea and vomiting that occur secondary to endocrine causes, such as experienced in early pregnancy, are likely to be central in origin, as is vomiting provoked by noxious odors, visual stimuli, somatic pain, or unpleasant tastes. Peripheral afferents can also trigger a vomiting response. This is especially the case when irritants are present in the gastric lumen, and some vagal afferents originating in the stomach and presumably linked to chemoreceptors project to the area postrema. Nausea also results in signals to the salivary glands to increase secretion; the bicarbonate thereby produced may serve in part to protect the esophagus from the injurious effect of gastric contents.

A second brain region, the nucleus tractus solitarius, also contributes to the emetic cascade, particularly following vagal activation (Figure 8–8). This region

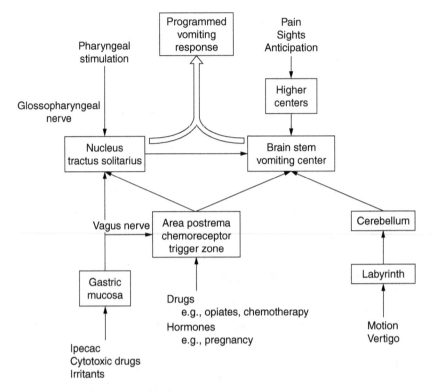

Figure 8-8. Neural pathways leading to the initiation of vomiting in response to various stimuli.

receives inputs from the area postrema, abdominal vagus, and labyrinths, and in turn coordinates the motor responses required. Emesis results from a stereotypical program of somatic muscle actions. First, the thoracic, diaphragmatic, and abdominal muscles contract concurrently against a closed glottis, resulting in the phenomenon of retching. The LES and crural diaphragm relax, and the high positive intraabdominal pressure forces the gastric contents into the esophagus. The brain then coordinates the synchronous contraction of inspiratory and expiratory muscles, resulting in a reversal of the thoracic pressure gradient. This high positive thoracic pressure acts in turn to drive expulsion of the vomitus. Simultaneously, respiration is suppressed and movement of laryngeal and pharyngeal structures prevents aspiration and, usually, passage of vomitus into the nasal cavity.

Intestinal motility is also regulated during vomiting. The BER is suspended and replaced by bursts of electrical activity that propagate orally. These result in a motility pattern referred to as a retrograde giant contraction, or the retroperistaltic contractile complex, that moves the gastric contents up and out of the esophagus. Despite the autonomy of the enteric nervous system in producing normal patterns of gastric and esophageal motility, the retrograde propulsion seen during

Table 8–1. Important causes of nausea and vomiting

Medications	GI disorders	CNS causes	Endocrine	Infections
Cancer chemotherapy	Mechanical obstruction	Increased intracranial pressure	Pregnancy	Viral/bacterial gastroenteritis
Analgesics	Gastroparesis	Emotional responses	Uremia	
Antibiotics	Radiation injury	Psychiatric conditions	Diabetic ketoacidosis	
Narcotics	Functional bowel disorders	Tumors		
	Intraperitoneal inflammation	Labyrinthine disorders		

emesis is entirely dependent on input from extrinsic nerves, coordinated by the brain centers that also regulate the functions of somatic muscles that support vomiting, as described earlier.

Vomiting can be a symptom of a vast number of diseases and iatrogenic conditions. Some of the causes of nausea and vomiting are summarized under various categories in Table 8–1. Motility disorders themselves, such as those we have discussed earlier, may be accompanied by vomiting, particularly if there is an element of functional obstruction, such as in pyloric stenosis. In fact, distension of all segments of the gastrointestinal tract, or the presence of irritant substances, can trigger the emetic cascade. In addition to being distressing for patients, vomiting can also have serious systemic consequences if it is intractable or involves large volumes. Significant fluid and electrolyte loss may result in dehydration and both electrolyte and acid–base imbalances, which may manifest as postural lightheadedness, a rapid heart rate, and a dry mouth.

KEY CONCEPTS

The stomach serves to receive the meal from the esophagus, and it displays motility functions that both initiate the process of digestion and control the delivery of nutrients to more distal segments.

Receptive relaxation of the proximal stomach allows the stomach to function as a reservoir and ensures that the pressure within the stomach changes little as its volume expands to receive the meal.

The distal stomach uses phasic contractions to grind and triturate the meal, moving only the smallest particles to the pylorus.

 In the fed state, the pylorus opens only partially and intermittently, permitting only small particles to move into the small intestine for further digestion and absorption.

 Emptying of the stomach involves tonic contractions of the proximal portions, and depends on both the physical and chemical characteristics of the meal. Liquids empty most rapidly; solids empty only after a lag phase. Nutrients, acidity, and the osmolarity of the meal feedback to retard gastric emptying once they reach the small intestine via both neural and humoral mechanisms.

 Fats leave the stomach especially slowly, which may be important for their adequate emulsification.

 During fasting, the stomach is the starting point for a motility pattern called the migrating motor complex (MMC) that serves to sweep undigested residues of the meal along the length of the GI tract.

 Phase III of the MMC results in large contractions that propagate aborally, while the pylorus relaxes maximally, allowing the exit of even large particles. This phase of the MMC is related to release of the GI hormone motilin.

 Disease can result from abnormal gastric emptying. Gastric emptying can be disturbed secondary to pyloric or gastric dysfunction, and may be disordered in systemic diseases, such as diabetes.

 Vomiting is a centrally mediated response to various noxious stimuli, inappropriate gastrointestinal distension, or hormonal influences. Vomiting requires a program of responses occurring in both somatic and gastrointestinal muscles, and involves retrograde propulsion of the gastric contents out of the body.

 STUDY QUESTIONS

8–1.   In an experiment, a balloon is inserted into the stomach of a human volunteer and gradually inflated while intraluminal pressures are monitored. Although the volume of the balloon increases considerably, pressures remain relatively constant. This remarkable pressure–volume relationship is thought to involve release of which of the following patterns of neurotransmitters?

	Acetylcholine	Vasoactive intestinal polypeptide	Nitric oxide
A.	Yes	Yes	Yes
B.	Yes	Yes	No
C.	No	Yes	Yes
D.	No	Yes	No
E.	Yes	No	Yes

8–2.   A mother brings her 2-year-old child to the emergency room, distressed because he has swallowed a quarter while the family was eating dinner at a restaurant. The physician reassures her that the quarter, which can be plainly seen in the stomach by fluoroscopy, will eventually pass in the stool. What physiological condition or response will be required to permit exit of the quarter from the stomach?

    A. Receptive relaxation

    B. Fasting

    C. Eating another meal

    D. Mixing and grinding by the stomach

    E. Relaxation of the lower esophageal sphincter

8–3.   Four medical students studying for their physiology final develop headaches and take either regular or enteric coated aspirin with either milk or water (enteric-coated pills will not dissolve until the pH is neutral). Assuming headache relief is proportional to blood aspirin concentrations, place the following conditions in order of headache relief (from fastest to slowest):

  1. Regular aspirin with water

  2. Enteric-coated aspirin with water

  3. Regular aspirin with milk

  4. Enteric-coated aspirin with milk

    A. 1> 2> 3> 4

    B. 4> 3> 2> 1

    C. 1> 3> 2> 4

    D. 2> 4> 1> 3

    E. 2> 4> 3> 1

8–4.   A patient receiving chemotherapy for treatment of breast cancer develops nausea and vomiting. Secretion of which of the following will be stimulated in response to nausea in this patient?

    A. Acid

    B. Pepsinogen

    C. Intrinsic factor

    D. Potassium

    E. Bicarbonate

8–5.   A 50-year-old woman who has suffered from type 1 diabetes for almost 40 years comes to the doctor complaining of epigastric pain and the sensation that her meals are regurgitating into her mouth. Imperfect control of blood glucose levels over the long-standing course of her primary disease will most likely have resulted in injury to which of the following?

    A. Enteric neurons

    B. Gastric circular muscle

    C. Gastric longitudinal muscle

    D. Lower esophageal sphincter

    E. Parietal cells

SUGGESTED READINGS

Hasler WL. Nausea, gastroparesis and aerophagia. *J Clin Gastroenterol.* 2005;39(suppl 5):S223–S229.

Hasler WL. The physiology of gastric motility and gastric emptying. In: Yamada T. Alpers DH, Kalloo AN, Kaplowitz N, Owyang C, Powell DW, eds. *Textbook of Gastroenterology.* 5th ed. Chichester: Wiley-Blackwell; 2009:207–230.

Khoo J, Rayner CK, Feinle-Bisset C, Jones KL, Horowitz M. Gastrointestinal hormonal dysfunction in gastroparesis and functional dyspepsia. *Neurogastroenterol Motil.* 2010;22:1270–1278.

Ranells JD, Carver JD, Kirby RS. Infantile hypetrophic pyloric stenosis: epidemiology, genetics and clinical update. *Adv Peds.* 2011;58:195–206.

Raybould HE. Nutrient tasting and signaling mechanisms in the gut. I. Sensing of lipid by the intestinal mucosa. *Am J Physiol Gastrointest Liver Physiol.* 1999;277:G751–G755.

Rayner CK, Hebbard GS, Horowitz M. Physiology of the antral pump and gastric emptying. In: Johnson LR, Ghishan FK, Kaunitz JD, Merchant JL, Said HM, Wood JD, eds. *Physiology of the Gastrointestinal Tract.* 5th ed. San Diego: Academic Press; 2012:959–976.

Smith DS, Ferris CD. Current concepts in diabetic gastroparesis. *Drugs.* 2003;63:1339–1358.

Tack J. Neurophysiologic mechanisms of gastric reservoir function. In: Johnson LR, Ghishan FK, Kaunitz JD, Merchant JL, Said HM, Wood JD, eds. *Physiology of the Gastrointestinal Tract.* 5th ed. San Diego: Academic Press; 2012:951–957.

Intestinal Motility

9

OBJECTIVES

▶ *Understand how the motility functions of the small intestine and colon contribute to the integrated response to a meal*
  ▶ Describe the muscle layers and their connections to the enteric nervous system that subserve intestinal motility
  ▶ Identify the sphincters that control movement of intestinal contents between segments, or out of the body
▶ *Define the motility patterns that characterize movements of the small and large intestines under fed and fasted conditions and their control mechanisms*
  ▶ Distinguish between mixing patterns and those that propel contents along the length of the intestine
  ▶ Describe reflexes that coordinate the motility functions of the small intestine and colon with the function of the stomach
  ▶ Understand the process whereby undigestible residues of the meal are eliminated from the body
▶ *Understand the pathophysiology of disease states where intestinal motility is abnormal*

BASIC PRINCIPLES OF INTESTINAL MOTILITY

The ability of the walls of the small and large intestines to contract and relax allows for the movement of intestinal contents from one site to another. Specific motility patterns subserve the functions of each intestinal segment. In addition, specialized muscle regions, or sphincters, retard the passage of intestinal contents in a controlled fashion at specific sites.

Role and Significance in the Small Intestine

As we have learned from previous chapters, the primary role of the small intestine is to digest the various components of the meal and to absorb the resulting nutrients into the bloodstream or lymphatic system. The motility patterns observed in the small intestine are profoundly altered by eating. The duration of such changes depends on the caloric load and the type of nutrients ingested, with lipids having the most durable effect. During the fed state, many of the motility patterns in the small intestine are designed not to propel the intestinal contents aborally, but rather to mix the contents with the various digestive secretions and prolong their exposure to the absorptive epithelium. The muscle layers of the small intestine interact to provide for "two steps forward and one step back," retaining the intestinal contents long enough to provide for efficient extraction of most or all useful substances. In general, therefore, the motility functions of the small intestine control the rate of nutrient absorption. The speed with which the contents are propelled also varies along the length of the small intestine. Movement is fastest in the duodenum and jejunum, providing for rapid mixing and propulsion of the contents both orally and aborally. Motility then slows in the ileum, providing additional time for the absorption of slowly permeable nutrients, and particularly, lipids. Then, once the meal is digested and absorbed, the small intestine converts to the migrating motor complex (MMC) we also discussed for the stomach, a pattern of relative quiescence punctuated by propulsive motility patterns that expel undigested residues through the small intestine and into the colon.

Role and Significance in the Colon

The functions of the colon are quite distinct from those of the small intestine. Thus, while the colon does engage in some limited digestion and salvage of nutrients from undigested residues, with the cooperation of its endogenous flora, the primary functions of the colon are to extract and reclaim water from the intestinal contents, and to process the feces for elimination. As a result, even in the fasted state, the motility functions of particularly the ascending and transverse colon are considerably more biased toward mixing the contents and retaining them for prolonged periods, and the colon does not participate in the MMC. On the other hand, periodically, large propulsive contractions sweep through the colon, transferring its contents to the rectum and ultimately promoting the urge to defecate.

FUNCTIONAL ANATOMY

Muscle Layers

The small intestine, a hollow tube approximately 600 cm in length in a normal adult, is surrounded by two overlapping muscle layers that together make up the muscularis externa. A layer of circular muscle is found closest to the mucosa, overlaid by a longitudinal muscle layer. Taken together, these muscle layers can produce most, if not all, of the stereotypical motility patterns of the small intestine. There is also a thin layer of muscle sandwiched between the mucosa and submucosa, the muscularis mucosa, but the contribution of this muscle layer to the bulk motility properties of the small intestine is unclear. Instead, it may confer specific motility functions on mucosal structures, such as the villi.

The functions of the circular and longitudinal muscle layers are closely integrated. In part, this derives from the fact that they engage in a high level of electrical coupling. Structures known as gap junctions, which permit small second messengers and electrical signals to be communicated between adjacent cells, mean that stimulation of one smooth muscle cell can rapidly be transmitted to its neighbors, without the need for additional neural input. The function of the two muscle layers is also coordinated by the activity of interstitial cells of Cajal. These cells undergo rhythmic cycles of depolarization, related to oscillations in intracellular calcium concentration. As in the stomach, these cells provide the pacemaker function that dictates the basal electrical rhythm, or slow waves, that ultimately control the rate and locations of phasic contractions of the smooth muscle. In the duodenum, the basal electric rhythm occurs at a rate of 12 cycles per minute (cpm), although this slows as one moves distally to 7–8 cpm in the distal ileum. Interstitial cells of Cajal are essential for the peristaltic reflex in the small intestine (and to a lesser extent in the colon) and their numbers may be reduced under conditions associated with slowed transit, such as constipation.

The large intestine also contains both circular and longitudinal muscle layers that regulate its motility, but the anatomic arrangement of these differs somewhat from that seen in the small intestine. In the ascending, transverse, and descending colon, the circular muscle layer is overlaid by three long nonoverlapping bands of longitudinal muscle oriented at 120° to each other, known as the *taeniae coli*. Electrical coupling between the circular muscle and taeniae coli is less effective than seen in between the corresponding muscle layers in the small intestine, which likely contributes to less effective propulsive motility. The circular muscle layer is also contracted intermittently to divide the colon into functional segments known as *haustra*. The speed of impulse propagation is faster in the circular muscle of the colon than in the longitudinal layers, allowing for these segmenting ring contractions. Note that the haustral segments are not permanent structures, however, and thus they can be smoothed out to permit propulsion of the colonic contents.

As one moves into the sigmoid colon and rectum, the intestine becomes completely enveloped by longitudinal muscle that is important to the specialized functions of this region, which include serving predominantly as a conduit and participating in defecation. The lumen of the rectum is also partially occluded by transverse folds, again formed by muscular contraction, which act as shelves to retard the passage of fecal material (Figure 9–1). Finally, the most distal portion of the gastrointestinal tract, the anal canal, is a specialized region that contains both smooth and striated muscle in its walls. In this respect, it can be compared with the most proximal gut segment, the esophagus, which is the only other segment of the gastrointestinal system whose motility is governed by both muscle types.

Enteric Nervous System

The primary determinant of motility function in both the small and large intestines derives from the activity of intrinsic neural circuits. The number of intrinsic nerves vastly exceeds that of extrinsic inputs, and the role of the latter is normally felt to be restricted largely to modulating motility

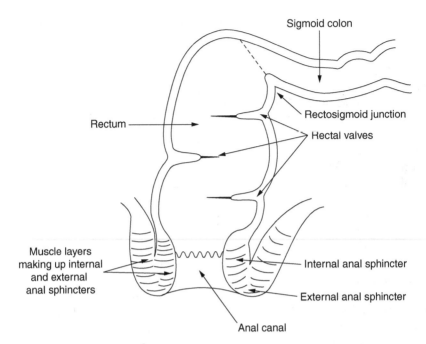

Figure 9–1. Anatomy of the rectum and anal canal.

patterns established by the "little brain" of the enteric nervous system, rather than independently initiating muscle activity. Enteric nerves contain a variety of neurotransmitters and may be responsible for smooth muscle contraction or relaxation. The major stimulatory neurotransmitters include acetylcholine (ACh), neurokinin A and substance P, whereas the inhibitory nerves express vasoactive intestinal polypeptide (VIP) and also produce nitric oxide on activation. There is also an abundant supply of sensory afferents that respond to the physicochemical characteristics of the luminal contents. Additional information about the coding of enteric nerves is provided in Chapter 2.

Modulatory influences of extrinsic nerves derive from a variety of sources depending on the intestinal segment in question. The vagus (parasympathetic) and splanchnic (sympathetic) nerves innervate the small intestine, ileocecal valve, and proximal colon. The pelvic nerves, on the other hand, are the conduits of extrinsic input to the remainder of the colon and the internal anal sphincter. Finally, the pudendal nerves provide input from the sacral region of the spinal cord to the external anal sphincter and the muscle layers of the pelvic floor. In fact, unlike the other gastrointestinal regions discussed earlier, voluntary input to these latter structures is vital to their function. The ability to contract the external anal sphincter and pelvic floor muscles, a behavior learned during toilet training, allows us to defer defecation until a time when it is socially convenient.

Sphincters

As alluded to earlier, the passage of contents along the length of the small intestine and colon is also regulated by sphincters. The *ileocecal valve*, or junction, is a localized zone of high pressure that cannot be abolished by neurotoxins, and which reflects the activity of the circular muscle layer. Unlike sphincters that we have encountered more proximally in the gastrointestinal tract, the primary function of the ileocecal valve does not appear to relate to the control of delivery of luminal contents to the next segment downstream, at least under normal conditions. Rather, the critical function of this valve is apparently to limit reflux of colonic contents into the ileum. This function is vital in maintaining the relative sterility of the small intestine, and injury to or dysfunction of this region can result in the overgrowth of bacteria in the small intestine. Indeed, the ileocecal valve contracts in response to colonic distension, a response that clearly can contribute to limiting reflux of the fecal stream. This reflex is mediated by sympathetic input from the splanchnic nerve. Under certain conditions, however, the ileocecal valve may also retard the aboral passage of the intestinal contents. This is thought to occur primarily under conditions of massively increased flow through this region, such as is seen in secretory diarrheal diseases that target the small intestine.

The elimination of waste matter from the colon is under the control of the internal and external anal sphincters. The internal anal sphincter consists of a thickened band of gastrointestinal circular muscle (Figure 9–1). This sphincter supplies approximately 70–80% of the tone of the anal canal at rest, and its regulation is entirely autonomous. If the rectum is suddenly distended, the sphincter relaxes in response to release of NO and VIP and then contributes only 40% of anal tone, with the remainder supplied by the external anal sphincter. At the same time, the external anal sphincter pressure is increased. This rectoanal inhibitory reflex, initiated by rectal distension, thus allows for efficient defecation while preventing accidental leakage. After a short period of time, however, the internal anal sphincter accommodates to the new rectal volume and regains its tone, unless defecation can conveniently be completed (Figure 9–2).

The external anal sphincter is comprised of striated muscle, and actually consists of portions of three different muscular structures in the pelvic cavity that wrap around the distal anal canal. Unlike the majority of striated muscles, it maintains a significant resting tone, although at baseline this only accounts for 20–30% of the overall tone of the anal canal. However, it can be contracted voluntarily, and also contracts reflexively in response to a sudden increase in abdominal pressure (such as when coughing or lifting a heavy object).

FEATURES OF INTESTINAL MOTILITY

We turn now to a discussion of the patterns of motility occurring in the small intestine and colon that subserve the functions of these segments, and the mechanisms whereby they are regulated.

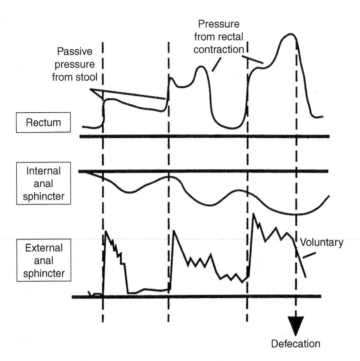

Figure 9–2. Motility of the rectum and anal sphincters in response to rectal filling and during defecation. Note that filling of the rectum with stool causes an initial decrease in internal anal sphincter tone, which is counterbalanced by a reflex contraction of the external anal sphincter. The internal sphincter then accommodates to the new rectal volume, allowing relaxation of the external anal sphincter. Finally, defecation occurs when the external anal sphincter is relaxed voluntarily. (From Chang EB, Sitrin MD, Black DD. *Gastrointestinal, Hepatobiliary and Nutritional Physiology.* Philadelphia: Lippincott-Raven; 1996.)

Fed versus Fasted Patterns of Motility

 For the small intestine, there is a marked distinction between motility observed in the postprandial versus fasting periods; however, colonic motility has far less temporal association with the ingestion of a meal. These differences are mirrored by the times taken for luminal contents to transit these two intestinal segments. In the small intestine, substances move from the mouth to the ileocecal valve in a little under 2 hours in healthy adults, on an average, with transit occurring most rapidly proximally. Transit is slowed in proportion to the number of calories presented to the intestine, providing for a relatively constant level of absorption across varying nutrient loads. In the colon, on the other hand, transit from the cecum to the rectum may take 1–2 days on an average, with considerable interindividual variability outside this range.

During fasting, the small intestine exhibits the migrating motor complex, or MMC, that we introduced in the previous chapter. When the meal has emptied from the small intestine, the MMC resumes with its characteristic three phases—phase I, quiescence; phase II, consisting of an increasing number of intermittent but rarely propulsive contractions; and phase III, a 5–10 minute burst of intense contractions that propagate aborally (Figure 9–3). As in the stomach, the purpose of the MMC, and of phase III in particular, appears to be to sweep the intestine clear of any remaining residues of the meal. Phase III of the MMC is produced by the action of the hormone, motilin, but the stimuli that generate release of this substance from enteroendocrine cells remains unclear. The MMC also cycles in phase with contractile activity of the gallbladder and relaxation of the sphincter of Oddi, as well as with periodic increases in secretory function of the intestine and organs draining into it, with these responses peaking just prior to the onset of phase III. It has been speculated that these additional responses are likewise important for the housekeeping function of the MMC. The MMC may additionally play a role in limiting reflux of colonic contents into the ileum, as illustrated by the fact that patients in whom the MMC is disrupted may display small bowel bacterial overgrowth.

After a meal is ingested, motility events in the small intestine become more frequent, with patterns designed to mix the meal with intestinal secretions and to maximize exposure of the digested nutrients to the absorptive mucosa. Many contractions during the fed state do not propel the contents at all, or are retrograde. In fact, up to 50% of the phasic contractions in the duodenum

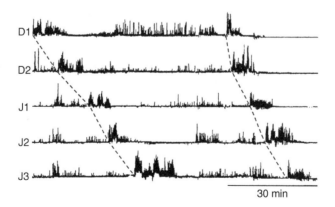

Figure 9–3. Migrating motor complexes in the duodenum and jejunum as recorded from a fasting human subject by manometry. D1, D2, J1, J2, and J3 indicate recording points along the length of the duodenum and jejunum. Note that the intense contractions occurring rhythmically during phase III propagate aborally. (From Soffer EE et al. Prolonged ambulatory duodeno-jejunal manometry in humans: normal values and gender effect. *Am J Gastroenterol.* 1998;93:1318–1323. Copyright American College of Gastroenterology.)

actually move the luminal contents orally. The ability of the intestine to display this fed pattern of motility, which will be discussed in more detail later, rests first on the basal electrical rhythm, generated by the intestinal pacemaker and propagated to surrounding smooth muscle cells. As in the stomach, however, the basal rhythm supplies only the nodes at which contractions can occur at any given moment, because the rhythmic changes in membrane potential that are induced in the muscle cells are insufficient to cause contraction. Rather, it is only when the effects of neurotransmitters and perhaps other neurohumoral regulators are superimposed on this rhythm that action potentials can take place. The result is a series of intermittent phasic contractions occurring along the length of the small intestine, peaking 10–20 minutes after eating. Acetylcholine is a critical mediator of such effects, and the enteric nervous system is the primary regulatory system. Vagotomy does not prevent the occurrence of the fed pattern, although this maneuver may shorten its duration as well as increase the latency for its initiation after the start of eating. Thus, vagal influences may contribute to the fact that changes in intestinal motility consistent with the fed pattern normally begin during the cephalic phase. On the other hand, the role for hormonal mediators is much less clear. Unlike the MMC, there is no role for motilin in generating the phasic contractions of the fed state. Indeed, circulating levels of motilin fall after the meal, and suppressed release of this hormone may in fact be needed to allow the fed motility pattern to take over from the MMC. CCK and neurotensin, among others, have been suggested to contribute to the fed pattern of motility. However, exogenous supply of CCK at levels that mimic those seen during digestion and absorption of a meal cannot independently reproduce all features of the fed pattern of motility.

The duration of the fed pattern of motility in the small intestine depends on the caloric content of the meal ingested as well as its composition. A 450 kcal mixed meal will disrupt MMC cycling for more than 3 hours. This effect is further enhanced if the meal contains greater quantities of long-chain triglycerides, although this effect is not seen with medium-chain triglycerides. As we will learn in Chapter 16, this corresponds nicely to the different kinetics and pathways for absorption of medium and long-chain fatty acids. The fed pattern also requires nutrients to be present in the gut lumen, since it cannot be reproduced by infusing nutrients parenterally. Thus implies a role for nutrient sensing in generating the response.

Mixing and Segmentation

During the fed state, the primary motility events observed in the small intestine are those that serve to mix the contents, and to propel it only slowly, if at all. An isolated contraction in the absence of others either proximal or distal to it will have the effect of mixing the contents of the lumen in the immediate vicinity of the contraction (Figure 9–4). Another common pattern seen is referred to as segmentation. In this pattern, a segment of small intestine is occluded by contractions at its proximal and distal ends, and then the segment is further subdivided by a contraction in its center, and so on (Figure 9–4). Segmenting contractions

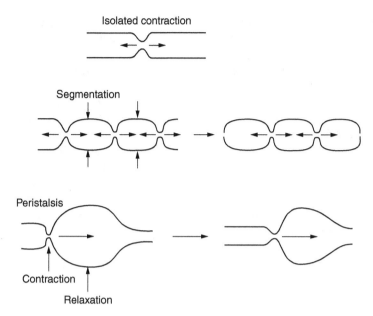

Figure 9–4. Patterns of intestinal mixing and propulsion. An *isolated contraction* moves contents both orally and aborally. *Segmentation* mixes contents over a short length of intestine, as indicated by the time sequence from left to right. In the diagram on the left, the vertical arrows indicate the points at which the next set of contractions is initiated. Finally, *peristalsis*, which involves both a contraction and a relaxation, propels the luminal contents aborally.

serve to move intestinal contents back and forth within a short segment of bowel. Some of the contents may move aborally coincidently as a result of this type of motility pattern, but it is almost as likely that they will move in a retrograde fashion, increasing their residence time in the small intestine. Significant propulsion is only achieved in the setting of peristalsis, as will be described in more detail later.

The relative contributions of the circular and longitudinal muscle layers to these motility patterns is unclear, although each is known to produce occlusive versus shortening effects, respectively, following contraction. Shortening of a segment may be important in hastening transit, whereas luminal occlusion can produce mixing by the mechanisms discussed earlier, but clearly this is an over-simplification. What is known is that the complex patterns of motility seen in the small intestine after a meal are the result of the almost autonomous effects of the enteric neural circuitry, and presumably reflect a stereotypical "programmed" response to a given set of physiologic conditions.

Peristalsis

Peristalsis produces aboral propulsion in both the small intestine and colon. It is a motility response that occurs predominantly in response to intestinal distension, or other events that deform the mucosa, such as the mechanical effects of passage of the food bolus along the wall of the gut. Rapid stretch of the intestine is most effective in triggering peristalsis.

As in the esophagus, where peristalsis is important in moving the bolus from the mouth to the stomach, intestinal peristalsis involves the influences of both an ascending contraction and a descending relaxation (Figure 9–4). Activation of stretch and possibly other mechano- receptors in the mucosa secondarily induce the release of 5-HT and calcitonin gene-related peptide. In turn, on the proximal side of the bolus, the circular muscle shortens and the longitudinal muscle relaxes, pushing the bolus forward. These responses have been attributed to the action of ACh and substance P from enteric nerve endings. On the distal side, the bolus is received by a segment of the intestine of increased caliber, brought about by shortening of the longitudinal muscle and relaxation of the circular muscle. These responses relate to the activity of VIP and nitric oxide. While peristalsis is a reflex that can wholly be accounted for by the activity of the enteric nervous system, it may be modified by extrinsic nerves. For example, it is well-known that the emotional state of an individual can modify bowel motility. Stress, for example, may slow transit secondary to the central effects of CRF.

Colonic Motility

The motility patterns of the colon are primarily concerned with mixing the contents and retaining them for a sufficient period to allow optimal salvage of the fluid utilized during the digestive process. The colon has the capacity to reabsorb even unusually large quantities of fluid, such as those produced by secretory diarrheal diseases that target the small intestine, provided there is adequate contact time with the mucosa. This is the principle of antidiarrheal drugs that target motility function; if propulsive motility patterns are disrupted, fluid absorption will be enhanced. However, periodically the colon also engages in a propulsive motility pattern that essentially moves the majority of the colonic contents into the rectum. In turn, this induces the need to defecate, which will be dealt with separately later.

During mixing, the colon shuttles both contents back and forth between its haustra, and progressively propels contents from one haustra to the next in a motility pattern referred to as segmental propulsion. These patterns are accomplished by two types of contraction that have been characterized in the colon: short- and long-duration contractions. Short-duration contractions arise in the circular muscle, and are stationary pressure waves lasting approximately 8 seconds on an average, which effect local mixing. Long-duration contractions, on the other hand, last for 20–60 seconds and may be stationary or may propagate for a short distance, and are attributed to contraction of the longitudinal muscles of the taeniae coli. Propagating contractions account for segmental propulsion. It is important to recognize that these long-duration contractions may propel the colonic contents in an oral direction as well as aborally. Retrograde oral migration is seen predominantly in the ascending and transverse colon, whereas these contractions in the distal colon typically propagate aborally.

High-amplitude propagating contractions are distinct from the motility patterns just described. They propagate exclusively aborally, and provide for mass movement of the feces over long distances. While they precede the urge to defecate, they in fact occur about ten times per day, and are associated with rising in the morning and with eating, in addition to occurring both prior to and in association with defecation. These contractions originate in the cecum and sweep throughout the colon to the rectum, also resulting in relaxation of the internal anal sphincter. They may be initiated by physiological stimuli, such as distension, or by medications or disease states (such as laxatives or inflammation, respectively). Evidence suggests that the propagation of these contractions is mediated by both cholinergic and neurokinin-dependent pathways.

Gastrocolic Reflex

Many individuals note an urge to defecate shortly after starting a meal. This response is produced by the *gastrocolic reflex*, which is a long reflex arc that is initiated by gastric distension. The reflex produces a generalized increase in colonic motility with mass movement of feces. Both mechano- and chemosensitive components of the gastrocolic reflex have been identified, and 5-HT and ACh appear to be important mediators of the response. There is also a more delayed aspect to this response that occurs once the meal reaches the ileum, and which is mediated by the release of peptide YY, neuropeptide Y, and neurotensin. Overall, however, the function of this reflex is to clear the colon to ready it to receive the residues of the new meal. In fact, the response is preserved, at least in part, even after gastrectomy, so it might more properly be referred to as the colonic response to eating. This response may also lead to post-prandial discomfort in patients suffering from irritable bowel syndrome.

Defecation

Defecation is the process of elimination of solid wastes from the gastrointestinal tract, and it involves several structures in and around the rectum and anus. The process of defecation is preceded by the mass movement of feces into the rectum, as discussed earlier. Filling of the rectum causes relaxation of the internal anal sphincter via the release of VIP and nitric oxide from intrinsic nerves, but this response is offset by a simultaneous action to increase the tone of the external anal sphincter (Figure 9–2). Overall, this reflex can permit efficient defecation while preventing leakage. Relaxation of the internal anal sphincter also permits the so-called anal sampling mechanism. Thus, while the rectum is relatively devoid of sensory nerve endings, the anus is amply supplied with these. The portion of rectal contents that enters the anal canal is identified as being gaseous, solid or liquid, and thereby initiates appropriate activity of the external anal sphincter to retain each of these, or to permit voluntary expulsion.

After toilet training, humans can choose to defer defecation until it is socially convenient, even if mass propulsion of feces has filled the rectal lumen. When defecation is desired, on the other hand, adopting a squatting position changes the relative orientation of the intestine and surrounding muscular structures to straighten the pathway for fecal exit. This is also assisted by relaxation of the puborectalis muscle, which results in a less acute rectoanal angle. Rectal contraction then produces the propulsive force to move the feces out of the body. Evacuation is enhanced by simultaneous contraction of the rectus abdominus, diaphragm, and other levator ani muscles, which increases intraabdominal pressure. The *valsalva* maneuver (attempting expiration against a closed mouth and nasal passage) can be used to assist evacuation still further. All of these events occur whether solid (in health) or liquid (in disease) feces are expelled, although less force is obviously needed to evacuate the latter. On the other hand, the voluntary expulsion of flatus involves the contractile functions listed, but the puborectalis muscle does not relax and there is no change in the rectoanal angle. This allows the flatus gas to be forced past the acutely angled anorectum without the simultaneous loss of feces.

PATHOPHYSIOLOGY AND CLINICAL CORRELATIONS

Ileus

Ileus refers to either a temporary or permanent state of inhibited GI motility. The symptoms of ileus are those that occur when the intestine becomes physically obstructed, but in the case of ileus, the obstruction is only a functional one. The best-known example of ileus is that following abdominal surgery, which likely involves the combined influences of neurogenic, myogenic, and humoral factors, as well as the release of inflammatory mediators and perhaps bacterial products. Surgical incisions into the peritoneal cavity can profoundly inhibit intestinal motility functions for several days, with changes in the colon taking the longest to subside. Part of the response likely reflects trauma, but anesthetic agents have also been shown to dampen motility patterns independently. The failure of motility leads to pain and distension as the gastrointestinal tract is unable to propel its contents appropriately, with accompanying malabsorption. Interestingly, a number of recent studies have suggested that post-operative ileus can be significantly ameliorated by the simple approach of asking patients to chew gum, underscoring the communication between proximal and distal segments of the gut.

Hirschsprung's Disease

Hirschsprung's disease, also known as congenital megacolon, is a developmental abnormality that results when the enteric nervous system fails to develop appropriately. During embryological development, neurons derived from the primitive neural crest migrate along the length of the intestine and progressively populate the enteric nervous system from the mouth to the anus. This neural development is under the control of several growth and trophic factors, including glial-derived neurotrophic factor and endothelin III. Mutations in these factors or their receptors (prominently, the RET receptor for GDNF) can result in premature cessation of neural migration, resulting in a segment of varying length at the end of the colon that lacks the ganglia of the enteric neural plexuses. A relative deficiency of interstitial cells of Cajal also occurs, further impairing motility function. The aganglionic segment, which invariably begins at the internal anal sphincter then extends upward to a varying extent, remains permanently contracted, presenting a functional barrier to the passage of fecal material. In turn, the intestinal segment proximal to this segment eventually becomes dilated.

Hirschsprung's disease is typically diagnosed in infancy, is more common in males, and occurs in 1 in 5000 live births, although milder cases may only be detected in adulthood. Neonates may present only with the symptoms of intestinal obstruction but infants and adults will also develop the megacolon that can be diagnosed radiographically. In either case, the symptoms of the disease can be related to eating. In most cases, the diseased segment is confined to the rectosigmoid, and extension to the remainder of the colon or further to the small intestine is rare. The symptoms of the disorder can be completely alleviated by surgical excision of the diseased segment. Recently, hope has also arisen that this and other disorders of enteric neural development (such as intestinal pseudo-obstruction) may be amenable to stem-cell therapy.

Functional Bowel Disorders

The terms functional bowel disorder and irritable bowel syndrome have been used to refer to disease entities where patients complain of abdominal pain, bloating, constipation, and/or diarrhea, but for which no organic cause can be found. Functional bowel disorders are the most common reason for patients to seek the help of a gastroenterologist, and are extremely common in the general population. Estimates of prevalence suggest that 10–30% of the population suffers from at least occasional symptoms, although many of these individuals will not seek medical assistance.

Functional bowel disorders are partially due to dysmotility, although consistent motor abnormalities have not been found, at least at baseline. In general, however, patients presenting with diarrhea as their chief complaint may have shortened transit times through the small intestine and colon, an exaggerated gastrocolonic response, and an increase in propulsive contractions in the colon. Patients with constipation-predominant functional bowel disorders, on the other hand, have slowed transit of intestinal contents.

Most researchers now agree that functional bowel disorders result from a condition of visceral hypersensitivity. That is to say, patients with these conditions respond abnormally to stimuli that would be perceived as innocuous by normal individuals. Normal physiologic events in the gut, such as distension, are perceived as painful by patients, and presumably lead to altered patterns of motility as a result. The prevailing hypothesis holds that such hypersensitivity results from sensitization of afferent neural pathways, which may occur idiopathically, as a result of certain stresses in childhood, or as the aftermath of pathological conditions such as GI infections or inflammation. The treatment of functional bowel disorders remains problematic, although symptomatic treatments (e.g., laxatives) or drugs intended to enhance motility can be effective. No current treatments, however, address the presumed underlying cause of disease.

Fecal Incontinence

The distressing condition of fecal incontinence occurs when the release of rectal contents occurs against one's wishes. As should be apparent from the previous discussion of defecation, failure of the external anal sphincter to maintain appropriate tone of the anal canal is the most likely culprit in causing disease. Under normal conditions, the external anal sphincter supplies only a minority portion of resting anal tone, but its contribution is markedly increased reflexively in response to sudden rectal distension, or when the pressure in the abdominal cavity is increased abruptly by coughing or lifting a heavy object. Damage to the external anal sphincter, therefore, may reduce its ability to contract at these critical times, and incontinence may result. Damage to the sphincter may result from trauma, obstetric or surgical injuries, prolapse of the rectum, or neuropathic disease that alters sphincter function without changes to its structure. In addition to the motility functions of the external anal sphincter in preventing incontinence, the ability of the puborectalis muscle to form an acute angle between the axes of the rectum and anal canal is a critical barrier to incontinence, and reverse peristalsis in the rectum also presents a subtle barrier to fecal flow. Finally, intact sensation in the anal canal is required to initiate a call to stool. In patients with long-standing diabetes, injury to sensory nerves (diabetic neuropathy) may impair such sensation, thereby also affecting continence.

Treatment of fecal incontinence may be challenging, and requires strengthening of the external anal sphincter muscle by exercise (biofeedback) therapy or by surgical intervention, particularly if incontinence is the direct result of injury to the external anal sphincter. Approaches to correct nerve damage in this region, on the other hand, are not readily available.

KEY CONCEPTS

Motility patterns in the small and large intestines serve not only to propel intestinal contents, but also to mix them with enzymes and other digestive juices, and to retain them in a given segment long enough for optimal absorption to occur.

Patterns of motility in both the small intestine and colon result primarily from the programmed activity of the enteric nervous system, which responds to the physicochemical characteristics of luminal contents to generate appropriate motility patterns for a given set of physiologic conditions.

Progress of intestinal contents along the small and large intestines is regulated in part by sphincters. The ileocecal valve appears to be important primarily to prevent the reflux of colonic contents into the ileum, thus maintaining the relative sterility of the small intestine.

 Movement of colonic contents out of the body is controlled by the internal and external anal sphincters, under involuntary and voluntary control, respectively.

 In the fed state, the small intestine engages primarily in segmentation and mixing motility patterns, with propulsion occurring both orally and aborally.

 After the meal has left the small intestine, the migrating motor complex (MMC) cycles to sweep the intestine clear of undigested residues. Phase III, the propulsive component of the MMC, is stimulated by the hormone motilin.

 Motility patterns can be modulated by humoral input, or by extrinsic neural activity. Motility and transit times are proportional to the caloric content of the meal.

 The colon serves predominantly a salvage and reservoir function, with slow transit of contents along its length and marked dehydration of luminal contents.

 Periodically, large propulsive contractions sweep through the colon and precede the urge to defecate.

 Induced or developmental abnormalities of the enteric nervous system, or traumatic injury to muscle layers, can lead to pathophysiologic effects on the ability to handle intestinal contents appropriately.

 STUDY QUESTIONS

9–1.   A healthy medical student enrolled in a study of intestinal motility ingests a solution of lactulose, and breath hydrogen measurements are made for the next 4 hours. On day 1 he ingests this solution alone, on day 2, together with a pint of ice cream, and on day 3, together with a glass of milk. No other items are consumed for the duration of the test. Place the test days in order of the most prompt appearance of breath hydrogen (from fastest to slowest).

A. Day 3 > Day 2 > Day 1

B. Day 1 > Day 2 > Day 3

C. Day 1 > Day 3 > Day 2

D. Day 2 > Day 3 > Day 1

E. There will be no difference between the days

9–2. Which of the following substances is not involved in mediating the fed pattern of intestinal motility?

A. Acetylcholine

B. Vasoactive intestinal polypeptide

C. 5-hydroxytryptamine (serotonin)

D. Nitric oxide

E. Motilin

9–3. The anal sampling mechanism allows for the voluntary passage of flatus without the elimination of solid stool, even if the rectal canal is filled with fecal material. Compared with defecation, which of the following does not occur during the passage only of flatus?

A. Increased intraabdominal pressure

B. Relaxation of the internal anal sphincter

C. Relaxation of the external anal sphincter

D. Activation of anal sensory nerve endings

E. Relaxation of the puborectalis muscle

9–4. A previously healthy 40-year-old executive suffers a bout of viral gastroenteritis on a business trip to Mexico. Some months after returning home, she begins to notice recurrent bouts of diarrhea, abdominal pain that is relieved by a bowel movement, and bloating. No weight loss or fever are present. She ascribes these symptoms to the stress of her job, but they fail to subside during a 6-month sabbatical. Her symptoms are most likely attributable to which of the following?

A. Inflammatory bowel disease

B. Chronic viral infection

C. Recurrent GI infection

D. Endometriosis

E. Postinfectious visceral hypersensitivity

9–5. Following a forceps delivery of her third child, a 36-year-old woman returns to her physician complaining of persistent, mild fecal incontinence when lifting her older children, without any urinary incontinence. Her symptoms are most likely attributable to dysfunction of which of the following?

A. Anal sensory nerves

B. Internal anal sphincter

C. External anal sphincter

D. Pudendal nerves

E. Puborectalis muscle

SUGGESTED READINGS

Bharucha AE, Brookes SJH. Neurophysiologic mechanisms of human large intestinal motility. In: Johnson LR, Ghishan FK, Kaunitz JD, Merchant JL, Said HM, Wood JD, eds. *Physiology of the Gastrointestinal Tract.* 5th ed. San Diego: Academic Press; 2012:977–1022.

Bornstein JC, Costa M, Grider JD. Enteric motor and interneuronal circuits controlling motility. *Neurogastroenterol Motil.* 2004;16(suppl 1):34–38.

Camilleri M, Szarka L. Dysmotility of the small intestine and colon. In: Yamada T, Alpers DH, Kalloo AN, Kaplowitz N, Laine L, Owyang C, Powell DW, eds. *Textbook of Gastroenterology.* 5th ed. Philadelphia, Chichester: Wiley-Blackwell; 2009:1108–1156.

Hasler WL. Motility of the small intestine and colon. In: Yamada T, Alpers DH, Kalloo AN, Kaplowitz N, Owyang C, Powell DW, eds. *Textbook of Gastroenterology.* 5th ed. Chichester: Wiley-Blackwell; 2009:231–263.

Jorge JM, Wexner SD. Etiology and management of fecal incontinence. *Dis Colon Rectum.* 1993;36:77–97.

Kehlet H, Holte K. Review of post-operative ileus. *Am J Surg.* 2001;182(suppl 5A):3S–10S.

Panza E, Knowles CH Graziano C, Thapar N, Burns AJ, Seri M, Stanghellini V, De Giorgio R. Genetics of human enteric neuropathies. *Prog Neurobiol.* 2012;96:176–189.

Sanders KM, Hwang SJ, Ward SM. Neuroeffector apparatus in gastrointestinal smooth muscle organs. *J Physiol.* 2010;588:4621–4639.

Functional Anatomy of the Liver and Biliary System

10

OBJECTIVES

▶ *Understand the role of the liver in whole-body homeostasis and the structural features that subserve its functions*

▶ *Understand the functions of bile secretion and the anatomy of the biliary system*

▶ *Describe the unusual circulatory features of the liver and the relationship of blood flow to bile flow*

▶ *Identify the parenchymal and nonparenchymal cell types of the liver, their anatomic relationships, and their respective functions*

▶ *Understand pathological conditions where structure and function of the liver and biliary system is compromised*

  ▶ Describe the role of liver transplantation in treating end-stage liver disease

  ▶ Describe the physiological rationale for commonly used tests of liver function, liver injury, and disease prognosis

OVERVIEW OF THE LIVER AND BILIARY SYSTEMS AND THEIR FUNCTIONS

The liver is the largest gland in the body, and conducts a myriad of vital metabolic and excretory functions. In addition, by virtue of its circulatory relationship to the absorptive surface of the gastrointestinal tract, the liver is the initial site where ingested nutrients, and other substances entering via the gastrointestinal tract, such as drugs and bacterial metabolites, are processed by the body. Thus, the liver is a gate-keeper that can process useful substances while detoxifying orally absorbed substances that are potentially harmful, such as toxic xenobiotics.

Metabolism and Detoxification

The liver contributes in a pivotal way to the biochemical status of the body as a whole. Indeed, a major portion of the discipline of biochemistry is concerned with the chemical reactions that take place in the cell type that makes up the majority of the hepatic mass, the hepatocyte. For this reason, it is beyond the scope of this text to provide a comprehensive analysis of all of the metabolic functions of the liver. Instead, we will focus our discussion on broad categories of metabolic functions of the liver that are relevant to the function of the gastrointestinal system, or are of particular importance to whole-body homeostasis.

First, the liver is an important repository of carbohydrate metabolism. The liver performs four specific functions in this regard: glycogen storage, conversion of galactose and fructose to glucose, gluconeogenesis, and the formation of many important biochemical compounds from the intermediate products of carbohydrate metabolism. Many of the substrates for these reactions derive from the products of carbohydrate digestion and absorption that travel directly to the liver from the gut, as will be described in more detail in Chapter 15. As a consequence, the liver plays a major role in maintaining blood glucose concentrations within normal limits, particularly in the postprandial period. The liver removes excess glucose from the blood and returns it as needed, in a process referred to as the *glucose buffer function* of the liver. This function is markedly impaired in an individual whose hepatic function has been reduced by disease, resulting in abnormally high postprandial glucose concentrations. However, because the liver also regulates the other aspects of glucose homeostasis described, in liver failure, hypoglycemia is seen. Indeed, hepatectomized animals rapidly develop fatal hypoglycemia.

The liver also contributes in a major way to fat metabolism. While many aspects of lipid biochemistry are common to all cells of the body, others are concentrated in the liver. Specifically, the liver supports an especially high rate of oxidation of fatty acids to supply energy for other body functions. Likewise, the liver converts amino acids and two-carbon fragments derived from carbohydrates to fats that can then be transported to adipose tissue for storage. Finally, the liver synthesizes most of the lipoproteins required by the body, as well as large quantities of cholesterol and phospholipids. Lipoproteins are used to transport various lipids to other sites in the body, whereas phospholipids and cholesterol are important structural components of plasma and intracellular membranes, as well as serving as substrates for the synthesis of other significant biochemicals. Indeed, about 50% of the cholesterol synthesized by the liver is converted to bile acids, which play important roles in the digestion and absorption of lipids, as will be discussed in greater detail in subsequent chapters.

The body also cannot dispense with the liver's capacity for protein processing for more than a few days. The liver contributes the following important aspects of protein metabolism: deamination of amino acids, formation of urea as a means to dispose of blood ammonia, formation of plasma proteins, and interconversion of various amino acids, as well as conversion of amino acids to other intermediates important in the body. Deamination of amino acids is an initial step in their conversion to carbohydrates or fats, and the liver conducts the vast majority of such reactions. Likewise, the liver can synthesize all of the so-called *nonessential amino acids* that need not be supplied in the diet in their native form (as will be discussed in more detail in Chapter 15).

The liver also synthesizes proteins that are critical to the circulatory system. With the exception of the immunoglobulins produced by cells of the immune system, the liver provides most of the plasma proteins. Following loss of a large portion of plasma proteins, such as following blood loss, the liver rapidly resynthesizes these such that they can be replaced in a matter of days to weeks. Likewise, the liver is also the major site of synthesis of proteins that contribute to blood clotting, including prothrombin and several clotting factors. These metabolic events depend on the availability of vitamin K.

The liver also serves to detoxify the blood of substances that originate from the gut or elsewhere in the body. In part, this detoxification function is a physical one, in that the liver is highly active in removing particulates from the portal blood, such as small numbers of colonic bacteria that may cross the wall of the intestine under normal circumstances and evade the lymph nodes, but would potentially be harmful if allowed access to the remainder of the circulation. The majority of this "blood cleansing" is provided for by specialized cells related to blood macrophages, known as Kupffer cells. These are highly effective phagocytes that are strategically located to be exposed to the majority of the blood flow originating from the gut.

Other detoxification functions of the liver are biochemical in nature. Hepatocytes express large numbers of cytochrome P450 and other enzymes that can convert xenobiotics, including drugs and toxins, to inactive, less lipophilic metabolites that can subsequently be excreted into the bile and thereby eliminated from the body. Indeed, the oral availability of many drugs is compromised by highly effective removal of such agents arriving in the portal blood, in a process known as *first-pass metabolism*, of which you will learn more in pharmacology lectures. In general, hepatic metabolism of xenobiotics is divided into phase I metabolism (oxidation, hydroxylation, and other reactions mediated by cytochrome P450s) followed by phase II esterification reactions that link the products to another molecule such as sulfate, glucuronic acid, amino acids, or glutathione. Occasionally, liver metabolism of specific drugs can lead to the production of toxic intermediates, particularly if an overdose is ingested, overwhelming normal pathways of safe metabolism. This scenario accounts for the liver injury that can ensue if patients ingest an overdose of acetaminophen (Tylenol). In addition to the metabolism of xenobiotics, the liver is responsible for the metabolism and excretion of a wide variety of hormones and other endogenous regulators that circulate in the bloodstream, thereby terminating their activity. In particular, the liver is responsible for essentially all of the metabolism of the various steroid hormones such as estrogen, cortisol, and aldosterone. As we saw for glucose homeostasis, liver disease can result in abnormal steroid metabolism and resulting overactivity of the associated hormonal systems.

Excretion of Lipid-Soluble Waste Products

The renal system is the major contributor to the excretion of water-soluble end products of metabolism in the body. However, the kidneys cannot dispose of lipophilic molecules and heavy metals that circulate in protein-bound form in the plasma, and as such cannot enter the glomerular filtrate. Instead, these are handled by the liver, and excreted in the bile. Hepatocytes express a family of specific transport proteins on their apical and basolateral domains. These recognize high-molecular-weight organic anions and cations, and mediate their vectorial transport into the bile, as will be discussed in more detail in Chapters 11 and 13. In turn, the biliary system is designed to convey these substances out of the liver and into the intestinal lumen, where they undergo little if any reabsorption and thus can be eliminated from the body in the feces.

ENGINEERING CONSIDERATIONS

Based on the foregoing discussion of the major functions fulfilled by the liver, we can begin to consider the design of the organ that is necessary to support these functions. Principally, these include the need for the hepatocyte mass, as well as the Kupffer cells, to be exposed to large volumes of blood, a design that provides for rapid exchange of solutes, including macromolecules, between the various cell types in the liver, and a ductular system to convey excreted substances out of the liver. The liver is also divided into various macroscopic divisions known as lobes, but these are distinguished only by their anatomy and blood supply. With respect to physiologic functions, all lobes of the liver are equivalent.

Blood Supply

HEPATIC MACRO- AND MICROCIRCULATION

The liver is unique among all of the organs of the body in that it receives the vast majority of its blood supply in the form of venous blood, especially in the postprandial period. Even at rest, blood flow to the liver via the portal vein is at a rate of 1300 mL/min, compared to only 500 mL/min supplied by the hepatic artery. Moreover, the proportion of blood flow supplied to the liver by the portal vein may increase to almost 90% in the period immediately after a meal. A schematic diagram of the splanchnic circulation is provided in Figure 10–1. Note that the portal vein is the confluence of the splenic, superior mesenteric and inferior mesenteric veins, and thus drains the spleen, stomach, pancreas, small intestine, and colon. It is also notable that while the splanchnic organs represent only 5% of adult body mass, they receive 25% of cardiac output, third in mass/perfusion mismatch behind only the brain and kidneys. Thus, the liver receives a blood supply that contains disproportionate amounts of both oxygen and nutrients compared with its weight.

At a microscopic level, blood perfuses the liver via a series of *sinusoids*, which are low-resistance cavities that receive blood supply both from branches of the portal vein and from the hepatic artery. At rest, many of these sinusoids are collapsed, whereas as portal blood flow to the liver increases coincident with ingestion and absorption of a meal, sinusoids are gradually recruited to allow the perfusion of the liver with a much greater volume per unit time but only a minimal increase in pressure. The liver also has a distinctive morphologic organization that underpins its functions. This organization is based on the so-called *hepatic triad* of branches of the portal vein, the hepatic artery, and

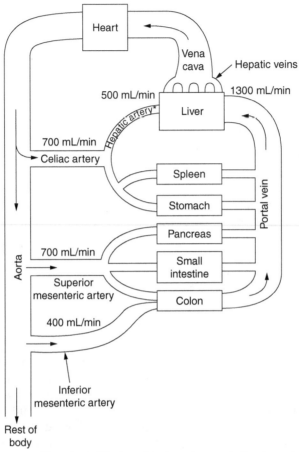

Figure 10-1. Schematic of the splanchnic circulation under fasting conditions. Note that even during fasting, the liver receives the majority of its blood supply via the portal vein.

the bile ducts. Blood flows into a branch of the portal vein in the center of portal areas, which are linked by anastomosing cords of cuboidal hepatocytes to a central venule that in turn drains into the hepatic vein. Branches of the hepatic artery likewise run close to the bile ducts, and likely play an important role in supplying energy and nutrients to the bile duct epithelial cells to support their transport functions. A diagram showing the interrelationships of the various cell types that make up the liver is shown in Figure 10-2.

ENTEROHEPATIC CIRCULATION

The circulatory features of the liver are also notable for the fact that some substances circulate continuously between the liver and intestine, in a circuit known

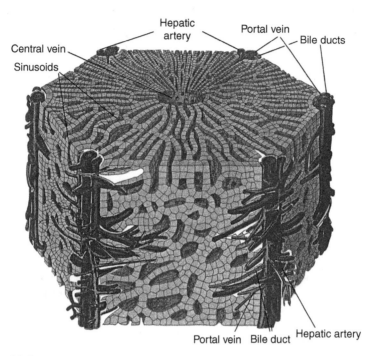

Figure 10–2. Arrangement of blood vessels, bile ducts, and hepatocytes to form the liver lobule. Branches of the portal vein and hepatic artery run parallel to bile ducts in the so-called *portal triads*. Blood percolates through sinusoids arranged between the hepatocytes, to be collected eventually in the central vein. (From Ross MH, Reith EJ. *Histology. A Text and Atlas.* New York: Harper and Row; 1985.)

as the enterohepatic circulation. The enterohepatic circulation in fact involves passage of solutes through three different environments—the portal vein and the sinusoids into which it empties, the biliary system, and the intestinal lumen (Figure 10–3). Thus, the requirement for a solute that enters into the enterohepatic circulation is that it be transported into hepatocytes and secreted into bile, then reabsorbed at an appreciable rate (either actively or passively) from the intestinal lumen. Most notably, this occurs for the bile acids that are utilized during intestinal lipid digestion and absorption, of which we will learn more later, but certain drugs and their metabolites may also circulate via this route, altering their pharmacokinetics. The physiological significance of this circuit is that it permits the secretion rate to greatly exceed the synthesis or input rate.

Hepatic Parenchyma and Sinusoids

The transport and metabolic functions of the liver center predominantly on the cells making up its parenchyma, the hepatocytes (80% of the total cells, approximately 100 billion in an adult human liver). Nevertheless, the nonparenchymal

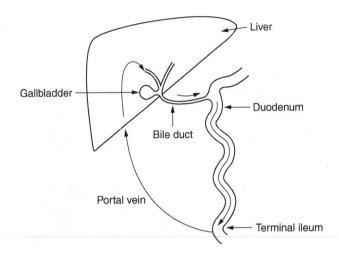

Figure 10–3. Schematic of the enterohepatic circulation of conjugated bile acids. Bile acids secreted by hepatocytes enter the bile and flow through the biliary system to the duodenum. Conjugated bile acids are selectively reabsorbed in the terminal ileum, and flow through the portal vein back to the liver to be reabsorbed by hepatocytes and resecreted.

cell types, including stellate cells, sinusoidal endothelial cells, and previously mentioned Kupffer cells, also play vital roles. In this section, we will review the distinctive structures of these cells and the extracellular environments in which they reside, as well as how their properties contribute to the physiological functions of the liver.

HEPATOCYTES

Hepatocytes are the metabolic "factories" of the liver, and are responsible for most of its characteristic functions. Hepatocytes are highly specialized polarized epithelial cells. Their apical membranes are in the form of grooves between adjacent cells, known as canaliculi (Figure 10–4). The canaliculi form a continuous network that drains eventually into the bile ductules (Figure 10–5). On the opposing pole of the hepatocyte, the basolateral membrane faces the bloodstream in the form of the hepatic sinusoids. Although the geometry of hepatocytes is more complex than that of a simple columnar epithelium, such as is found lining the intestine, it may nevertheless be helpful to consider both in similar functional terms. Thus, the hepatocyte apical membranes are formally contiguous with the outside world, analogous to the continuous plate of the apical membrane presented by enterocytes. Also as seen in a simple columnar epithelium, the apical and basolateral membranes of hepatocytes are separated by tight junctions that define the canaliculi. These junctions are relatively permeable, however, permitting the passage of glucose and other small solutes.

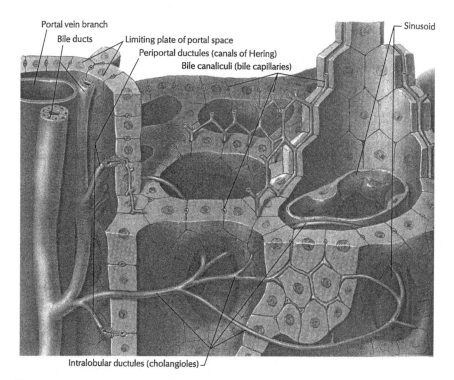

Figure 10-4. Structure of the intrahepatic biliary system. The bile canalicili, which are actually made up of the apical membranes of adjacent hepatocytes, empty into intra-lobular ductules and eventually into the bile ducts of the portal triad. (From Hansen JT, Koeppen BM. Netter's *Atlas of Human Physiology*. New Jersey: Icon Learning Systems; 2002.)

Hepatocytes all possess the capacity for a similar set of metabolic and transport functions. However, there is evidence to suggest that their actual functions, as expressed *in vivo*, may represent a continuum that relates to their position relative to the portal and hepatic veins. This concept of *zonation* holds that hepatocytes closest to the portal vein, which are referred to as "zone 1" or "periportal" cells and receive blood that is relatively rich in oxygen and nutrients, are responsible for the majority of detoxification and secretory functions under normal circumstances. However, if liver function is compromised, cells in zones 2 and 3, progressively closer to the hepatic vein, can be recruited, analogous to the "anatomic reserve" we will consider in the intestine. Thus, the liver recapitulates the general truism that the gastrointestinal system normally displays excess capacity for its essential functions. The zonation of hepatocyte functions also impacts on their susceptibility to injury. For example, if blood supply to the liver is compromised, hepatocytes in zone 3 are most sensitive to hypoxia, whereas oxidant injury produced by reperfusion of a previously ischemic organ is usually most marked in zone 1. Inspection

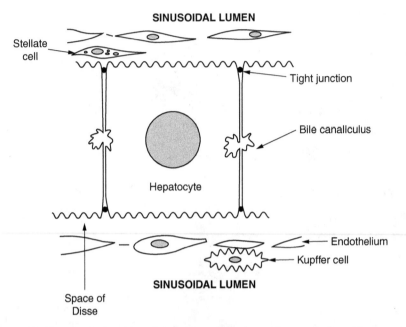

SINUSOIDAL LUMEN

Stellate cell

Tight junction

Bile canaliculus

Hepatocyte

Endothelium

Kupffer cell

SINUSOIDAL LUMEN

Space of Disse

Figure 10–5. Interrelationships of the major cell types making up the liver. Hepatocytes are arranged in plates joined by tight junctions, and their apical membranes make up the bile canaliculi. Hepatocytes are segregated from the blood-filled sinusoids by fenestrated endothelial cells without a basement membrane, and by a loose connective tissue layer known as the space of Disse. Kupffer cells reside in the sinusoidal lumen, whereas stellate cells are found in the space of Disse.

of the pattern of hepatocyte injury relative to liver structure may therefore provide clues about the etiology of liver disease.

A final striking property of hepatocytes is their ability to regenerate if a portion of the liver is lost or removed surgically. In fact, if a segment of the liver is removed, over a period of only days, the remaining hepatocytes will proliferate by undergoing mitosis once or twice to replace the lost tissue mass until an equivalent weight has been accomplished. In animal models, up to 70% of total liver mass can be regenerated in this way, even in adult animals. The cues that drive this remarkable regenerative process, and indeed those that arrest it once the original liver size has been accomplished, are topics of active investigation. Both humoral factors released secondary to the increased metabolic demands imposed on the liver remnant, and hemodynamic cues related to the more generous blood supply per unit mass, have been suggested. In any case, hepatic regeneration has the very practical implication that liver transplantation can often be accomplished with the transfer of only a segment of donor liver, including from a living donor, which has obvious beneficial effects when the supply of donor organs is insufficient to meet demands.

KUPFFER CELLS

Kupffer cells arise from the macrophage lineage, and line the sinusoidal epithelium on the bloodstream side (Figure 10–5). They are presumed to play a major role in host defense, by virtue of their highly active phagocytic properties. Their location is such that they are exposed to virtually all of the portal blood flow, where they serve as a sentinel for particulates arising from the intestine, such as bacteria. Kupffer cells also express cell-surface receptors for altered proteins, such as Fc immunoglobulin receptors that can be used to internalize foreign proteins or microorganisms that have been coated with host antibodies. Activation of Kupffer cells may result in the production of cytokines and other inflammatory mediators that potentially can contribute to liver injury, especially to the adjacent sinusoidal endothelial cells.

SINUSOIDAL ENDOTHELIUM

The endothelial cells that line the hepatic sinusoids have two characteristic properties that distinguish them from endothelial cells in most other organs of the body. First, they are extensively perforated by large intracellular pores known as fenestrae, which are 100–200 nm in diameter. These are designed to permit the passage of even quite large macromolecules out of the blood, including albumin with bound ligands (such as various lipids) as well as lipoproteins, while preventing the passage of formed elements (red blood cells, white blood cells, and platelets) as well as intact chylomicrons. Second, sinusoidal endothelial cells in the healthy liver are not invested with a basement membrane. Like their fenestrae, the lack of a basement membrane is a design feature that increases endothelial permeability to solutes arising from the bloodstream. In total, therefore, the sinusoidal endothelium presents virtually no barrier to the efflux of albumin and other similarly sized molecules from the vascular space.

Passage of macromolecules, such as albumin and chylomicron remnants derived from ingested lipids, out of the bloodstream is also enhanced in the sinusoids by a process known as *forced sieving*. Thus, fast-moving blood cells physically press molecules against endothelial fenestrae, forcing them out into the space of Disse (Figure 10–6). This further enhances the ability of hepatocytes to be exposed to a high proportion of the substances in the blood flow received by the liver. However, fenestrae are not fixed structures. Sinusoidal endothelial cells are contractile and responsive to various hormones and neurotransmitters, which may acutely alter the diameter of the fenestrae. Evidence suggests that maintenance of the fenestrae also requires the input of cellular energy, and a variety of hepatotoxins may result in their disappearance, with effects on the ability of the liver to perform normal transport of solutes. In fact, fenestrae are regulated by the actin cytoskeleton, and in the absence of key factors that scaffold cytoskeletal reorganization, the liver cannot develop properly due to hepatocyte injury. Likewise, in liver diseases that are associated with activation of fibrotic changes, a basement membrane may be laid down, further impairing endothelial permeability.

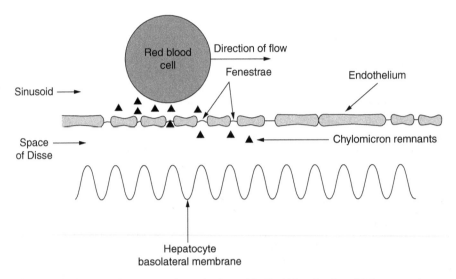

Figure 10–6. Forced sieving in hepatic sinusoids. Red blood cells, which are too large to pass through endothelial fenestrations, force smaller particles such as chylomicron remnants into the space of Disse where they can interact with the basement membranes of hepatocytes.

SPACE OF DISSE

The space of Disse (pronounced Diss-eh), named after a German anatomist who first described it in the late 1800s, is a space containing a layer of loose connective tissue that lies between the sinusoidal endothelium and the basolateral membrane of hepatocytes. It is notable for the fact that it contains a simpler set of extracellular matrix molecules than found in other epithelial tissues, rendering the space highly permeable to the bidirectional exchange of solutes between the sinusoidal blood flow and hepatocytes. Indeed, by virtue of the fenestrations in sinusoidal endothelial cells, it is functionally contiguous with the plasma for molecules up to and including small proteins. However, in disease, excess collagen may be deposited in the space of Disse, reducing the rate at which macromolecules can traverse it.

HEPATIC STELLATE CELLS

Hepatic stellate cells, previously also referred to as Ito cells, are star-shaped cells that reside in the space of Disse. They play an important role in the normal liver by storing a variety of lipids, most notably vitamin A in esterified form. Hepatic stellate cells have been calculated to store approximately 80% of the body's complement of retinoids. In addition, these cells are contractile, and may be involved in the regulation of sinusoidal diameter, although their precise physiological significance in health is unknown. However, it is clear that stellate cells play a critical role in liver injury. In response to inflammatory cytokines and other stimuli, they undergo a morphological and functional transformation referred to as activation, which involves the loss of stores of vitamin A and a dramatic upregulation in the production of extracellular matrix materials, such as collagen. This collagen is deposited in the space of Disse and impairs hepatic function.

Biliary Tract and Gallbladder

The third functional division of the liver is concerned with the production and transport of bile out of the liver and into the gastrointestinal lumen. The functional anatomy of the biliary system is depicted in Figure 10–7. Bile drains from the liver via the right and left hepatic ducts that join to form the common hepatic duct. A cystic duct diverts bile for storage into the gallbladder. The anastomosis of the common hepatic duct and the cystic duct forms the common bile duct, which transfers bile to the sphincter of Oddi. Here, biliary secretions mix with those coming from the pancreas, and flow into the duodenal lumen in a controlled fashion when the sphincter relaxes in response to neurohumoral influences discussed previously.

At a functional level, the biliary system can be divided into four components. First, the canaliculi, which are comprised of the adjacent apical membranes of hepatocyte couplets, actually form the initial biliary secretion. This secretion is then modified as it flows along the biliary ductules, which are analogous to pancreatic ducts. The ductules are made up of columnar epithelial cells ("cholangiocytes") and both absorb and secrete various substances into and out of the bile. The ductules are perfused by a capillary network arising from the hepatic artery, rather than from the sinusoids. The majority of this periductular capillary plexus drains into the sinusoids. Flow in the periductular capillary plexus is in the opposite direction to bile flow, which has implications for the modification of bile

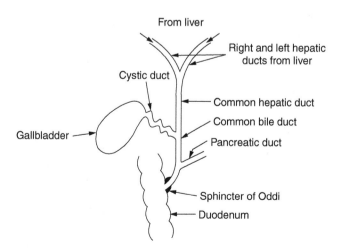

Figure 10–7. Functional anatomy of the biliary system.

composition as it flows along the ductules. For example, glucose, which enters the bile across the canalicular tight junctions, is actively scavenged as the bile flows through the smallest bile ductules, and can then be returned to the sinusoids. The larger bile ductules dilute and alkalinize the bile, again analogous to the function of the pancreatic ducts.

The bile ducts serve simply as conduits for the bile without modifying its composition significantly, other than by adding mucus from peribiliary glands. Mucus secretion presumably serves to protect the ductular epithelium from potentially injurious surfactant effects of the bile itself, and may also protect against bacterial invasion of the biliary tract. It is also notable that the cystic duct has a spiral lumen. This is believed to increase the level of turbulence in ductular flow, thereby decreasing the risk that concentrated bile will precipitate and form stones. Finally, between meals, bile is stored in the gallbladder, which is a blind sac lined by highly absorptive epithelial cells linked by well-developed tight junctions. The gallbladder serves not only to store bile, but also to concentrate it, via mechanisms that we will discuss in Chapter 12. However, the gallbladder is not essential to life and can be removed without compromising nutrition. In this case, the bile acid pool is relocated to the small intestine, which may cause a minor impairment in fat digestion. Patients who lack their gallbladder therefore tolerate large, fatty meals with great difficulty.

PATHOPHYSIOLOGY AND CLINICAL CORRELATIONS

 Based on the foregoing discussion of liver anatomy, we now turn to a consideration of several conditions where the architecture of the liver is deranged, leading to impaired hepatic function.

ACUTE LIVER FAILURE

As might be predicted by our discussions of the myriad vital roles played by the liver in normal homeostasis, a sudden and significant loss in the metabolic capacity of the liver for detoxification and bile secretion has profound consequences for the patient. The majority of cases of acute liver failure in the United States are caused by reactions to drugs, either in response to inappropriately high doses (overdoses or suicide attempts) or as idiosyncratic reactions in uniquely sensitive individuals. Infections (e.g., acute viral hepatitis) or environmental toxins are also recognized causes of liver failure. While many etiologies for drug-induced acute liver failure are possible, overall there is usually direct hepatocyte necrosis and/or apoptosis, either produced by a toxic drug metabolite, or as a result of immunologic injury in response to adducts of drug metabolites and cytochrome P450 enzymes. Some drugs can be specifically toxic toward the bile ducts or canaliculi, resulting in acute cholestasis (a failure of bile to reach the duodenum); the bile acids and other biliary constituents that thereby accumulate in the liver in turn exert toxic effects.

Patients suffering from acute liver failure typically present initially with jaundice (a yellow coloration of the skin ascribable to retained bilirubin); this then progresses rapidly to altered mentation, confusion, and coma (due to increases in plasma ammonia and hypoglycemia), together with disorders of blood coagulation. Liver failure is also predictably accompanied by problems with a host of body systems, including cardiovascular and renal abnormalities. In most cases, treatment is mostly supportive, particularly if the causative agent has been identified and discontinued. In the specific case of liver failure associated with acetaminophen overdose (the most common single cause of acute liver failure in the United States), administration of N-acetylcysteine given soon after the overdose is associated with therapeutic benefit, most likely by increasing the capacity of the liver to convert toxic metabolites of the drug to glutathione conjugates that can safely be eliminated. Overall, the only definitive treatment for worsening acute liver failure is transplantation, although experimental extracorporeal liver support devices ("artificial livers" that can reproduce some, if not all, of the metabolic functions of the liver) may yield new therapeutic options in the future.

Hepatitis, Fibrosis, and Cirrhosis

Hepatitis refers to liver inflammation. Fibrosis and cirrhosis refer to reversible and irreversible deposition of excess collagen in the liver, respectively, reducing the effective hepatic mass, compressing sinusoids, and causing an increase in resistance to blood flow that in turn causes portal hypertension. The two major causes of all of these outcomes in adults are chronic alcohol abuse and viral hepatitis.

ALCOHOLIC CIRRHOSIS

Chronic ingestion of excessive quantities of alcohol can have insidious effects on hepatic function, as fibrotic hardening of the liver alters several aspects of structure and function. Indeed, alcohol abuse is one of the most important causes of chronic liver disease, and cirrhosis accounts for the majority of all medical deaths among alcoholics. While liver injury is related to the cumulative amount of alcohol consumed, it remains an unsolved mystery as to why only a subset of alcoholics develops hepatitis and cirrhosis. There are strong data suggesting a genetic component to the development of alcoholism but much less evidence that genetic factors play a role in the risk of alcoholic liver disease.

The majority of ingested ethanol is metabolized rapidly in the liver. Products of ethanol metabolism, most notably acetaldehyde, impair several aspects of hepatocyte metabolic function, as well as producing oxidative stress and forming protein adducts that may trigger adverse immune reactions that lead to cell death. In its initial stages, alcoholic liver disease involves the accumulation of fat in the liver. Ultimately, hepatic stellate cells are activated to produce collagen, and this occurs chronically if ingestion of excessive amounts of alcohol continues. Activation of the stellate cells apparently results from the activity of cytokines produced by Kupffer cells, in response to toxins arriving from the gut as well as oxidative stress and immunologic activation. In a subset of patients, hepatitis and fibrosis will progress to cirrhosis, characterized by fibrous bands connecting the portal triads with central veins, and small, regenerative nodules.

Patients with alcoholic liver disease that has progressed at least to hepatitis and fibrosis present with a spectrum of symptoms of chronic liver failure, including jaundice, nausea, and malaise. Male patients may have hypogonadism and feminization, ascribable both to the direct toxic effects of ethanol on testicular Leydig cells as well as effects on estrogen production and reduced estrogen breakdown. In severe cases, there can be ascites (often infected), hepatic encephalopathy, renal failure, and eventually death. The primary treatment is to secure abstinence from alcohol, although some liver changes may be irreversible even after drinking has stopped. Most liver-transplant programs will now consider alcoholics as candidates for transplantation after a minimum period of abstinence, although this remains controversial in the setting of inadequate organ supply and evidence for rising rates of recidivism with longer follow-up.

VIRAL HEPATITIS

Infections with a series of viruses that are trophic for the liver are increasingly important causes of chronic liver disease. Infection with the hepatitis C virus, in particular, is expected to produce an epidemic of liver disease in the coming years, since it has been estimated that 2% of the world's population is chronically infected. A subset of these patients will also be expected to progress to the development of hepatocellular carcinoma. While some patients infected with hepatitis viruses will develop an acute illness, in some cases severe enough to precipitate acute liver failure, most are asymptomatic in the early stages of infection, developing hepatitis and the sequelae of fibrosis and cirrhosis only later as a consequence of immune cell activation. Of the five known hepatitis viruses that infect humans, hepatitis B, C, and D viruses appear to have the propensity to progress to chronic hepatitis, with hepatitis A and E viruses causing acute viral hepatitis. In general, hepatitis viruses may have direct cytopathic effects on the hepatocytes they infect, but more likely the most important factor in the generation of liver injury is the immune response provoked by the infection. The clinical consequences in the subset of patients who progress to cirrhosis are similar to those seen in other causes of chronic liver failure, such as discussed earlier for alcoholic liver disease. Most patients, however, may develop nothing more than a chronic, asymptomatic elevation in liver enzymes, without markers of liver disease. Newly available directly acting antiviral agents offer hope for higher rates of viral clearance, particularly in patients infected with hepatitis C virus.

Portal Hypertension

Portal hypertension refers to conditions where the resistance to blood flow across the liver is increased, which can have several causes and results in a variety of problems. As we have already discussed, the liver has a very low resistance vasculature in health, and pressures increase little as flow increases as additional sinusoids can be recruited. However, in several liver diseases, inflammatory responses trigger hepatic stellate cells to increase collagen production, reducing permeability across the sinusoidal endothelium and space of Disse and impairing liver function due to the associated fibrosis. The hardening of the liver impedes flow through the sinusoids. Some of the sinusoids and liver parenchyma may also be destroyed and replaced by fibrous tissue, further impairing liver function.

The most obvious clinical consequence of portal hypertension is a condition known as ascites. Because the hepatic sinusoids and space of Disse are very permeable and allow albumin to pass, large quantities of lymph are produced by the liver even in health, and are collected by a series of lymph ducts that eventually return the fluid to the blood via the thoracic duct. However, when portal hypertension develops, plasma transudation increases and overwhelms the hepatic lymphatics, which may themselves be compromised by liver fibrosis. The resulting fluid, which contains almost as much albumin as the plasma, weeps from the surface of the liver and accumulates in the peritoneal cavity. In advanced liver disease, many liters of fluid may be found, and such patients are treated with diuretics and sodium restriction, or if refractory, by periodically removing the fluid percutaneously. Although liver disease can also result in hypoalbuminemia due to reduced synthetic function of hepatocytes, albumin infusions are not a useful treatment for ascites because the major driving force for fluid loss from the liver is the increased pressure in a highly permeable vascular bed, rather than a fall in plasma oncotic pressure. The development of ascites is a serious complication of chronic liver disease and reflects decompensation. Approximately 50% of patients with cirrhotic ascites will die in 2 years if they do not receive a liver transplant.

Another consequence of portal hypertension is the development of collateral blood vessels to surrounding structures. These form in an attempt to bypass the blockage to portal flow posed by the hardened liver, and reconnect to the systemic circulation. If the collateral vessels link to the esophagus, they are referred to as "esophageal varices" and are vulnerable to erosion and rupture, particularly if their internal pressure is high. Rupture of such varices represents a major medical emergency due to the challenges involved in reestablishing hemostasis, which is usually done endoscopically by ligating the varices. Ruptured varices are also at high risk for rebleeding. Variceal pressures can be reduced by constructing a surgical shunt between the portal vein and the systemic circulation, although doing so diverts portal blood from any remaining functional liver parenchyma, and thus increases complications associated with the loss of the detoxifying functions of hepatocytes.

Liver Transplantation

 The definitive treatment for end-stage liver disease is transplantation. In the 50 years since this surgery was first successfully accomplished, it has become a highly effective treatment for patients with advanced disease. The majority of patients undergoing liver transplantation will survive for more than 5 years, and many recover sufficiently to resume active lives and paid employment. The success of liver transplantation, however, is markedly limited by a crisis in the availability of donor organs; many more patients are added to transplant waiting lists every year than are transplants performed, leading to an increasing proportion of patients dying while waiting for a liver. Advances in the application of partial liver transplants from either cadaveric or living donors, taking advantage of the liver's capacity to regenerate itself to match its final size to body mass, is gradually increasing the number of transplants that can be performed. Indeed, transplantation from a living related donor has become almost standard for pediatric recipients, although there remain ethical issues around living-related liver transplantation because it carries inherent risks for the healthy donor.

Liver transplantation involves removal of the diseased liver from the recipient, followed by implantation of the donor organ and reconnection of its vascular and biliary systems to those of the recipient. Many patients who undergo this surgery experience dramatic improvement in their hepatic function and overall quality of life, although this comes at the price of life-long immunosuppression and attendant risks. Likewise, many patients will experience acute episodes of graft rejection, although increasingly these can be managed medically and do not seem to impact on long-term survival of the graft. Other complications of liver transplantation include vascular thrombosis (which may require retransplantation), biliary complications such as leaks and strictures, or recurrent disease in the graft, especially if the indication for transplantation has been viral hepatitis or hepatocellular carcinoma. Nevertheless, rapid improvements in therapeutic approaches to the complications of liver transplantation have markedly increased survival rates, and the success of this treatment strongly underscores the physiological role of the liver in a multitude of important body systems and functions.

Methods for Assessment of Liver Injury and Liver Function

Blood tests remain a mainstay for the diagnosis of a patient with suspected liver disease or to stage patients with known liver disease. In general, the goal of such tests is to detect the release of products that are characteristic of the liver into the bloodstream, thereby indicating liver cell injury. Similarly, accumulation of molecules normally excreted via the biliary system is indicative of a failure in liver function, although further tests are necessary to assess the site at which the defect is occurring.

Two enzymes referred to as transaminases are easily measured in the serum, and are sensitive markers of liver cell injury. Alanine aminotransferase (ALT) is produced by hepatocytes, and when these cells are injured, its circulating levels are increased. Aspartate aminotransferase (AST) is similarly increased in the setting of hepatocellular injury, although it is less specific for liver disease because it is also produced by other tissues. For example, AST levels are increased following cardiac injury, such as a myocardial infarction. Nevertheless, measurement of AST remains useful in the setting of clinical symptoms consistent with liver disease, particularly because it appears to be disproportionately elevated in patients whose liver injury is related to alcohol abuse. Measurements of ALT and AST over time are also used to assess the progress of established liver disease. It is important to remember, however, that elevations in transaminases can only occur if there is ongoing hepatocellular death. In cirrhosis, where large portions of the liver may be replaced by fibrous tissue, little new cell injury may be occurring and thus ALT and AST levels may not be elevated.

Two other enzymes are useful markers of injury to the biliary system. Alkaline phosphatase, while not specific to the liver (being produced also by bone, the intestine and placenta), is expressed as a membrane protein in the canaliculus. In the setting of localized obstruction to the biliary tree, alkaline phosphatase levels in the serum are increased. Similarly, gamma glutamyltranspeptidase (GGT) is localized predominantly to the apical membrane of cholangiocytes, although some is also expressed in the bile canaliculi. Serum elevations in GGT are therefore largely reflective of cholangiocyte injury.

The foregoing tests, while often referred to as "liver function" tests, are not strictly measures of actual hepatic function. To assess whether liver function is impaired, other tests are needed. One such test that is very important clinically is the measurement of bilirubin. Handling of bilirubin by the liver will be discussed in greater detail in Chapter 13, but for now, suffice to say that accumulation of bilirubin in the circulation indicates cholestasis, which can result from injury to either hepatocytes or cholangiocytes, or obstruction within the biliary system. Based on the discussion of the synthetic functions of the liver, it should be easy to understand that liver function can also be assessed by measuring levels of its various products in the circulation. The most useful tests are to measure serum albumin, and a blood clotting parameter, the prothrombin time. Tests of coagulation are not specific for liver disease and thus must be interpreted in the context of other findings. Patients with suspected liver disease are also often evaluated for serum glucose and ammonia levels, since hypoglycemia and hyperammonemia are major problems in the setting of liver failure.

Biopsies and imaging tests also play a major role in the evaluation of liver disease. Liver biopsies, which are usually obtained by inserting a needle into the liver percutaneously, can be used to evaluate the extent of liver fibrosis, or to search for evidence of rejection in a previously transplanted liver. A widely applied imaging technique is referred to as ERCP, which stands for endoscopic retrograde cholangiopancreatography. In this procedure, a special endoscope is introduced into the duodenum via the mouth, and used to insert a small tube through the sphincter of Oddi, through which contrast medium is injected. Subsequent x-rays can then visualize the drainage routes from the biliary system and pancreas, which permits the diagnosis of obstructions (such as by a gallstone) or strictures. Other imaging modalities, such as magnetic resonance imaging, are also assuming an increasing role in assessing liver disease and the architecture of the biliary system.

The prognosis of end-stage liver disease, and by extension the urgency of transplantation, has commonly been assessed by calculating the so-called Child–Pugh score, which takes into account 5 measures of hepatic function—bilirubin, serum albumin, prothrombin time, and the presence and severity of both ascites and hepatic encephalopathy. The Child–Pugh score was originally designed as a predictor of surgical mortality in liver disease patients. More recently, the Child–Pugh score has been supplemented by the Model for End-Stage Liver Disease (MELD) score, which weights serum bilirubin, creatinine, and prothrombin time to predict survival. Patients awaiting liver transplantation in the United States are now prioritized on the basis of their MELD score, which results in the allocation of organs first to those who are sickest. This has reduced waiting-list mortality without impairing post-transplant outcomes.

KEY CONCEPTS

 Functions of the liver and biliary system include glucose storage and release, protein synthesis, detoxification of xenobiotics and ammonia, metabolism of endogenous hormones, initial handling of substances absorbed from the intestine, and excretion of lipophilic molecules and heavy metals in the bile.

 Functions of the liver are facilitated by its unique circulatory features. Blood arrives at the liver via two routes: the portal vein, which drains blood from the intestine, and the hepatic artery.

 Blood percolates through the liver via a low-resistance system of sinusoids that maximizes exposure of hepatocytes to the blood's contents.

 The functions of the liver are also subserved by specific cell types that assume specific anatomic relationships. Hepatocytes conduct the majority of the metabolic functions of the liver and produce the initial biliary secretion.

 Kupffer cells line the sinusoids and cleanse the blood of particulates, such as bacteria.

 The endothelial cells of the liver have large fenestrations that allow small proteins and other molecules to leave the circulation, but retain blood cells and intact chylomicrons.

 Hepatic stellate cells are contractile and likely regulate sinusoidal caliber. In health, they also store retinoids. In disease, they play an important role in generating fibrosis.

 Liver failure due to damage to the liver cells or to the biliary system, or blockade of biliary drainage, results in a host of systemic problems.

 The definitive treatment for end-stage liver failure is transplantation, although poor availability of donor organs limits the effectiveness of this treatment. The liver has a remarkable regenerative capacity that allows partial transplants and also can restore liver function after an acute insult.

 Biochemical tests of specific serum components can be used to assess either liver injury or liver function. Combinations of these measures predict the prognosis of end-stage liver disease to allocate organs for transplantation. Imaging techniques also play important roles in diagnosis and management.

STUDY QUESTIONS

10–1. In a patient with end-stage liver disease, which of the following combinations of findings would be expected in the plasma?

	Albumin	**Glucose**	**Ammonia**
A.	Increased	Increased	Increased
B.	Decreased	Decreased	Decreased
C.	Increased	Decreased	Increased
D.	Decreased	Increased	Decreased
E.	Decreased	Decreased	Increased

10–2. A 60-year-old man comes to his physician complaining of a progressive increase in girth over several months, despite attempts to diet. He is suffering from jaundice and also complains of nausea and malaise. When a large needle is inserted into his abdomen, several liters of tan fluid drain out. An increase in which of the following does not account for this accumulation of fluid?

A. Portal pressure

B. Hepatic collagen

C. Plasma albumin

D. Stellate cell activity

E. Plasma transudation

10–3. The liver is responsible for removing the small numbers of bacteria that enter the portal circulation from the intestines. Which cell type fulfills this function?

A. Sinusoidal epithelial cells

B. Cholangiocytes

C. Hepatocytes

D. Kupffer cells

E. Stellate cells

10–4. A gallstone lodged in which of the following sites will result in increased bile acid flux through the hepatocytes making up the left side of the liver?

A. Cystic duct

B. Common hepatic duct

C. Right hepatic duct

D. Left hepatic duct

E. Common bile duct

10–5. What structure in the liver permits chylomicron remnants to access the basolateral membranes of hepatocytes?

A. Canaliculi

B. Sinusoidal fenestrae

C. Kupffer cells

D. Bile ducts

E. Tight junctions

SUGGESTED READINGS

Abshagen K, Eipel C, Vollmar B. A critical appraisal of the hemodynamic signal driving liver regeneration. *Langenbecks Arch Surg.* 2012;397:579–590.

Adam R, Hoti E. Liver transplantation: the current situation. *Semin Liver Dis.* 2009;29:3–18.

Battaller R, Brenner DA. Liver fibrosis. *J Clin Invest.* 2005;115:209–218.

Fraser R, Cogger VC, Dobbs B, Jamieson H, Warren A, Hilmer SN, Le Couteur DG. The liver sieve and atherosclerosis. *Pathology.* 2012;44:181–186.

Kanel GC. Liver: anatomy, microscopic structure and cell types. In: Yamada T, Alpers DH, Kalloo AN, Kaplowitz N, Owyang C, Powell DW, eds. *Textbook of Gastroenterology.* 5th ed. Chichester: Wiley-Blackwell; 2009:2057–2072.

Ross MH, Reith EJ. *Histology—A Text and Atlas.* New York: Harper and Row; 1988:472–482.

Tazaki T, Sasaki T, Uto K, Yamasaki N, Tashiro S, Sakai R, Tanaka M, Oda H, Honda Z, Honda H. p130Cas, Crk-associated substrate plays essential roles in liver development by regulating sinusoidal endothelial cell fenestration. *Hepatology.* 2010;52:1089–1099.

Watkins PB. Drug metabolism and transport in the liver and intestine. In: Yamada T, Alpers DH, Kalloo AN, Kaplowitz N, Owyang C, Powell DW, eds. *Textbook of Gastroenterology.* 5th ed. Chichester: Wiley-Blackwell; 2009:645–657.

Bile Formation and Secretion 11

OBJECTIVES

- ▶ *Understand the physiologic functions of bile as a route for excretion and in aiding in the digestion and absorption of dietary lipids*
- ▶ *Understand how bile acids are formed from cholesterol, how they are modified during gut passage, and their role in driving bile secretion*
  - ▶ Describe the mechanisms that regulate the rate of conversion of cholesterol into bile acids
- ▶ *Describe the major biliary lipids and how they are transported into the canaliculus*
- ▶ *Describe how the composition of bile is modified as the bile moves through the biliary ductules*
  - ▶ Define the cellular transport mechanisms that render bile alkaline
- ▶ *Understand the consequences of a failure to secrete bile, and conditions that cause this problem*

BASIC PRINCIPLES OF BILIARY EXCRETION AND SECRETION

Role and Significance

The liver fulfills its excretory function by producing bile, a lipid-rich solution designed to promote the elimination of hydrophobic solutes. Bile consists of a micellar solution in which bile acids, products of hepatocytes produced by the metabolism of cholesterol, form mixed micelles with phosphatidylcholine. These mixed micelles solubilize molecules that would otherwise have minimal aqueous solubility, such as cholesterol itself and a variety of xenobiotics. In addition to its role in providing for excretion of hydrophobic waste products, bile also plays an important role in the digestion and absorption of lipids ingested in the diet. Bile acids form mixed micelles with the products of lipid digestion, increasing the rate at which they can diffuse across the aqueous environment of the gastrointestinal lumen. While bile acids are not essential for the uptake of most fatty acids, which have appreciable aqueous solubility, they do markedly increase the efficiency of this process. On the other hand, insoluble dietary lipids, such as saturated long-chain fatty acids and fat-soluble vitamins, are almost entirely dependent on micellar solubilization for absorption. In patients suffering from cholestasis, deficiencies of fat soluble vitamins can occur. Bile acids also influence bacterial populations in the gut, both by being (in micellar form) directly antimicrobial, and by inducing the expression of genes that protect against bacterial overgrowth.

BILE ACID METABOLISM

Bile secretion in the liver is driven primarily by the active, ATP-dependent efflux of conjugated bile acids out of the hepatocyte into the canaliculus. In some animals, there is also a variable component of bile acid-independent bile flow, although the solutes that drive this secretion are not fully understood. But in humans, canalicular bile flow is almost entirely dependent on the secretion of bile acids. Thus, in this section, we will consider how bile acids are synthesized, and subsequent modifications to their structure that promote their role as biological detergents.

Formation of Bile Acids from Cholesterol

Bile acids are amphipathic end products of cholesterol metabolism. The term amphipathic refers to the fact that bile acids have both a hydrophobic and hydrophilic face, and form micelles. This is essential to their physiologic function, as will be discussed later.

Synthesis of bile acids from cholesterol occurs in the hepatocytes, and pericentral hepatocytes are believed to be most active in this regard. Changes to both the steroid nucleus of cholesterol, as well as to its alkyl side chain, are required to convert the highly insoluble cholesterol to the water-soluble bile acid product. Bile acid synthesis in healthy humans is at a rate of approximately 200–400 mg/day. The initial, and rate-limiting, step in bile acid formation is the hydroxylation of cholesterol at the 7 position of the steroid nucleus via the enzyme cholesterol 7α hydroxylase (CYP7A1) (Figure 11–1). Note that cholesterol already contains a hydroxyl group at the 3 position, and this is retained in all of the bile acids. However, the 3-hydroxy group in cholesterol is in the β-orientation, and this is converted to the α-position by a process known as epimerization. After these initial reactions, downstream pathways diverge to yield the two primary bile acids of humans. Thus, 7α hydroxycholesterol can be acted upon by a C27 hydroxylase and several other peroxisomal enzymes, which shorten the alkyl side chain and add a carboxylic acid function to yield the bile acid chenodeoxycholic acid. In the alternate pathway, activity of the C27 hydroxylase is preceded by that of 12α hydroxylase (CYP8B1), which adds a third hydroxyl group to the steroid nucleus, ultimately yielding the tri-hydroxy bile acid, cholic acid. Changes in the expression of CYP8B1, while not rate-limiting for bile formation, result in changes in the ratio of cholic to chenodeoxycholic acid, and may thereby alter the functional properties of the resulting bile. Note that all of the hydroxyl groups in the mature bile acids are in the form of α-epimers, and are thus oriented to the same face of the molecule. Cholesterol is a flat molecule, insoluble and a major membrane constituent. In contrast, bile acids are kinked molecules that are highly water soluble when ionized.

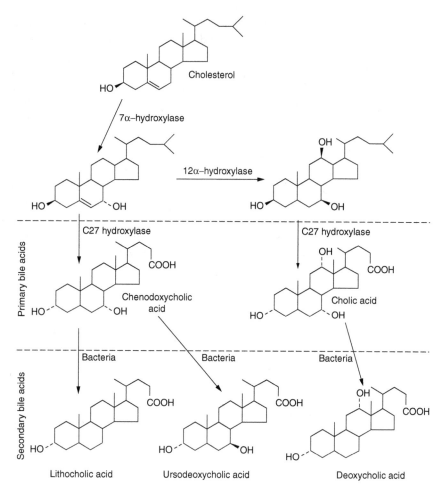

Figure 11–1. Structures of primary and secondary bile acids and their precursors. Primary bile acids are synthesized in the liver whereas secondary bile acids are produced in the colon by bacterial enzymes.

Primary and Secondary Bile Acids

In humans, the only bile acids generated directly from cholesterol by endogenous enzymes are the primary bile acids, chenodeoxycholic acid and cholic acid. However, when these bile acids enter the distal small intestine or the colon, they can be acted on by bacterial enzymes to yield secondary bile acids. The most important conversion is dehydroxylation of the 7 position of the steroid nucleus, to yield lithocholic acid from chenodeoxycholic acid, and deoxycholic acid from cholic acid. Trace amounts of a third secondary bile acid, ursodeoxycholic acid (so called because it is a prominent bile acid in bears), are also generated in humans by epimerization of the 7α hydroxyl group. Although only very little ursodeoxycholic acid is formed in humans, it is important to know about this compound because it is used therapeutically. The secondary bile acids are less water soluble than the primary bile acids. Lithocholic acid, in particular, is cytotoxic if present at high concentrations, and physiologic mechanisms have developed to limit its toxicity, particularly in the bile ductules, as will be described in more detail later.

Bile Acid Conjugation

Following hepatic synthesis, both chenodeoxycholic acid and cholic acid are then further modified in the hepatocyte by conjugating them to the amino group of either glycine or taurine in a stable amide linkage (Figure 11–2). Likewise, secondary bile acids that return to the liver are also conjugated with glycine or taurine in the hepatocyte. It is these conjugated bile acids that are the substrates for active transport across the canalicular membrane. Conjugation also renders the bile acids more water-soluble, and alters their physicochemical properties as will be discussed further later.

In addition to bacterial conversion of primary to secondary bile acids, bacteria can deconjugate both primary and secondary bile acids, making them more lipophilic. Unconjugated bile acids can be considered "damaged" and can be passively absorbed across the wall of the intestine. They then travel through the portal vein

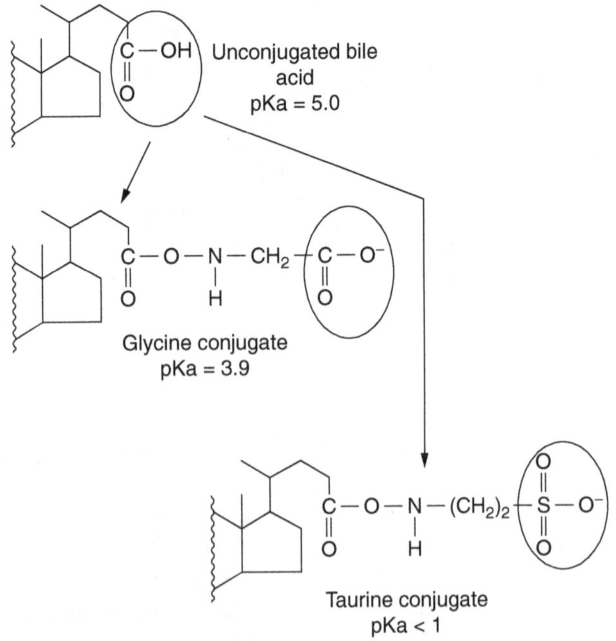

Figure 11–2. Conjugation of bile acids with either glycine or taurine reduces their pKa.

back to the liver, where they are reconjugated in the hepatocyte. Thus, all bile acids secreted by the hepatocyte are in their conjugated forms.

Special handling applies to the potentially toxic bile acid, lithocholic acid. In addition to conjugation with glycine or taurine, lithocholic acid is sulfated, particularly if present in abnormally high concentrations. This increases the hydrophilicity of the molecule and is therefore believed to reduce its cytotoxic effects, which might otherwise lead to liver injury, especially if bile flow is reduced. The sulfated conjugates of lithocholic acid also cannot be absorbed by the intestine, which results in their elimination from the pool of bile acids that circulate enterohepatically (of which more will be learned later).

Physicochemical Properties of Bile Acids

The reactions involved in bile acid biosynthesis yield amphipathic molecules with both hydrophobic and hydrophilic faces. This characteristic is vital to the physiologic function of these molecules. Although they have an appreciable solubility in water as monomers, above a certain concentration (called the critical micellar concentration, or CMC), bile acid molecules spontaneously self-associate into structures known as micelles, in which the hydrophobic faces are masked from the surrounding aqueous environment (Figure 11–3). However, simple micelles composed of bile acids alone do not exist in bile or intestinal content. In bile, bile acids form *mixed micelles* with phosphatidylcholine. In turn, these mixed micelles can serve as the "solvent" for hydrophobic molecules such as cholesterol or products of lipid digestion.

As noted earlier, conjugation also alters the physicochemical properties of bile acids. Most importantly, the process of conjugation decreases the pKa of bile acids from approximately 5 to 4 for glycine conjugates, or less than 2 for taurine conjugates (Figure 11–2). As a consequence, at physiologic pH, conjugated bile acids are fully ionized and are present in both bile and intestinal contents as anions. Due to this charge, conjugated bile acids are incapable of crossing cell membranes by passive means, needing instead an active transport mechanism for their secretion or uptake (Figure 11–4). This becomes important in allowing for appropriate enterohepatic circulation of bile acids in a manner coordinated with the period when they are needed to help digest the meal.

BILE COMPOSITION

Bile undergoes various alterations in its composition as it moves through the biliary system. These changes reflect both active and passive transport events and the activity of specific enzymes.

Canalicular Bile

 The secretion of bile begins when bile acids are actively secreted across the canalicular membrane. Because the bile acids constitute osmotically active particles, canalicular bile is transiently hyperosmotic. However, the

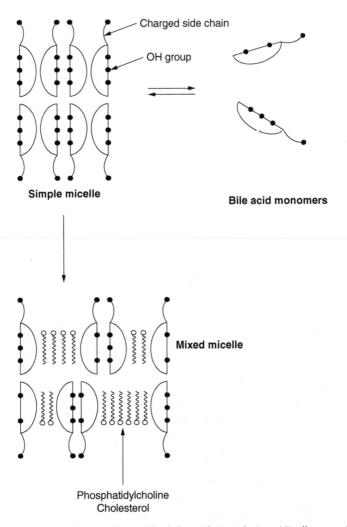

Figure 11–3. Physical forms adopted by bile acids in solution. Micelles are shown in cross-section, and are actually thought to be cylindrical in shape. Mixed micelles of bile acids present in hepatic bile also incorporate cholesterol and phosphatidylcholine.

tight junctions that delineate the canaliculus are relatively permeable, and so water is drawn into the canaliculus to balance this, along with plasma cations to maintain electrical neutrality. Of these cations, calcium, which is present at concentrations that approximate those in plasma (1 mM), is particularly important from a pathophysiologic standpoint because it can form insoluble precipitates with certain bile solutes, such as unconjugated bilirubin, under adverse conditions. Other secondary solutes also enter bile passively from the plasma, including glutathione, glucose, amino acids, and urea.

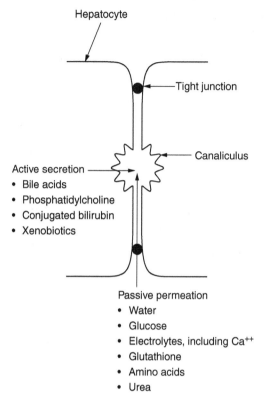

Hepatocyte

Tight junction

Canaliculus

Active secretion
- Bile acids
- Phosphatidylcholine
- Conjugated bilirubin
- Xenobiotics

Passive permeation
- Water
- Glucose
- Electrolytes, including Ca^{++}
- Glutathione
- Amino acids
- Urea

Figure 11–4. Pathways for solute entry into bile by either active secretion or passive permeation through the tight junctions linking adjacent hepatocytes.

The composition of canalicular bile is also modified by the active secretion of additional substrates from the hepatocyte itself. Phosphatidylcholine, a component of the hepatocyte membrane, enters the bile and forms mixed micelles with the secreted conjugated bile acids. The ratio of phosphatidylcholine to bile acids is approximately 0.3. Although phosphatidylcholine is only one of the phospholipids present in the hepatocyte plasma membrane, it is selectively secreted into bile. We now know that this occurs by the activity of a specific protein called multidrug resistance protein 3 (MDR3; MDR2 in mice), which serves as a "flippase," meaning that it "flips" molecules of phosphatidylcholine from their normal position in the inner leaflet of the canalicular membrane, and forms them into hemivesicles that are detached by secreted bile acids to form mixed micelles. Along with several other canalicular transporters, MDR2 is a member of a large family of ATP-dependent membrane transporters termed ABC transporters (for ATP-binding cassette), which also includes CFTR.

Table 11–1. Hepatocyte transporters

Name	Location	Substrate/function
Sodium taurocholate cotransporting polypeptide (NTCP)	Basolateral membrane	Uptake of conjugated bile acids from blood
Organic anion transporting proteins (OATP)	Basolateral membrane	Uptake of bile acids and xenobiotics from blood
Bile salt export pump (BSEP)	Canalicular membrane	Secretion of conjugated bile acids into bile
Multidrug resistance protein 3 (MDR3)	Canalicular membrane	"Flippase" that adds phosphatidylcholine to bile
Multidrug resistance protein 1 (MDR1)	Canalicular membrane	Secretion of hydrophobic cationic drugs into bile
ABC5/ABC8	Canalicular membrane	Secretion of cholesterol into bile
Multiple organic anion transport protein (cMOAT, MRP2)	Canalicular membrane	Secretion of sulfated lithocholic acid and conjugated bilirubin into bile

Cholesterol itself is also secreted into the bile, particularly in humans, at a ratio of approximately 0.3 to the amount of phosphatidylcholine (or one tenth of the amount of bile acids). Such secretion appears to be mediated, at least in part, by a heterodimer of two ABC transporters, ABC5 and ABC8. Canalicular bile, in health, also contains conjugated bilirubin, which gives bile its characteristic brown color and is water soluble, and a variety of other organic anions and cations that arise from the biotransformation of xenobiotics and endogenous hormones in the hepatocyte. In recent years, there has been an explosion of our molecular understanding of the membrane transporters that allow these various latter molecules to enter the bile, and details of the known molecules are shown in Table 11–1.

Ductular Bile

As the bile moves out of the canaliculi, it is transferred to the smallest bile ductules via structures known as the canals of Hering. The bile ductules are lined by cholangiocytes, which are columnar epithelial cells specialized to modify bile composition. The tight junctions linking the cholangiocytes are much less permeable than those linking hepatocytes. They are freely permeable to water, but are only selectively permeable to electrolytes and impermeant to larger solutes. Because of their permeability to water, bile rapidly becomes isotonic. Hormonal stimulation of cholangiocytes also activates the apical insertion of aquaporin water channels, further contributing to bile dilution.

The ductules also serve to scavenge solutes that were filtered into the bile at the leaky canaliculus. In particular, glucose is actively reabsorbed and returned to the bloodstream. Likewise, glutathione is hydrolyzed to its constituent amino acids by the apically fixed enzyme, gamma glutamyltranspeptidase (GGT), which we encountered as a serum marker of cholangiocyte injury in the preceding chapter. The reuptake of glucose and amino acids is likely important in preventing bacterial overgrowth in the biliary tree, by limiting nutrient availability. Overgrowth of bacteria in the bile ductules has potentially serious consequences because bacterial enzymes can deconjugate bilirubin, yielding a product that can form a highly insoluble salt with the calcium that is present in the bile.

The function of the bile ductules is also coordinated with ingestion of a meal. In particular, in a manner analogous to the cells of the pancreatic ducts, the cholangiocytes secrete bicarbonate in response to secretin, via a process involving the coupled activity of the CFTR chloride channel and chloride/bicarbonate exchangers at the apical membrane. Bile acids themselves may also stimulate CFTR by binding to a membrane receptor termed TGR5, which, like the secretin receptor, is linked to increases in intracellular cAMP. This may be an important mechanism to limit the toxic effects of bile acids, particularly for lithocholic acid, by driving fluid secretion that results in bile acid dilution. In either case, sodium ions follow paracellularly to maintain electrical neutrality, in turn drawing additional water into the bile and increasing its volume and flow. Thus, bile becomes slightly alkaline. In patients suffering from cystic fibrosis, biliary secretion is impaired and some patients will develop liver injury as a result of retained biliary constituents.

Finally, the ductules secrete IgA molecules into the bile, by virtue of their expression of the polymeric IgA receptor that we discussed in Chapter 6. The secretory IgA present in bile presumably contributes to host defense, and again helps to maintain the sterility of the bile.

Hepatic Bile

Hepatic bile refers to the bile that emerges from the liver in the common hepatic duct, prior to further modification by gallbladder storage as will be discussed in the next chapter. The large bile ducts are thought to have little ability to modify bile composition, other than by adding mucus that presumably serves a protective and lubricating role. Thus, the composition of hepatic bile reflects that which emerges from the ductules, as can be studied experimentally by cannulating the hepatic duct. Hepatic bile is isoosmotic with plasma, slightly alkaline, and contains appreciable quantities of IgA but essentially no glucose or amino acids.

ENTEROHEPATIC CIRCULATION OF BILE ACIDS

At several points in the foregoing discussion, we have alluded to the fact that bile acids enter into the so-called *enterohepatic circulation*. Here, we will consider the physiologic utility of this circuit, and the means by which it is accomplished.

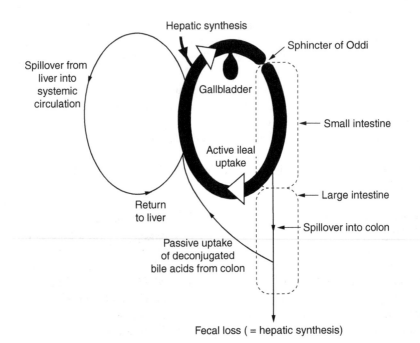

Figure 11–5. Quantitative aspects of the circulation of bile acids. The majority of the bile acid pool circulates between the small intestine and liver. A minority of the bile acid pool is in the systemic circulation (due to incomplete hepatocyte uptake from portal blood) or spills over into the colon and is lost to the stool. Fecal loss must be equivalent to hepatic synthesis of bile acids at steady state.

Unlike the digestive enzymes arising from the pancreas, which contribute to nutrient digestion catalytically, bile acids contribute to lipid digestion and absorption by mass action. This means that considerable quantities of bile acids are needed to solubilize the quantities of products of fat digestion that are derived from a typical diet on a daily basis. We have learned that the liver synthesizes 200–400 mg of bile acids per day. However, the concentration of bile acids in the small intestinal lumen during digestion of a meal is likely of the order of 10–30 mM, because bile acid secretion with a meal is about 2000–3000 mg/h.

This is achieved by recycling the majority of the bile acids secreted during a meal, such that a large pool (about 2000 mg) of these molecules is constantly cycling between the intestine and liver (Figure 11–5).

Intestinal Uptake Mechanisms

Bile acids secreted into the gut lumen are initially entirely in conjugated form. Because these bile acids are ionized, they cannot cross the wall of the intestine passively. Rather, there is a specific transporter that recognizes bile acid conjugates and reabsorbs them via a process of secondary active transport. The uptake of the conjugated bile acids is coupled to that of sodium, and thus bile acid uptake across intestinal epithelial cells takes advantage of the low intracellular sodium concentration that is established in the epithelial cells by the activity of the basolateral Na, K-ATPase. The transporter that mediates this uptake is referred to as the *apical sodium-dependent bile salt transporter*, ASBT. Importantly for its role in lipid digestion, ASBT expression in the intestine is limited to epithelial cells in the terminal ileum. Thus, conjugated bile acids remain with the meal in the lumen until the nutrients are absorbed, whereupon they are reclaimed from the lumen and enter the portal circulation to be returned to the liver. A second heterodimeric sodium-independent bile acid transporter, OSTα/β, is present at the basolateral domain of ileal epithelial cells to accomplish this. Only a minor portion of the bile acid pool spills over into the colon in health. Moreover, conjugated bile acids that enter the colon are deconjugated by the resident bacteria. Because deconjugated bile acids have a higher pKa, they are largely nonionized at luminal pH and thus can be absorbed passively. This further reduces bile acid loss, such that the amount of bile acids found in the feces balances daily synthesis from cholesterol at a steady state (Figure 11–5).

Bile acids are carried in the portal circulation bound to albumin. However, the efficiency of albumin binding varies depending on the physicochemical characteristics of the bile acid. Trihydroxy-bile acids are less efficiently bound than their dihydroxy-counterparts.

Hepatocyte Transport Mechanisms

Bile acids returned to the liver, either in conjugated or unconjugated form, leave the portal circulation in the sinusoids bound to albumin and then are specifically taken up across the basolateral membrane of the periportal hepatocytes. The hepatocytes are highly efficient at taking up bile acids from the blood. Depending on the specific bile acid, 50–90% of the bile acid pool presented to the hepatocyte enters the cytosol. A variety of specific transporters for both conjugated and unconjugated bile acids have been identified in hepatocyte basolateral membranes (Table 11–1). Probably the most well-characterized is the sodium taurocholate cotransporting polypeptide (NTCP), a sodium-coupled transporter for the taurine conjugate of cholic acid (and likely other conjugated bile acids) that shares homology with ASBT. Unconjugated bile acids are transported by the 1B1 and 1B3 members of the organic anion transporting polypeptide (OATP) family, which transport bile acids into the hepatocyte in a sodium-independent fashion.

Bile acids that enter the hepatocyte likely associate with binding proteins that traffic them across the hepatocyte cytosol. Unconjugated bile acids are reconjugated with either taurine or glycine, and overall the recycled bile acids are handled in much the same way as bile acids that have been newly synthesized from cholesterol. Bile acids are actively transported into the bile canaliculus via the activity of another transport protein known as the bile salt export pump (BSEP). The only exception applies to secretion of the sulfated forms of conjugated lithocholic acid, which enter the bile via a protein called the canalicular multiple organic anion transporter (cMOAT), also referred to as MRP2. This pump is also the means whereby conjugated bilirubin enters the bile, as we will discuss in Chapter 13.

Because hepatocyte uptake of bile acids is efficient, only a small amount of these molecules spills over into the general circulation in health. The concentration of bile acids in the portal circulation after a meal is approximately 25–50 μm, whereas that in the systemic plasma is less than 10 μm. Nevertheless, bile acids are measurable in the serum and their concentration demonstrates predictable peaks immediately after meals. Moreover, because bile acids are largely bound to albumin, only small quantities enter the glomerular filtrate. Those that do are efficiently reabsorbed in the proximal tubule by the same transporter that mediates their uptake in the terminal ileum, ASBT. Thus, under normal conditions, the concentration of bile acids in the urine is negligible.

Regulation of Bile Acid Synthesis and Transport

The enterohepatic cycling of bile acids also controls the rate at which they are synthesized and transported. Bile acids exert feedback inhibition on cholesterol 7α-hydroxylase, such that when return of bile acids from the intestine is high, the synthesis of new primary bile acids is reduced. This feedback is mediated predominantly by the ability of bile acids to bind to the farnesoid X nuclear receptor (FXR) in ileal epithelial cells, which induces the expression of fibroblast growth factor 19 (FGF19). FGF19 then mediates gut–liver signaling by binding to its heterodimeric receptor on hepatocytes, comprised of the proteins βKlotho and FGF receptor 4. This receptor signals to repress CYP7A1 expression (Figure 11–6). Mutations in any of these proteins interrupt the down-regulation of bile acid synthesis. Conversely, interruption of the ileal uptake of bile acids for any reason will relieve this feedback inhibition, increasing the rate at which cholesterol is converted to bile acids. It has been calculated that normal rates of bile acid synthesis can increase 10- to 20-fold under these conditions. This increased synthetic rate may or may not be sufficient to maintain the size of the circulating bile acid pool, depending on the extent of fecal losses.

Bile acids also regulate their own transport. FXR activation by bile acids in the hepatocyte upregulates the synthesis of BSEP. By related mechanisms, bile acids also repress expression of NCTP. The net effect is to decrease uptake of bile acids from the portal circulation and to increase their export into bile, reducing cytosolic levels. Likewise, increased amounts of bile acids in the intestinal lumen decrease the expression of ASBT.

Bile acid synthesis should also be considered in the context of whole body cholesterol metabolism (Figure 11–7). Cholesterol is a vital component of cell membranes and the myelin sheath of nerves. The body's cholesterol pools reflect hepatic and extrahepatic synthesis (the majority; typically 1 g/day on average) as well as a small component derived from absorption of dietary cholesterol (approximately 0.2 g/day, depending on diet). At steady state, cholesterol input must be balanced by elimination. Cholesterol is lost from the body in two forms—by being secreted intact into the bile (approximately 0.8 g/day) or after conversion

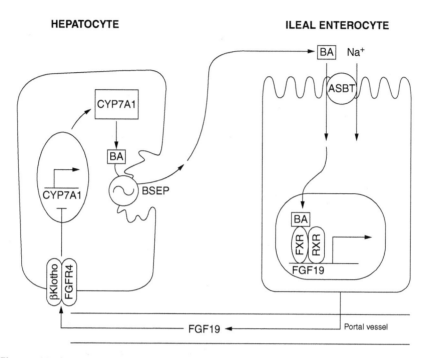

HEPATOCYTE   **ILEAL ENTEROCYTE**

Figure 11–6. Cross-talk between ileal epithelial cells and hepatocytes that leads to the feedback suppression of bile acid (BA) synthesis when levels of conjugated bile acids rise in the lumen of the terminal ileum. Bile acids transported into epithelial cells in the terminal ileum via the apical sodium-coupled bile salt transporter, ASBT, bind to the farnesoid X receptor (FXR), which translocates to the nucleus with its partner, the retinoid X receptor (RXR). This dimer acts as a transcription factor that increases expression of fibroblast growth factor 19 (FGF19), which is secreted into the portal circulation and can thus access its receptor (βKlotho/FGFR4) on the basolateral pole of hepatocytes. This results in signaling that limits the expression of CYP7A1, the rate-limiting enzyme in the bile acid synthetic pathway. BSEP, bile salt exit pump.

to bile acids (0.2–0.3 g/day). In either case, the sole excretory pathway in health is via the bile as no cholesterol or bile acids are excreted in urine. Interrupting the enterohepatic circulation of bile acids has been exploited as a therapeutic strategy in hypercholesterolemia, since it will increase demand for cholesterol biosynthesis in the hepatocyte. In turn, this upregulates receptors for low-density lipoprotein (LDL) and lowers plasma levels of LDL cholesterol.

PATHOPHYSIOLOGY AND CLINICAL CORRELATES

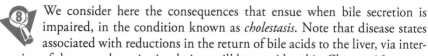 We consider here the consequences that ensue when bile secretion is impaired, in the condition known as *cholestasis*. Note that disease states associated with reductions in the return of bile acids to the liver, via interruption of the enterohepatic circulation, will be considered in Chapter 16.

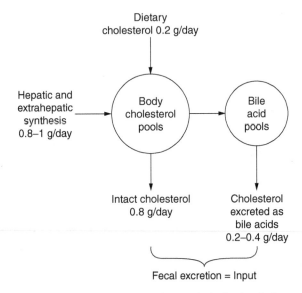

Figure 11–7. Relationship of bile acid pools to whole body cholesterol homeostasis in health. The combined fecal excretion of cholesterol and bile acids is equivalent to input of cholesterol from the diet plus endogenous synthesis of cholesterol. (From the Undergraduate Teaching Project of the American Gastroenterological Association, Unit 11. Copyright 2002.)

Cholestasis

 Cholestasis refers simply to a condition where the production of bile is impaired or bile flow is obstructed. Cholestasis may arise from defects within the liver, or more distally in the biliary tree. Depending on the etiology of the condition, the precise consequences that ensue vary.

PRIMARY BILIARY CIRRHOSIS AND PRIMARY SCLEROSING CHOLANGITIS

PBC and PSC are distinct conditions that affect different groups of patients. PBC refers to a slowly progressive, inflammatory destruction of the cholangiocytes lining small to medium-sized intralobular bile ductules. It is more common in women and is believed to have an autoimmune pathogenesis, although evidence for this remains circumstantial. PBC may have a long asymptomatic period where only modest biochemical changes can be detected. However, once symptoms of cholestasis develop, most patients will progress to develop cirrhosis. PSC, on the other hand, is characterized by inflammation and fibrosis of both the intra and extrahepatic bile ducts. At least some series find greater incidence of this condition in men, and it is often seen in conjunction with the inflammatory bowel disease of ulcerative colitis. Like PBC, the pathogenesis of PSC is not fully understood, although it appears to relate to both genetic and immunologic defects.

Despite the presumed differences in their etiology, the consequences of both PBC and PSC are similar. As bile ducts become destroyed, bile cannot exit the liver and the lipid components of bile regurgitate into the plasma. This leads to the classical symptoms of cholestasis, including pruritus, or itching, which is thought to be an effect of increased plasma levels of bile acids. Hypercholesterolemia also occurs, since, as we have learned, cholesterol cannot be eliminated in the urine. With increasing concentrations of the biliary lipids in the bloodstream, chenodeoxycholic acid becomes a substrate for hepatocyte sulfation, as seen under normal conditions for lithocholic acid. Sulfated bile acids are not substrates for ASBT, and can be filtered at the glomerulus because they are not so tightly bound to albumin. Thus, a portion of retained bile acids enter the urine, and are not reabsorbed in the proximal tubule and thus can be excreted. Thus, some of the body's cholesterol can likewise be eliminated in the form of bile acids, however, it is also important to recognize that bile acid synthesis can be suppressed by the effect of high concentrations of bile acids in the plasma on hepatocyte synthesis of these molecules. Thus, cholesterol accumulates in the plasma where it is found in bilayers with phospholipids and albumin referred to as "lipoprotein X." Retained bile acids also are toxic to the liver and worsen the damage and fibrosis caused by the primary disease process, impairing the metabolic functions of the liver. In later stages, patients will also display jaundice due to the failure to excrete adequate amounts of bilirubin. Patients with either condition will also display symptoms related to a lack of adequate bile acids to provide for the absorption of fat-soluble vitamins and dietary fat. Patients accordingly develop prolonged prothrombin times and steatorrhea (loss of fat to the feces).

Eventually, patients with either condition may need a liver transplant. In its early stages, PBC can also be treated effectively with ursodeoxycholic acid, which displaces more cytotoxic bile acids from the recirculating bile acid pool. However, most trials of ursodeoxycholic acid therapy in PSC have been disappointing. The reason for this difference between the conditions is unclear.

CONGENITAL BILIARY ATRESIA

Congenital biliary atresia is a pediatric condition in which the intrahepatic bile ducts do not form properly. The molecular basis of this disease is unknown, but infants born with this condition rapidly become jaundiced and have no ability to excrete cholesterol or other biliary constituents via bile. The consequences are similar to those described earlier for PBC and PSC, but treatment is more urgent because of the rapid onset of disease. The only effective treatment at present is a liver transplant, often performed as a donation of a portion of the liver from a living-related donor.

OBSTRUCTIVE JAUNDICE

A more common cause of biliary obstruction is blockage of one of the extrahepatic bile ducts with a gallstone. The pathogenesis of gallstones will be discussed in the next chapter; here we will consider the consequences that ensue when such a stone becomes lodged in a bile duct segment. The outcome of such blockade depends on the point at which the stone is found. If the blockage is in the right or left hepatic duct, bile flow from the opposite side of the liver will increase. If left untreated, the side of the liver no longer drained will eventually atrophy because of the cytotoxic effect of retained bile acids. If a stone occludes the common hepatic duct, bile flow from the entire liver will be blocked and the symptoms will be comparable to those described for the conditions discussed earlier. Similar findings will be seen in a patient with a gallstone blocking the common bile duct, and additionally the gallbladder will become distended if the obstruction is acute. Finally, a gallstone blocking the cystic duct will not cause cholestasis, as the bile can still exit the liver and the bile acid pool will be stored in the small intestine. Physiologically, this is analogous to the situation that pertains in a patient whose gall bladder has been removed surgically. On the other hand, with acute obstruction of the cystic duct, the painful condition of cholecystitis (inflammation of the gallbladder) may occur and may require surgery.

In some cases, obstructive jaundice due to gallstones in the common bile duct can be treated endoscopically. Using the same endoscopic configuration used for ERCP, stones can be broken apart and removed from the biliary tree if they are physically accessible, or the sphincter of Oddi can be cut to widen its diameter. At the very least, ERCP is useful to localize the obstruction. However, since most gallstones develop initially in the gallbladder, patients with recurrent symptomatic gallstones are usually treated by surgical removal of the gallbladder. Medical therapies to dissolve or fragment gallstones are also available, but with the advent of laparoscopic gallbladder surgery (cholecystectomy), which is rapid and safe, medical treatments are now usually reserved for patients who are poor surgical candidates.

HEREDITARY CHOLESTASIS SYNDROMES

It has been known for many years that inherited defects can also lead to clinically significant cholestatic liver disease, of varying severity. With the advent of a molecular understanding of the transport mechanisms that are needed to pump solutes into canalicular bile, some of these inherited conditions have been attributed to mutations in specific transport proteins. We will mention just two such syndromes here on the basis of the insights they have provided into the molecular basis of bile secretion. First, type II progressive familial intrahepatic cholestasis (PFIC II) is an autosomal recessive disorder that presents with progressive cholestasis but limited evidence of bile ductule injury (i.e., serum GGT levels are low). The underlying defect has been mapped to a mutation in BSEP, and there is an almost total absence of bile acids in the bile. Patients therefore develop liver injury as a result of the cytotoxic effects of bile acids accumulating in hepatocytes. This syndrome can be contrasted with PFIC III, which is a more aggressive disease in which cholestasis is accompanied by early jaundice and increased levels of serum GGT. The syndrome has been ascribed to mutations in MDR3, and an almost total absence of phosphatidylcholine in the bile. This disorder nicely illustrates the importance of phosphatidylcholine secretion into bile in protecting the biliary ductules from the injurious effects of bile acids. When phosphatidylcholine is absent, mixed micelles cannot form and thus the concentration of monomeric bile acids in the biliary system is increased. Milder mutations in MDR3 have likewise been associated with cholestatic syndromes that arise in adulthood, and perhaps may also be responsible for at least a portion of hereditary susceptibility to cholesterol gallstones.

KEY CONCEPTS

 Bile is secreted by the liver as a vehicle to excrete lipid-soluble waste products of metabolism as well as xenobiotics, and it also aids in fat digestion and absorption.

 The major solutes driving the primary secretion of bile are the bile acids, which are amphipathic molecules synthesized from cholesterol in the hepatocyte.

 Bile acids can be modified by intestinal bacteria to yield compounds known as secondary bile acids. One of these, lithocholic acid, is relatively toxic, and so mechanisms exist to promote its elimination from the body.

 Bile acids are actively secreted into the bile canaliculus in conjugated forms by an energy-dependent transporter.

 Bile also contains cholesterol and phosphatidylcholine, which are actively transported into the primary secretion, as well as solutes filtered from the plasma, such as calcium and glucose.

 Glucose is actively reabsorbed from the bile as it passes through the biliary ductules, which also add IgA and render the bile alkaline.

 Bile acids recycle several times daily from the intestine to the liver in the enterohepatic circulation; in their conjugated forms, they are actively reabsorbed in the terminal ileum, thereby generating a recycling pool of bile acids.

 Bile flow can be deficient because of injury to or an absence of bile ducts, a deficiency of canalicular transporters, or physical obstructions such as gallstones or tumors.

 Cholestasis is associated with malabsorption of fat-soluble vitamins, as well as with other symptoms.

 When bile flow is interrupted, biliary lipids accumulate in the plasma and the only route for cholesterol excretion is the urinary excretion of bile acids.

STUDY QUESTIONS

11–1. A patient with Crohn's disease undergoes surgical resection of her diseased terminal ileum. After recovering from the surgery, she is noted to have moderate steatorrhea. What level of bile acid synthesis by the patient's hepatocytes would be
expected compared to a normal individual?

A. Tenfold higher

B. 10% higher

C. Unchanged

D. 10% less

E. Tenfold less

11–2. The composition of bile is modified as it flows through the biliary ductules. Which
of the following is expected to increase in concentration during this transit?

A. Glucose

B. Bile acid monomers

C. Alanine

D. Glutathione

E. IgA

11–3. Bile acids are conjugated in the hepatocyte to increase their aqueous solubility
and decrease their pKa. In addition to conjugation with taurine or glycine, which
of the following bile acids is alternatively sulfated in health?

A. Chenodeoxycholic acid

B. Deoxycholic acid

C. Cholic acid

D. Ursodeoxycholic acid

E. Lithocholic acid

11–4. A newborn baby is suffering heavily from jaundice and produces only pale stools.
Tests reveal a total absence of bile secretion. Increased concentrations of which
of the following will be expected in the urine of this baby compared to a healthy
neonate?

A. Glucose

B. Cholesterol

C. Phosphatidylcholine

D. Chenodeoxycholic acid

E. Albumin

11–5. A scientist studying the enterohepatic circulation measures the portal concentration of conjugated bile acids in rats treated with various drugs. An inhibitor of which of the following ion transport proteins would be expected to reduce the uptake of sodium taurocholate from the small intestinal lumen?

A. *Na⁺, K⁺ ATPase*

B. *CFTR*

C. *ENaC*

D. *NKCC1*

E. *Chloride/bicarbonate exchanger*

SUGGESTED READINGS

Carlton VE, Pawlikowska I, Bull LN. Molecular basis of intrahepatic cholestasis. *Ann Med.* 2004;36: 606–617.

Dawson PA. Bile formation and the enterohepatic circulation. In: Johnson LR, Ghishan FK, Kaunitz JD, Merchant JL, Said HM, Wood JD, eds. *Physiology of the Gastrointestinal Tract.* 5th ed. San Diego: Academic Press; 2012:1461–1484.

Hay DW, Carey MC. Chemical species of lipids in bile. *Hepatology.* 1990;12:6S–14S.

Hofmann AF. Bile acids: trying to understand their chemistry and biology with the hope of helping patients. *Hepatology.* 2009;49:1403–1418.

Kullak-Ublick GA, Steiger G, Meier P. Enterohepatic bile salt transporters in normal physiology and liver disease. *Gastroenterology.* 2004;126:322–342.

Mack C, Sokol RJ. Unraveling the pathogenesis and etiology of biliary atresia. *Pediatr Res.* 2005.

Russell DW. The enzymes, regulation, and genetics of bile acid synthesis. *Annu Rev Biochem.* 2003;72: 137–174.

Weinman SA, Jalil S. Bile secretion and cholestasis In: Yamada T, Alpers DH, Kalloo AN, Kaplowitz N, Laine L, Owyang C, Powell DW, eds. *Textbook of Gastroenterology.* 5th ed. Philadelphia, Chichester: Wiley-Blackwell; 2009:401–428.

Gallbladder Function

OBJECTIVES

▶ *Understand the role of the gallbladder in concentrating bile and coordinating its secretion with ingestion of a meal*
  ▶ Describe the molecular mechanisms whereby bile is concentrated during storage
  ▶ Discuss the mechanism and significance of gallbladder secretion
  ▶ Understand how bile remains isoosmolar during concentration
  ▶ Explain how contraction of the gallbladder is regulated
▶ *Explain why the gallbladder is vulnerable to the formation of cholesterol gallstones*
  ▶ Describe the physiologic consequences of surgical removal of the gallbladder
▶ *Understand the role of the sphincter of Oddi in regulating bile outflow into the intestine*

BASIC PRINCIPLES OF GALLBLADDER FUNCTION

Role and Significance

The gallbladder serves to store and concentrate bile coming from the liver in the period between meals. Gallbladder function therefore permits coordination of the secretion of a bolus of concentrated bile with the entry of dietary lipids into the small intestine. It is important to be aware, however, that the gallbladder is not essential to normal digestion and absorption of a meal. In the absence of a functioning gallbladder, the bile acid pool continues to cycle through the enterohepatic circulation and the majority of the bile acid pool is stored in the small intestine.

FUNCTIONAL ANATOMY OF THE GALLBLADDER

The gallbladder is a muscular sac located just below the liver and lying adjacent to the liver's surface. Its capacity is approximately 50 mL in adult humans. It is linked to the biliary system via the cystic duct, a bidirectional conduit for bile flow. During periods of fasting, bile secreted by the liver is diverted into the gallbladder on the basis of pressure relationships in the biliary system, as will be discussed in more detail later. On the other hand, when the gallbladder receives neurohumoral cues that fats are present in the small intestine, it contracts and bile flows out of the gallbladder and into the intestine via the cystic and common bile ducts.

Epithelium

The gallbladder has two functional layers. The innermost of these, facing the bile, is a columnar epithelium that participates actively in bile concentration. The tight junctions that link adjacent epithelial cells are among the most well-developed anywhere in the body, making the epithelium highly resistant to the passive flux of solutes. This "tight" epithelium prevents the passive loss of bile acid molecules and thus is essential to the ability of the gallbladder to concentrate the bile. It is likely also important in limiting the potentially deleterious effects of amphipathic bile acids. To this end, the epithelium also contains abundant goblet cells that secrete mucus, which is also believed to protect the epithelium from injury.

Musculature

The epithelial layers are underlaid by smooth muscle that can alter the caliber of the gallbladder lumen according to the presence of neurohumoral stimuli. The muscle cells receive input from branches of the vagus nerve, and express cholinergic receptors to respond to released acetylcholine (ACh). They also express receptors for gastrointestinal hormones, and in particular for cholecystokinin (CCK_1). As we learned earlier, this hormone is actually named for its ability to contract the gallbladder. However, the majority of the action of CCK on gallbladder motility is believed to be indirect, and mediated by the effects of this hormone on nerves that innervate the gallbladder, as well as on vagal afferents that travel from the duodenum and coordinate gallbladder emptying with the presence of nutrients in the gut lumen (Figure 12–1).

GALLBLADDER STORAGE OF BILE

Effects on Composition

Hepatic bile emerging from the biliary ducts is isotonic with plasma, with sodium as its major cation and chloride as its major anion. Bile acids are typically present at a concentration of approximately 30–50 mM; there are small amounts of potassium, calcium, and approximately 20–50 mM bicarbonate. After gallbladder storage, water is removed from the lumen and the concentration of bile acids is increased by approximately tenfold, whereas chloride and bicarbonate concentrations fall dramatically. On the other hand, the concentrations of all cations in the bile increase, although to a lesser degree than that of the bile acids indicating that cations are also subject to net absorption by the gallbladder epithelium. The concentration of calcium ions, which remains low, nevertheless increases disproportionately compared to that of sodium and potassium because of a phenomenon known as the *Gibbs–Donnan equilibrium*,

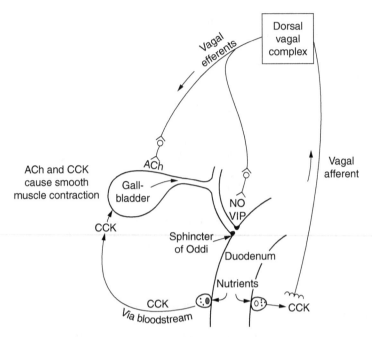

Figure 12–1. Neurohumoral control of gallbladder contraction and biliary secretion. Nutrients in the duodenum lead to the release of cholecystokinin (CCK), which acts through both endocrine and neurocrine routes to activate gallbladder contraction and relax the sphincter of Oddi, resulting in the secretion of a bolus of concentrated bile into the duodenal lumen. Secondary neurotransmitters released by the enteric nervous system in response to a vago-vagal reflex include the excitatory neurotransmitter acetylcholine (ACh) and the inhibitory transmitters vasoactive intestinal polypeptide (VIP) and nitric oxide (NO).

where divalent cations are retained in a given compartment containing proteins more avidly than are monovalent anions. You may recall this concept from previous discussions of how plasma oncotic pressure is established, or the rules establishing the ionic composition of plasma versus the interstitial fluid. A figure comparing the composition of hepatic and gallbladder bile is shown as Figure 12–2.

Despite the dramatic increase in the sum of anions and cations during gallbladder storage of bile, bile remains isotonic. How is this possible? The answer lies in the fact that the majority of the bile acid molecules are physically in the form of mixed micelles that also contain cholesterol and phosphatidylcholine. Once the critical micellar concentration is reached, the monomeric concentration of bile acids does not change. Any additional bile acid molecules are immediately incorporated into existing micelles. Osmolality is a colligative property, which means that each particle in a solution contributes the

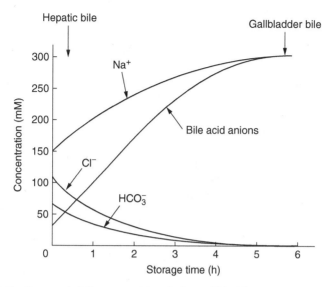

Figure 12–2. Changes in bile composition during gallbladder storage.

same amount of osmotic force, be it a molecule, ion, or micelle. This allows the osmolality of bile to remain constant despite its concentration. In addition, counterion binding to micelles may also further decrease the osmolality of the stored bile.

Bile also changes from being slightly alkaline (a result of bicarbonate secretion in the ductules) to slightly acidic. This may be important in reducing the risk of calcium precipitation, since calcium bicarbonate is more soluble than calcium carbonate. Bile acidification results from the activity of gallbladder epithelial cells, as will be discussed in more detail later.

We should also address the effect of gallbladder storage on the concentration of the other biliary lipids, cholesterol and phosphatidylcholine. The solubility of cholesterol in bile, in particular, depends on its concentration relative to that of the bile acids and phosphatidylcholine that form the mixed micelles. As bile is concentrated, bile acids cannot leave the gallbladder since they are too large to pass through the tight junctions linking adjacent epithelial cells, and they are also not actively transported by the gallbladder epithelium. Accordingly, the proportion of bile acids to cholesterol plus phosphatidylcholine does not change, or even increases slightly, because the gallbladder can absorb cholesterol. As a result, bile becomes slightly less saturated in cholesterol as it is stored. Theoretically, this should lessen the chance of cholesterol precipitation during fasting. However, this beneficial effect needs to be viewed in light of the fact that adult humans are unusual in that they secrete high concentrations of cholesterol into the bile. Indeed cholesterol is supersaturated in the hepatic bile of many older individuals (precipitation is usually limited by the presence of proteins that reduce "nucleation," or the initiation of a focus around which a cholesterol precipitate can be laid down). The longer that bile is stored, the greater the risk that nucleation will occur and thus the greater the risk for formation of gallstones. Indeed, the high concentration of cholesterol in bile likely accounts for the relatively high prevalence of cholesterol gallstones in humans. A case can be made, therefore, for avoiding prolonged fasts and not skipping breakfast if one wants to minimize one's risk of gallstone disease.

Mechanism for Bile Concentration

Bile is concentrated in the gallbladder via the active transport of ions across the tight gallbladder epithelium (Figure 12–3). The primary transport process that has received attention occurs at the apical membrane of the epithelial cells, where sodium in the bile is exchanged for protons either transported from the bloodstream, or (more likely) generated in the cytosol of the epithelial cells via the activity of carbonic anhydrase. The protein(s) that mediate this sodium/hydrogen exchange are members of the NHE family of exchangers that we encountered in the gastrointestinal tract, although the precise isoform(s)

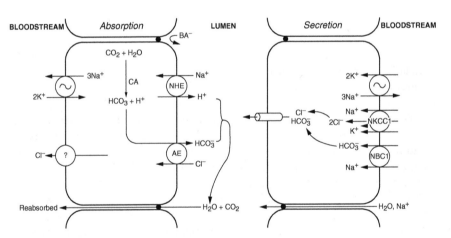

Figure 12–3. Ion transport by gallbladder epithelial cells. During bile concentration (left), sodium is reabsorbed via a sodium–hydrogen exchanger on the apical membrane (NHE), in exchange for protons generated intracellularly by carbonic anhydrase (CA). Chloride is absorbed in exchange for bicarbonate by a coupled chloride–bicarbonate exchanger (AE). The driving force for absorptive transport is the basolateral Na,K-ATPase. Gallbladder epithelial tight junctions have extremely low permeability, and resist the passage of bile acid anions (BA⁻) out of the lumen, allowing for bile concentration. After the gallbladder empties, there is evidence for active secretion of chloride and/or bicarbonate (right) by the CFTR chloride channel. Chloride is taken up across the basolateral membrane by NKCC1, and bicarbonate is generated intracellularly by carbonic anhydrase (not shown) and/or is taken up basolaterally by a sodium-coupled bicarbonate cotransporter, NBC1. Sodium and water follow paracellularly to flush the gallbladder lumen.

involved have not yet been fully elucidated; gallbladder epithelial cells express NHE1, NHE2, and NHE3. However, it is known that the ability of the gallbladder to concentrate bile is markedly reduced by amiloride, a broad-spectrum inhibitor of most NHE proteins. Protons that are secreted into the stored bile react with bicarbonate ions, yielding CO_2 and water. The CO_2 diffuses out of the gallbladder lumen passively and water can be reabsorbed via the mechanisms discussed later.

In addition to sodium absorption, chloride is also actively absorbed by the gallbladder epithelium during the period of bile storage. This is likely accomplished by a chloride–bicarbonate exchanger. The molecular identity of this transporter is not yet clear, although at least one chloride–bicarbonate exchanger isoform, AE2, has been found in the gallbladder. Finally, water leaves across the gallbladder epithelium to follow the osmotic effect of absorbed sodium chloride. The relative contribution of paracellular and transcellular movement of water in this concentrating process is not well understood. The gallbladder epithelium expresses the AQ1 aquaporin water channel, but mice lacking this protein had no obvious defect in biliary or gallbladder function despite other abnormalities in the handling of dietary fat.

In the period immediately after bile ejection from the gallbladder, there is emerging evidence that active chloride and bicarbonate secretion into the lumen occurs, mediated by the CFTR chloride channel that is defective in patients with cystic fibrosis. This secretory response may be triggered by bile acids via the ability of TGR5 to elevate cAMP, and may serve to clear the lumen of debris and/or to facilitate mucus secretion to protect the mucosa. In any event, at least some patients with cystic fibrosis have impaired bile secretion with gallbladder injury. In sum, it is clear that the gallbladder is both an absorptive and a secretory epithelial organ by turn, depending on physiological requirements relative to food intake.

MOTOR FUNCTIONS OF THE GALLBLADDER AND BILIARY SYSTEM

Determinants of Gallbladder Pressure and Filling

Whether hepatic bile will enter the gallbladder, or be secreted directly into the intestine, depends on the interrelationships between three pressures, as shown in Figure 12–4. Firstly, bile is secreted from the liver at a relatively high pressure (25–30 mmHg). This arises both from the hydrostatic pressure produced by bile flow, as well as, perhaps, the effect of contractile elements of the liver (such as stellate cells and myofibroblasts surrounding bile ductules) that constrict portions of the biliary tree. Sphincter of Oddi pressure is also relatively high between meals (11–30 mmHg). Finally, pressure in the gallbladder is low at rest, in part because the gallbladder displays receptive relaxation, and also because there may be active stimulation of gallbladder filling. Humoral factors released in the interprandial period that contribute to active gallbladder filling

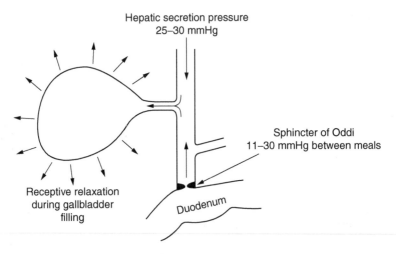

Figure 12–4. Motility responses of the fasting gallbladder. Between meals, gallbladder filling is promoted by hepatic secretion pressure, high pressure at the sphincter of Oddi, and receptive relaxation of gallbladder smooth muscle.

include FGF19, released from ileal enterocytes in response to bile acid uptake (see Figure 11–6) and also bile acids in the gallbladder lumen, which can trigger gallbladder filling by binding to apical TGR5. In addition, because the diameter of the gallbladder is considerably greater than that of the bile ducts, the pathway of least resistance is for bile to flow into this organ, an influence that only increases further as the gallbladder fills. The consequence of these various pressure relationships is that newly secreted bile will be directed toward the gallbladder when the sphincter of Oddi is closed.

Gallbladder Contraction

Postprandial gallbladder contraction coincides with gastric emptying. The entry of the meal into the duodenum triggers the release of a series of neurohumoral messengers that increase gallbladder tone (Figure 12–1). Cholecystokinin released from cells lining the duodenal lumen travels through the bloodstream, and binds directly to CCK_1 receptors on gallbladder smooth muscle cells. In addition, CCK sensitizes preganglionic terminals in gallbladder vagal efferent pathways, and also activates vagal afferents in the wall of the duodenum. The latter, in turn, initiate a vago-vagal reflex that releases ACh at gallbladder synapses, further increasing contractile activity. The importance of both CCK and ACh as gallbladder agonists can be demonstrated experimentally in animals, where neural blockade significantly reduces postprandial gallbladder contractions. Likewise, patients that have undergone nonselective vagotomy also have gallbladders that empty relatively poorly, which may predispose them to the development of gallstones. Patients who have undergone liver transplantation where the donor gallbladder is also transferred may also have diminished gallbladder contractile function due to the lack of the relevant neural circuitry. However, fortunately, there is evidence that, over time, the denervation of the gallbladder in both vagotomized patients and transplant recipients may lead to sensitization of the smooth muscle cells to CCK, such that the cells contract to lower concentrations of the hormone than would normally be required.

Sphincter of Oddi Function

Of course, even if the gallbladder contracts fully, this will not allow for bile secretion into the duodenum if pressure at the sphincter of Oddi remains high. Perhaps not surprisingly, therefore, in health, relaxation of the sphincter is coordinated with gallbladder contraction. The reduction in sphincter of Oddi tone is primarily brought about by the neurohumoral activity of CCK. Evidence supports the concept that CCK activates predominantly a neural mechanism to initiate this physiologic response, transmitted through the enteric nervous system. Postprandial relaxation of the sphincter, or that induced by administration of CCK exogenously, can be blocked by the muscarinic antagonist, atropine, or by total neural blockade with a nerve toxin such as tetrodotoxin. Evidence also exists to support the contention that the mediators acting at the level of the sphincter smooth muscle are VIP and nitric oxide, released from sphincter of Oddi nerve ganglia.

In the period between meals, the sphincter of Oddi directs bile to the gallbladder as well as preventing the backflow of duodenal contents into the biliary tree. Phasic contractions of the sphincter are superimposed on a basal tone, but the precise neurotransmitters responsible have not been established. It is known, on the other hand, that the sphincter of Oddi relaxes periodically, even when nutrients are absent from the lumen, in concert with the migrating motor complex that we encountered in Chapter 9. The physiologic significance of these periodic increases in bile secretion into the gut during fasting is unknown, but such secretion may be important to allow flushing of the system, perhaps secondary to the secretory responses discussed above, and to limit stasis in the biliary tree.

PATHOPHYSIOLOGY AND CLINICAL CORRELATIONS
Cholesterol Gallstones

The formation of stones in the gallbladder is a disease that has afflicted humans for millennia. Autopsies of Egyptian and Chinese mummies show that gallstones have existed for at least 35 centuries, and today, more than 20 million Americans have gallstones. Gallstone-related symptoms and complications are among the most common gastroenterologic disorders requiring hospitalization, at great cost to the healthcare system. Gallstones are of two types, related to the deposition of either cholesterol (cholesterol stones) or bilirubin (pigment stones). Cholesterol stones account for the majority of gallstones in most western countries and will be considered here; the pathogenesis of pigment stones will be discussed in the next chapter.

As discussed in the previous chapter, human bile is unusually rich in cholesterol. In cholesterol gallstone disease, the balance between the normal ratio of cholesterol to the other biliary lipids is disrupted, either due to cholesterol hypersecretion, relative hyposecretion of bile acids or phospholipids, or some combination of these. Obesity, the use of oral contraceptives, estrogen, old age, sudden weight loss, and genetic factors may lead to cholesterol hypersecretion. Conversely, a diminished bile acid pool can occur if the enterohepatic circulation is interrupted. In either case, patients are at risk for supersaturation of cholesterol and thus for the development of gallstones. Supersaturation is not necessarily sufficient for stone formation, however; nucleation must also occur. Some patients may be genetically predisposed to secrete proteins that can act as nucleating agents, whereas other proteins in bile may retard nucleation. Further, in some patients, frank stones are not seen, but rather there is simply a precipitate in bile that is referred to as biliary sludge, consisting of calcium bilirubinate and cholesterol crystals embedded in a mucus gel. Biliary sludge is usually asymptomatic and only seen incidentally during imaging studies, but it may be a precursor to the development of actual gallstones. The gallbladder has a special role to play in the development of gallstones, likely due to long residence times of bile in the interprandial period.

The majority (two-thirds) of patients with gallstones will have no associated symptoms. Others present with episodic pain in the epigastric region. In most patients, the pain is *biliary colic*, thought to reflect a tonic spasm resulting from transient obstruction of the cystic duct by a stone, and sometimes precipitated by eating a large meal. Biliary colic, while severe, usually subsides within a few hours, which serves to distinguish it from acute cholecystitis, where obstruction of the cystic duct leads to inflammation of the gallbladder. In some patients, acute inflammation may progress to chronic cholecystitis, resulting in a thickened and fibrotic gallbladder. If stones or sludge obstruct other parts of the biliary tree, and particularly the common bile duct, obstructive jaundice and ascending cholangitis (which can be fatal if untreated) can ensue as discussed in the preceding chapter.

The definitive treatment for symptomatic gallstone disease is cholecystectomy, which is usually simple, safe, and curative, particularly with the advent of laparoscopic approaches. Endoscopic approaches may also be used to remove gallstones from the common bile duct if the sphincter of Oddi is widened (a sphincterotomy). However, in this case, the gallbladder is left in place and gallstones often recur. Sphincterotomy may likewise be associated with a later risk for biliary complications.

Consequences of Cholecystectomy

The gallbladder is not essential for normal digestive function, and large studies have shown that its removal has no effect on life expectancy or metabolic status. Because the residence time for bile in the biliary tree is markedly decreased, there is much less risk for the development of gallstones of either type. Cholecystectomy also has no effect on cholesterol composition of hepatic bile, although the balance of specific bile acids may change because the bile acid pool is resident predominantly in the small intestine. This results in an increase in bile acid deconjugation and dehydroxylation by enteric bacteria, and thus may enrich the bile in the secondary bile acid, deoxycholic acid (recall that the other secondary bile acid, lithocholic acid, undergoes specific conjugation with sulfate to limit its accumulation in the bile acid pool).

The only significant consequence of removal of the gallbladder relates to the inability to form concentrated bile and to secrete it in a coordinated fashion when the meal enters the duodenum. Thus, patients who have undergone a cholecystectomy may find that they are less able to tolerate large fatty meals. However, most would agree that this is a small price to pay for the absence of pain and other symptoms related to gallstone disease.

Sphincter of Oddi Dysfunction

After cholecystectomy, some patients have persistent pain suggestive of biliary cholic that cannot be ascribed to gallstones, tumors, or biliary strictures. In some cases, the pain will be accompanied by mildly elevated liver function tests and/or evidence of dilation of the common bile duct. A high frequency of such patients will have a condition known as sphincter of Oddi dysfunction, which refers to a benign, noncalculous obstruction to the flow of bile and/or pancreatic juice. The pathogenesis of this condition may relate to a motor abnormality resulting in a hypertonic sphincter, referred to as sphincter of Oddi dyskinesis, or a structural abnormality, likely secondary to inflammation and fibrosis, referred to as sphincter of Oddi stenosis. Both conditions result in similar symptoms and are difficult to distinguish. Evaluation of such patients is most effectively accomplished by manometry of the sphincter (i.e., measurement of the pressures existing across the sphincter), but this is technically difficult to accomplish, and noninvasive imaging tests may be used to infer dysfunction. It is assumed that dysfunction of the sphincter causes pain by impeding the flow of bile and pancreatic juice, although ischemia arising from spastic contractions may also contribute. A few patients may develop sphincter of Oddi dysfunction without having had their gallbladder removed. Sphincter of Oddi dysfunction may also contribute to recurrent pancreatitis due to retained pancreatic juice and autodigestion.

Treatment of sphincter of Oddi dysfunction is suboptimal at present. If symptoms are severe and manometric abnormalities are present, relief may be obtained by cutting the sphincter either surgically or endoscopically. But as described earlier, patients who undergo a sphincterotomy may be at increased risk for subsequent biliary complications. Medical therapy with smooth muscle relaxants is also tried, particularly in patients with less severe symptoms, but drawbacks exist in terms of side effects and incomplete efficacy, particularly if a structural abnormality of the sphincter exists.

KEY CONCEPTS

 The gallbladder serves to store bile between meals and to coordinate the release of a concentrated bolus of bile with the presence of the meal in the duodenum.

 Gallbladder storage of bile results in changes in its composition, such that bile acids become the dominant anions.

 Bile remains isotonic during this process as bile acid monomers are rapidly incorporated into mixed micelles.

 The relative proportion of biliary lipids is largely unchanged, although the high concentration of cholesterol in human bile makes us vulnerable to cholesterol precipitation and thus to gallstones.

 Concentration of bile results from active transport processes taking place in the lining epithelial cells.

 Gallbladder filling and emptying are dynamic processes that depend on the pressures existing in the biliary tree and are regulated by neurohumoral cues.

 Cholesterol gallstones are common in humans, and may cause pain and cholestasis.

 The gallbladder is not essential to normal digestion, and symptomatic gallstone disease can often be cured by removal of the gallbladder.

STUDY QUESTIONS

12–1. In an experiment, imaging techniques were used to measure gallbladder volumes in human volunteers after a test meal. Which of the following drugs would be expected to maintain gallbladder volume in this study?

A. Muscarinic cholinergic antagonist

B. Nicotinic cholinergic antagonist

C. Nitric oxide synthase inhibitor

D. Adrenergic agonist

E. Cholinergic agonist

12–2. A 40 year-old-woman undergoes a laparoscopic cholecystectomy for recurrent gallstone disease. Two months after the surgery, what changes in the daily volume and fractional composition of hepatic bile will be expected compared to a normal subject?

	Volume	Primary bile acids	Secondary bile acids
A.	Increased	Increased	Decreased
B.	Increased	Decreased	Increased
C.	Unchanged	Decreased	Increased
D.	Decreased	Increased	Decreased
E.	Decreased	Decreased	Increased
F.	Unchanged	Increased	Decreased

12–3. Compared to hepatic bile, bile that has been stored in the gallbladder for several hours would be expected to display which of the following changes in composition?

	Cholesterol	pH	Calcium
A.	Increased	Increased	Increased
B.	Decreased	Decreased	Decreased
C.	Increased	Decreased	Increased
D.	Decreased	Increased	Decreased
E.	Decreased	Decreased	Increased
F.	Increased	Increased	Decreased

12–4. A 45-year-old-woman is brought to the emergency room complaining of a 3-day history of colicky epigastric pain that suddenly increased in severity after a meal. Tests reveal that she has a gallstone blocking her sphincter of Oddi. Of the following substances, which would not be expected to be increased in her circulation?

A. Unconjugated bile acids

B. Conjugated bile acids

C. Cholesterol

D. Phosphatidylcholine

E. Amylase

12-5. *Sphincter of Oddi relaxation is normally coordinated with gallbladder contraction to allow bile outflow into the duodenum. Which of the following mediators circulates through the bloodstream to mediate this coordination when the meal is in the duodenum?*

A. *Gastrin*

B. *Motilin*

C. *Acetylcholine*

D. *Cholecystokinin*

E. *Nitric oxide*

SUGGESTED READINGS

Chathadi KV, Elta GH. Motility and dysmotility of the biliary tract. *Semin Gastrointest Dis.* 2003;14:199–207.

Debray D, Rainteau D, Barbu V, Rouahi M, el Mourabit H, Lerondel S, Ray C, Humbert L, Wendum D, Cottart C, Dawson P, Chignard N, Housset C. Defects in gallbladder emptying and bile acid homeostasis in mice with cystic fibrosis transmembrane conductance regulator deficiencies. *Gastroenterology.* 2012;142:1581–1591.

Ko CW, Lee SP. Gallstones. In: Yamada T, Alpers DH, Kalloo AN, Kaplowitz N, Owyang C, Powell DW, eds. *Textbook of Gastroenterology.* 5th ed. Chichester: Wiley-Blackwell; 2009:1952–1977.

Li T, Holmstrom SR, Kir S, Umetani M, Schmidt DR, Kliewer SA, Mangelsdorf DJ. The G protein-coupled bile acid receptor, TGR5, stimulates gallbladder filling. *Mol Endocrinol.* 2011;25:1066–1071.

Mawe GM, Lavoie B, Nelson MT, Pozo MJ. Neuromuscular function in the biliary tract. In: Johnson LR, Ghishan FK, Kaunitz JD, Merchant JL, Said HM, Wood JD, eds. *Physiology of the Gastrointestinal Tract.* 5th ed. San Diego: Academic Press; 2012:847–859.

Mawe GM, Moses PL, Saccone GTP, Pozo MJ. Motility of the biliary tract. In: Yamada T, Alpers DH, Kalloo AN, Kaplowitz N, Owyang C, Powell DW, eds. *Textbook of Gastroenterology.* 5th ed. Chichester: Wiley-Blackwell; 2009:264–282.

Moser AJ, Gangopadhyay A, Bradbury NA, Peters KW, Frizzell RA, Bridges RJ. Electrogenic bicarbonate secretion by Prarie dog gallbladder. *Am J Physiol Gastrointest Liver Physiol.* 2007;292:G1683–G1694.

Bilirubin Formation and Excretion by the Liver

13

OBJECTIVES

- ▶ *Understand the origins of bilirubin in the plasma, and the need to excrete this substance*
  - ▶ Describe how bilirubin is transported through the body
- ▶ *Describe the pathway of bilirubin handling, and further metabolic modifications that occur*
  - ▶ Describe the mechanism and consequences of bilirubin conjugation
  - ▶ Delineate the mechanism of bilirubin secretion into the bile
  - ▶ Understand how enteric bacteria modify bilirubin and the fate of the metabolic products produced
- ▶ *Explain the difference between conjugated and unconjugated hyperbilirubinemia, and diseases that can cause these conditions*
  - ▶ Outline treatments that are effective in resolving the symptoms of hyperbilirubinemia
  - ▶ Explain the mechanisms that can lead to pigment gallstones

BASIC PRINCIPLES OF BILIRUBIN METABOLISM

 Bilirubin is a metabolite of heme, a compound that serves to coordinate iron in various proteins. Very recently, bilirubin has been shown to possess important functions as an antioxidant, but it also serves simply as a means to excrete unwanted heme, derived from various heme-containing proteins such as hemoglobin, myoglobin, and various P450 enzymes. Bilirubin and its metabolites are also notable for the fact that they provide color to the bile and stool, as well as, to a lesser extent, the urine.

Role and Significance

It is important for the body to be able to excrete bilirubin as it is potentially toxic. As we will discuss at the end of this chapter, certain disease states that involve excessive levels of bilirubin in the bloodstream can lead to accumulation of bilirubin in the brain due to its ability to cross the blood–brain barrier, a condition known as *kernicterus* (meaning "yellow-stained nucleus"). The development of this condition impairs brain function by mechanisms that are not well-understood, but it can be fatal if left untreated. Bilirubin is also notable for its yellow coloration. Accumulation of this substance in the blood is the basis for *jaundice*, or a yellow discoloration of the skin and eyes which is a common symptom of liver diseases. Thus, measurement of bilirubin in the plasma can be a useful marker of such conditions.

PATHWAYS OF BILIRUBIN SYNTHESIS AND METABOLISM

Bilirubin derives from two main sources. The majority (80%) of the bilirubin formed in the body comes from the heme released from senescent red blood cells. The remainder originates from various heme-containing proteins found in other tissues, notably the liver and muscles.

Cellular Heme Metabolism

Bilirubin is produced by a two-stage reaction that occurs in cells of the reticulo-endothelial system, including phagocytes, the Kupffer cells of the liver, and cells in the spleen and bone marrow. Heme is taken up into these cells and acted on by the enzyme heme oxygenase, liberating the chelated iron from the heme structure and releasing an equimolar amount of carbon monoxide, which is excreted via the lungs. The reaction yields a green pigment known as biliverdin (Figure 13–1). Biliverdin is then acted on by the enzyme biliverdin reductase, again releasing a molecule of carbon monoxide and producing the yellow bilirubin. Although it contains two propionic acid side chains, the structure of bilirubin is highly compacted by hydrogen bonding. This renders the molecule essentially insoluble in aqueous solutions at neutral pH.

Bilirubin is released into the plasma and is taken up by albumin, which serves to transport this molecule throughout the body. The binding affinity of this unconjugated bilirubin for albumin is extremely high, and under normal conditions, there is essentially no free unconjugated bilirubin in the plasma. When the bilirubin-laden albumin reaches the liver, the high permeability of the hepatic microcirculation, as discussed in Chapter 10, allows the complex to enter the space of Disse such that it encounters the basolateral aspect of hepatocytes. At this site, bilirubin is taken up by a specific transport mechanism to enter the hepatocyte. However, this process is relatively inefficient, with the first pass clearance of bilirubin being approximately 20%. As a result, there is always a measurable concentration of unconjugated bilirubin, bound to albumin, in the venous circulation leaving the liver.

Hepatic Transport Mechanisms

 The transporters responsible for uptake of unconjugated bilirubin into the hepatocyte are not fully understood, and uptake may not require a protein carrier given bilirubin's lipid solubility. However, there is some

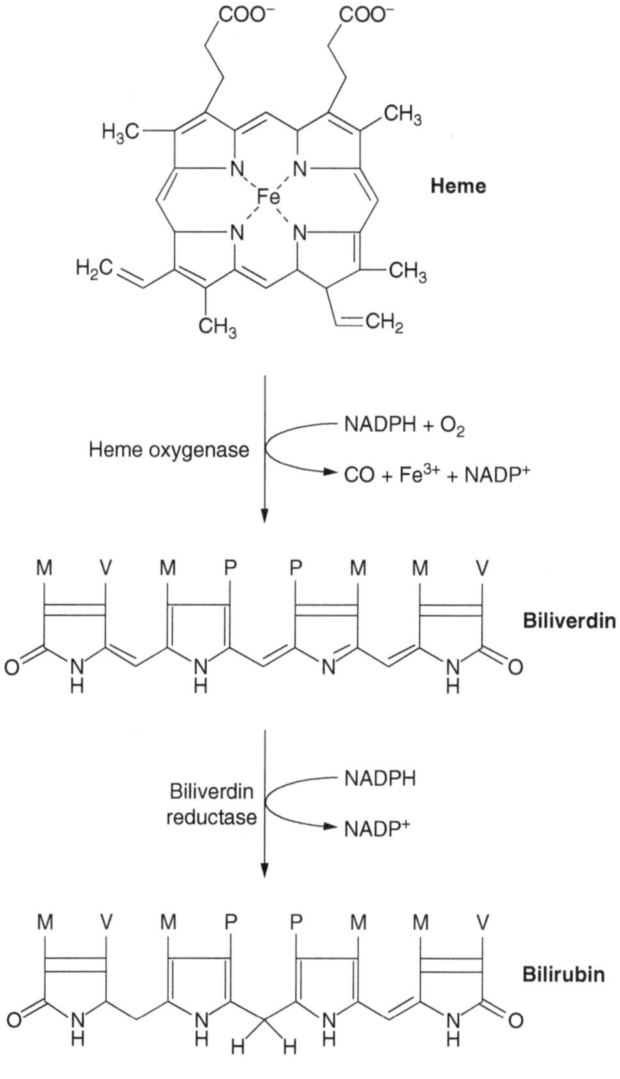

Figure 13–1. Conversion of heme to bilirubin is a two-step reaction catalyzed by heme oxygenase and biliverdin reductase. M, methyl; P, propionate; V, vinyl.

evidence to suggest its uptake may be mediated in part by the 1A and 1B members of the organic anion transporting polypeptide (OATP) family (Figure 13–2). These transporters may also take up any conjugated bilirubin that refluxes to the plasma. Once inside the hepatocyte, bilirubin requires special handling to maintain its solubility and traffic it appropriately. Thus, it is believed to be bound to a variety of intracellular proteins, including fatty acid binding proteins, that direct the molecule to the microsomal compartment for conjugation, as we will discuss

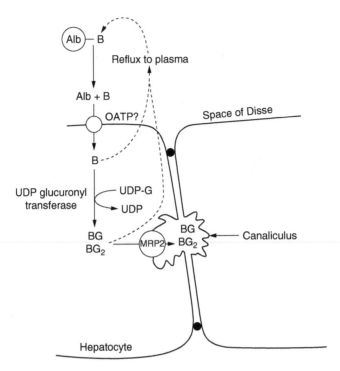

Figure 13–2. Handling of bilirubin by hepatocytes. Albumin (Alb)-bound bilirubin (B) enters the space of Disse and bilirubin is transported into the hepatocyte (either actively or (not shown) passively). In the hepatocyte, bilirubin is either mono- or di-conjugated with glucuronic acid (G). The conjugates are secreted into bile via the multidrug resistance protein 2 (MRP2). Some unconjugated and conjugated bilirubin may also reflux into the plasma, from where they can be reabsorbed into the hepatocyte or, in the case of conjugated bilirubin, excreted via the urine. OATP, organic anion transporting polypeptide.

later. These proteins are likely also responsible for vectorial transport of the conjugated bilirubin to the canalicular membrane for transport into the bile.

Following its conjugation, bilirubin exits the hepatocyte into the bile via a member of the ATP-binding cassette family of membrane transport proteins known as MRP2. While this transporter has a relatively broad specificity, transporting additional metabolic products as well as some drug conjugates, it appears that its main physiological substrate is conjugated bilirubin. Insights into the role and significance of this transporter have been gained from a genetic disorder known as Dubin–Johnson syndrome, which will be discussed in more detail later. However, even in health, transport of either unconjugated or conjugated bilirubin through the hepatocyte cytosol is not entirely efficient, and some escapes back into the plasma where it binds once more to albumin and can be transported around the body. On the other hand, only conjugated bilirubin is able to enter the bile via MRP2. It is primarily present in the aqueous fraction of the bile and is not believed to associate to any significant extent with the mixed micelles formed by the biliary lipids. Conjugated bilirubin is also neither further metabolized nor absorbed during its passage along the biliary tree.

Hepatocyte Conjugation

As alluded to earlier, the hepatocyte plays an important role in bilirubin handling by conjugating the molecule to glucuronic acid. This reaction is catalyzed by the enzyme UDP glucuronyl transferase, or UGT, and results in the sequential esterification of two glucuronide moieties to the propionic acid side chains of bilirubin (Figure 13–2). Under normal conditions, most molecules of bilirubin are modified with two glucuronide groups, forming bilirubin diglucuronide. This proportion can, however, be changed if the conjugation system is overwhelmed under conditions of excessive bilirubin synthesis, or if it is defective, when bilirubin monoglucuronide will become the major species found in the bile.

Conjugation has several important effects on the physicochemical properties of bilirubin. First, it markedly increases its water solubility, allowing it to be transported in the bile without a protein carrier. Second, as a result of this increase in hydrophilicity, and increased molecular size, conjugated bilirubin cannot be passively reabsorbed from the intestinal lumen. There are also not thought to be specific transporters for the uptake of conjugated bilirubin in the intestine, unlike the situation for conjugated bile acids. Thus, conjugation serves to promote the elimination of a potentially toxic metabolic waste product. Finally, conjugation modestly decreases the affinity of bilirubin for albumin. This has diagnostic implications in the setting of hyperbilirubinemia.

Overall, plasma bilirubin in health comprises both conjugated and unconjugated bilirubin. These two forms of bilirubin can be distinguished in the clinical laboratory, and their relative proportions in the diseased state provide important clues about the level of any dysfunction in the bilirubin export pathway. Conjugated bilirubin is also referred to as "direct" bilirubin, based on the original clinical test for this molecule where the molecule would react with a specific reagent without further treatment. Total bilirubin, on the other hand, is measured after the addition of chemicals designed to disrupt the hydrogen bonds of unconjugated bilirubin. The amount of unconjugated (or "indirect") bilirubin can then be obtained by subtraction. Normal levels of total bilirubin are approximately 1–1.5 mg/dL in human adults, consisting of approximately 90% unconjugated and 10% conjugated bilirubin.

BILIRUBIN HOMEOSTASIS

Bacterial Metabolism

In the small intestine, there appears to be little deconjugation or additional metabolism of bilirubin in the healthy gut. However, when conjugated bilirubin enters the colon, it can be rapidly deconjugated by the enteric flora, releasing it for further metabolism by anaerobic bacteria (Figure 13–3).

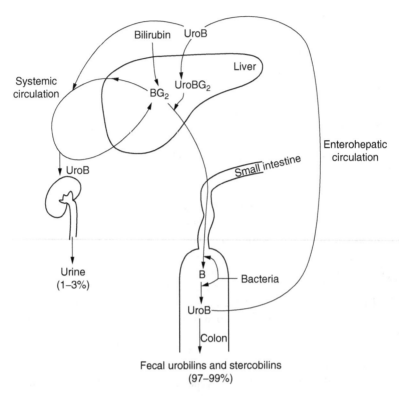

Figure 13–3. Cycling of bilirubin and its products through the liver, intestines, portal and systemic circulations, and kidneys. B, bilirubin; UroB, urobilinogen; G, glucuronide.

Bilirubin is extensively metabolized at this site, producing molecules known as urobilinogens and stercobilinogens. These are further metabolized to urobilins and stercobilins, which give color to the stool.

Enterohepatic Circulation

Bilirubin is not felt to circulate enterohepatically to any great degree, likely because it cannot be taken up from the intestinal lumen in its conjugated form, and once unconjugated in the colon, it is rapidly metabolized to other products. Under some circumstances, unconjugated bilirubin is absorbed from the distal intestine, and then reconjugated in the liver. However, bilirubin in the colon is converted to urobilinogen, which is able to cross the colonic epithelium passively, and thereby also enters an enterohepatic circulation. Urobilinogen, in turn, can be conjugated by the hepatocyte and secreted into bile (Figure 13–3).

Urinary Elimination

Even under conditions of hyperbilirubinemia, little if any unconjugated bilirubin is able to enter the urine because its tight binding to albumin means that it is unable to enter the glomerular filtrate. Urobilinogen, on the other hand, has appreciable aqueous solubility, and a small fraction (typically less than 5% of the urobilinogen pool) is lost to the urine on a daily basis, and is thought to contribute to urine's color.

PATHOPHYSIOLOGY AND CLINICAL CORRELATIONS

Hyperbilirubinemia

 As discussed earlier, hyperbilirubinemia simply refers to excessive levels of bilirubin in the blood. This can be detected during clinical examination by the coloration it imparts to the skin, and is an important marker of several disease states, some of which center on the liver. It is important to distinguish whether the plasma contains increased levels of conjugated bilirubin, unconjugated bilirubin, or both, in order to define the mechanism of disease. This can be assessed directly, but clues can also be provided by the presence of bilirubin in the urine, which imparts a brown coloration. Because of its less avid binding to albumin, an increase in urinary bilirubin involves almost exclusively the conjugated molecule. In general, because conjugated bilirubin can be excreted in the urine, increases in plasma levels represent a less serious state than those associated with severe unconjugated hyperbilirubinemia. An algorithm for the differential diagnosis of hyperbilirubinemia that takes account of these factors is presented in Figure 13–4.

UNCONJUGATED BILIRUBINEMIA

 In a patient with severe jaundice yet no bilirubin in the urine, the increase in circulating bilirubin is due to the unconjugated form. Based on the foregoing discussion of the mechanisms responsible for bilirubin conjugation, it should be easy to appreciate that such an increase must be due to a

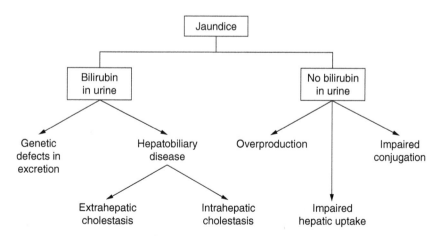

Figure 13–4. Differential diagnosis of jaundice depending on whether bilirubin is or is not present in the urine.

increase in heme production that overwhelms the conjugation pathway, diminished or absent conjugation, or, at least in principle, a failure in hepatocyte uptake (although the latter has not been identified as a mechanism of a specific human disease). Increased heme production occurs in the setting of a massive increase in hemolysis, such as is seen when a child is born to a mother with an Rh incompatibility. Under these circumstances, the liver cannot handle the increased bilirubin load, and unconjugated bilirubin regurgitates back into the plasma where it circulates bound to albumin. An absolute deficiency in the ability to conjugate bilirubin, on the other hand, is found in the rare type I Crigler–Najjar syndrome, where a congenital mutation in the UGT gene results in the total lack of this enzyme. In either case, bilirubin levels can rise precipitously, and entail the risk of neurologic injury if untreated. A milder form of Crigler–Najjar syndrome, type II, is the product of less serious mutations that reduce UGT levels to approximately 10% of normal levels, with correspondingly milder symptoms. In a related vein, Gilbert syndrome, which is a common disorder affecting 3–8% of the population, reflects a variety of mutations that reduce UGT levels somewhat from normal levels, and is a relatively benign condition that manifests as mild, episodic jaundice that may be exacerbated by stress. Similarly, mild jaundice is relatively common in newborns because there is a developmental delay in the maturation of the UGT enzyme, which may take several days to accumulate to levels adequate for bilirubin handling.

Therapy for unconjugated bilirubinemia is dictated by the severity of the condition. In cases of severe hemolysis, exchange transfusions are used to cleanse the body of the excessive heme and bilirubin. The only definitive therapy for type I Crigler–Najjar syndrome is liver transplantation, whereas the hyperbilirubinemia associated with milder forms or with Gilbert syndrome can be treated with phototherapy, where blue light converts the bilirubin circulating through the skin into more soluble forms that are less highly bound to albumin, and hence can be excreted via the urine. Tin protoporphyrin, a potent inhibitor of heme oxygenase, can also be used to reduce overproduction of bilirubin.

CONJUGATED BILIRUBINEMIA

In conjugated hyperbilirubinemia, bilirubin is found in the urine because a portion is able to dissociate from the albumin, and its increased aqueous solubility allows it to be filtered at the glomerulus. The condition implies that conjugated bilirubin is being formed in the hepatocyte, but that it cannot be transported adequately into the bile. This can arise from defective canalicular transport, intra- or extrahepatic cholestasis (as discussed in more detail in Chapter 11), or hepatocyte injury. In the latter case, however, there is likely to be an increase in both conjugated and unconjugated bilirubin circulating in the bloodstream, since liver injury will likely also impair the ability of the hepatocyte to perform conjugation, resulting in regurgitation of both forms into the plasma.

An interesting, albeit largely benign, form of conjugated bilirubinemia is the Dubin–Johnson syndrome. This condition allowed elucidation of the mechanism of canalicular transport of conjugated bilirubin, since it has been shown to arise from mutations that lead to defective expression of MRP2. Patients affected by Dubin–Johnson syndrome develop a black coloration of their liver tissue that can be detected on liver biopsy, but are otherwise normal. There is believed to be a compensatory upregulation of alternative MRP transporter family members in the sinusoidal membrane of hepatocytes, allowing bilirubin conjugates to be regurgitated into the plasma and eliminated via the renal system.

The most common neonatal cause of conjugated hyperbilirubinemia is congenital biliary atresia. Not only will this absence of mature bile ducts result in the retention of biliary lipids, as discussed in Chapter 11, but it will also cause the accumulation of conjugated bilirubin in the plasma. However, unlike cholesterol and phosphatidylcholine, conjugated bilirubin can be eliminated via the urine and thus is not a major source of morbidity in this disease.

As in the case of unconjugated hyperbilirubinemia, therapy for conjugated hyperbilirubinemia depends on the pathogenesis of the condition. If the condition is due to hepatocyte injury or dysfunction, it can be corrected by treating the underlying liver disease. Likewise, in obstructive cholestasis, removal of the obstruction (such as a common duct stone) will likewise resolve the hyperbilirubinemia. In some cases, however, such as congenital biliary atresia, the only effective therapy is a liver transplant.

Pigment Gallstones

As we learned in the preceding chapter, most gallstones are composed of precipitated cholesterol, which is supersaturated in the bile of most humans. However, a minority of gallstones are comprised not of cholesterol, but rather of precipitated unconjugated bilirubin. These are referred to as pigment gallstones, and as the name implies, are dark in color as a result of their composition.

Under normal circumstances, unconjugated bilirubin is not present in the bile since only conjugated bilirubin is a substrate for canalicular transport by MRP2. However, if the biliary tract becomes infected, bacteria can deconjugate bilirubin glucuronides to form the much less soluble unconjugated form. Since bile does not contain albumin, there is no carrier for these compounds. Likewise, bile contains relatively high concentrations of calcium, which complexes with bilirubin to form insoluble calcium bilirubinate. In turn, a pigment gallstone can form. If such stones occur in the gallbladder, the bilirubin polymerizes, forming a black stone. Such stones cannot be dissolved with organic solvents, and also are not influenced by strategies designed to alter the lipid composition of bile. Their formation is, however, limited by the same proteins present in the bile that also limit the nucleation of cholesterol gallstones, and the symptoms they produce are identical.

KEY CONCEPTS

Bilirubin is a highly insoluble antioxidant produced by the metabolism of heme. It is derived mostly from senescent red blood cells and circulates with albumin. Bilirubin and its metabolites provide color to the bile, feces, and urine and account for discoloration of the skin in jaundice.

Bilirubin is potentially toxic, particularly in the central nervous system, and thus pathways have evolved for its elimination from the body.

Bilirubin is taken up into hepatocytes, conjugated with glucuronide, and transported across the bile canaliculus by MRP2.

Only conjugated bilirubin is transported into the bile, but both conjugated and unconjugated bilirubin may regurgitate from the hepatocyte into the plasma.

Conjugation increases the solubility of bilirubin and prevents its reuptake from the intestinal lumen.

Bilirubin is deconjugated and further metabolized by colonic bacteria; some of the products may circulate enterohepatically—notably urobilinogen, which also enters the urine.

Hyperbilirubinemia can arise from an increase in the plasma levels of conjugated bilirubin, unconjugated bilirubin, or both, and often reflects liver disease.

Unconjugated hyperbilirubinemia also results when there is massive hemolysis.

Bilirubin conjugates can be eliminated in the urine if biliary outflow is blocked.

Bilirubin can also form gallstones if the biliary tract becomes infected by bacteria, leading to bilirubin deconjugation and the formation of insoluble precipitates.

STUDY QUESTIONS

13–1. A newborn infant is noted to be suffering from mild jaundice, but no bilirubin is found in the urine. The child's symptoms are most likely attributable to a developmental delay in the expression or establishment of which of the following?

A. Colonic bacterial colonization

B. MDR2

C. UDP glucuronyl transferase

D. Heme oxygenase

E. Biliverdin reductase

13–2. An otherwise healthy medical student notices that his skin and eyes develop episodic mild yellow discoloration around the time of exams. His urine remains normal in color. He does not drink alcohol. The most likely diagnosis is which of the following?

A. Excessive hemolysis

B. Gilbert syndrome

C. Crigler–Najjar syndrome Type I

D. Cirrhosis of the liver

E. Dubin–Johnson syndrome

13–3. A 2-year-old boy is bought to the pediatrician because his mother has noted a persistent, dark brown coloration of his urine. He is otherwise healthy, and his mother notes that a cousin displayed similar symptoms. Tests reveal conjugated hyperbilirubinemia. Bile produced by this child would be expected to display which of the following changes in composition compared to a normal child?

	Bilirubin	Urobilinogen	Bile acids
A.	Decreased	Decreased	Decreased
B.	Increased	Increased	Increased
C.	Decreased	Increased	Decreased
D.	Increased	Decreased	Increased
E.	Decreased	Decreased	Unchanged
F.	Increased	Increased	Unchanged

13–4. In the patient described in question 3, what is the most likely diagnosis?

A. Crigler–Najjar syndrome Type I

B. Crigler–Najjar syndrome Type II

C. Congenital biliary atresia

D. Dubin–Johnson syndrome

E. Gilbert syndrome

13-5. *A second baby is born to a woman with Rh incompatibility, and suffers from severe jaundice within hours. No bilirubin is detected in the urine. What is the most appropriate therapy to reduce the hyperbilirubinemia?*

   A. *Exchange transfusion*

   B. *Liver transplantation*

   C. *Phototherapy*

   D. *Tin protoporphyrin*

   E. *Ursodeoxycholic acid*

SUGGESTED READINGS

Chowdhury JR, Chowdhury NR. Conjugation and excretion of bilirubin. *Semin Liver Dis.* 1983;3:11–23.

Iusuf D, van de Steeg E, Schinkel AH. Functions of OATP1A and 1B transporters *in vivo*: insights from mouse models. *Trends Pharmacol Sci.* 2012;33:100–108.

Nowicki MJ, Poley JR. The hereditary hyperbilirubinemias. *Ballieres Clin Gastroenterol.* 1998;12:355–367.

Sedlak TW, Snyder SH. Bilirubin benefits: cellular protection by a biliverdin reductase antioxidant cycle. *Pediatrics.* 2004;113:1776–1782.

Vitek L, Carey MC. New pathophysiological concepts underlying pathogenesis of pigment gallstones. *Clinics Res Hepatol Gastroenterol.* 2012;36:122–129.

Wolkoff AW. Mechanisms of hepatocyte organic anion transport. In: Johnson LR, Ghishan FK, Kaunitz JD, Merchant JL, Said HM, Wood JD, eds. *Physiology of the Gastrointestinal Tract.* 5th ed. San Diego: Academic Press; 2012:1485–1506.

Ammonia and Urea **14**

OBJECTIVES

▶ *Define the contributors to the level of ammonia in the circulation, and explain why a mechanism for disposal of this metabolite is needed*
  ▶ Outline the pathways that lead to ammonia production in the intestinal lumen
  ▶ Describe extraintestinal sources of ammonia
▶ *Describe the metabolic steps involved in the conversion of ammonia to urea in the hepatocyte*
▶ *Understand the routes for eventual disposal of urea*
▶ *Explain the consequences of excessive ammonia in the circulation, and the disease states that can lead to this outcome*
  ▶ Discuss treatments for hepatic encephalopathy

BASIC PRINCIPLES OF AMMONIA METABOLISM

 Ammonia (NH_3) is a small metabolite that results predominantly from protein and amino acid degradation. It is highly membrane-permeant and readily crosses epithelial barriers in its nonionized form.

Role and Significance

Ammonia does not have a physiologic function. However, it is important clinically because it is highly toxic to the nervous system. Because ammonia is being formed constantly from the deamination of amino acids derived from proteins, it is important that mechanisms exist to provide for the timely and efficient disposal of this molecule. The liver is critical for ammonia catabolism because it is the only tissue in which all elements of the urea cycle, also known as the Krebs–Henseleit cycle, are expressed, providing for the conversion of ammonia to urea. Ammonia is also consumed in the synthesis of nonessential amino acids, and in various facets of intermediary metabolism.

AMMONIA FORMATION AND DISPOSITION

Ammonia in the circulation originates in a number of different sites. A diagram showing the major contributors to ammonia levels is shown in Figure 14–1. Note that the liver is efficient in taking up ammonia from the portal blood in

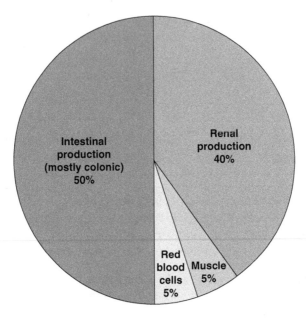

Figure 14–1. Sources of ammonia production.

health, leaving only approximately 15% to spill over into the systemic circulation (Figure 14–2).

Intestinal Production

The major contributor to plasma ammonia is the intestine, supplying about 50% of the plasma load. Intestinal ammonia is derived via two major mechanisms. First, ammonia is liberated from urea in the intestinal lumen by enzymes known as ureases. Ureases are not expressed by mammalian cells, but are products of many bacteria, and convert urea to ammonia and carbon dioxide. Indeed, this provides the basis for a common diagnostic test, since *H. pylori*, which colonizes the gastric lumen and has been identified as a cause of peptic ulcer disease, has a potent urease. Therefore, if patients are given a dose of urea labeled with carbon-13, rapid production of labeled carbon dioxide in the breath is suggestive of infection with this microorganism.

Second, after proteins are digested by either host or bacterial proteases, further breakdown of amino acids generates free ammonia. Ammonia in its unionized form crosses the intestinal epithelium freely, and enters the portal circulation to travel to the liver; however, depending on the pH of the colonic contents, a portion of the ammonia will be protonated to ammonium ion. Because the colonic pH is usually slightly acidic, secondary to the production of short-chain fatty acids, the ammonium is thereby trapped in the lumen and can be eliminated in the stool (Figure 14–2).

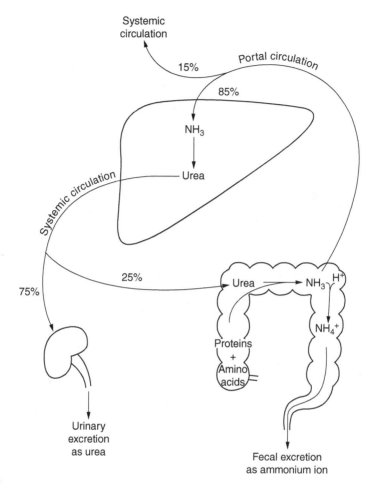

Figure 14–2. Whole-body ammonia homeostasis in health. The majority of ammonia produced by the body is excreted by the kidneys in the form of urea.

Extraintestinal Production

The second largest contributor to plasma ammonia levels is the kidney. You will recall from renal physiology that ammonia transport by tubular epithelial cells is an important part of the response to whole-body acid–base imbalances. Ammonia is also produced in the liver itself during the deamination of amino acids. Minor additional components of plasma ammonia derive from adenylic acid metabolism in muscle cells, as well as glutamine released from senescent red blood cells.

Urea Cycle

 As noted earlier, the most important site for ammonia catabolism is the liver, where the elements of the urea cycle are expressed in hepatocytes. A depiction of the urea cycle is provided as Figure 14–3. Ammonia derived

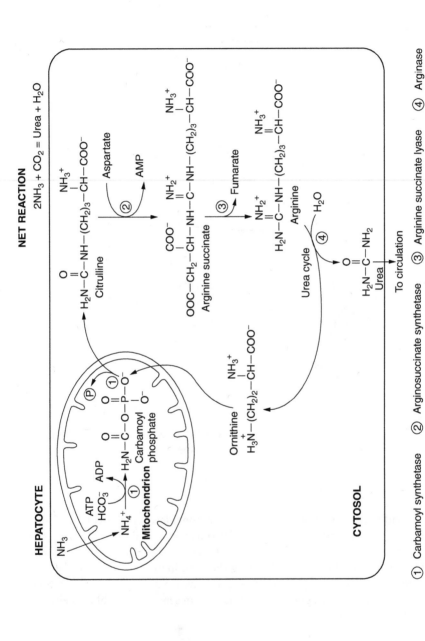

Figure 14–3. The urea cycle, which converts ammonia to urea, takes place in the mitochondria and cytosol of hepatocytes.

from the sources described earlier is converted in the mitochondria to carbamoyl phosphate, which in turn reacts with ornithine to generate citrulline. Citrulline, in turn, reacts in the cytosol with aspartate, produced by the deamination of glutarate, to yield sequentially arginine succinate then arginine itself. The enzyme arginase then dehydrates arginine to yield urea and ornithine, which returns to the mitochondria and can reenter the cycle to generate additional urea. The net reaction is the combination of two molecules of ammonia with one of carbon dioxide, yielding urea and water.

Urea Disposition

A "mass balance" for the disposition of ammonia and urea is presented in Figure 14–2. As a small molecule, urea can cross cell membranes readily. Likewise, it is filtered at the glomerulus and enters the urine. While urea can be passively reabsorbed across the renal tubule as the urine is concentrated, its permeability is less than that of water such that only approximately half of the filtered load can be reabsorbed. Because of this, the kidney serves as the site where the majority of the urea produced by the liver is excreted. However, some circulating urea may also passively back diffuse into the gut, where it is acted on by bacterial ureases to again yield ammonia and water. Some of the ammonia generated is excreted in the form of ammonium ion; the remainder is again reabsorbed to be handled by the liver once more.

PATHOPHYSIOLOGY AND CLINICAL CORRELATIONS

Hepatic Encephalopathy

When ammonia degradation is reduced, it can accumulate in the plasma to levels that become toxic to the central nervous system. Remember that ammonia, as a small, neutral molecule, is relatively permeant across cell membranes and can easily traverse the blood–brain barrier. If ammonia levels rise abruptly, in acute liver failure, coma and death can rapidly ensue. More commonly, as in the setting of chronic liver disease, patients will experience a gradual (and sometimes relapsing and remitting) decline in mental status with confusion and dementia, followed eventually by coma if the condition is untreated. The increase in plasma ammonia in liver disease occurs by two mechanisms. First, if hepatocyte function is compromised, there is less capacity to degrade ammonia coming from the intestine and extraintestinal sites. Second, if blood flow through the liver is impaired by cirrhosis and portal hypertension has set in (see also Chapter 10), collateral blood vessels may form that shunt the portal blood flow around the liver, bypassing the residual capacity of the liver to degrade ammonia (the same is true if a shunt is placed surgically to relieve portal hypertension). It is likely that both mechanisms contribute to the rise in plasma ammonia in the setting of long-standing liver disease.

8 Because the intestine supplies the largest load of ammonia to the circulation, treatments for hepatic encephalopathy focus primarily on reducing the delivery of ammonia into the portal circulation. A common technique is to give a sugar, lactulose, which cannot be degraded by mammalian digestive enzymes but is broken down by bacteria in the colon to form short-chain fatty acids. In turn, the pH of the colonic lumen is decreased and more of the ammonia being formed at that site is protonated and "trapped" as ammonium ion to be lost to the stool. Similarly, patients can be given a nonabsorbable antibiotic such as neomycin (or now, more commonly, rifaximin), which reduces the level of bacterial colonization in the intestine, thereby reducing ammonia production. Conversely, probiotics are being used as second-line treatment options. These may increase the proportion of urease-negative bacteria in the gut, and, if lactic acid-producing strains are used, further reduce colonic pH. Patients with liver disease were previously advised to follow a low-protein diet in an effort to reduce ammonia production in the intestine, but this is no longer recommended in chronic disease because of the deleterious effect of a long-term negative nitrogen balance on other body systems. Nevertheless, short-term protein restriction may be of considerable value in treating an acute episode of hepatic encephalopathy. Ultimately, however, the only lasting treatment for hepatic encephalopathy is a liver transplant, and mental symptoms often are completely reversible if they have not been too long-standing.

9 While ammonia is clearly toxic to the central nervous system, it is important to note that it is probably not the only contributor to hepatic encephalopathy. For example, manganese, normally excreted via the bile, has been implicated as a cause of some of the brain structural changes that are seen in cirrhotic patients. Indeed, while plasma ammonia levels are commonly measured in patients with severe liver disease and altered mental status, they do not always correlate well with the degree of encephalopathy nor are they a reliable index of the effectiveness of treatment. It is likely that other substances normally detoxified by the liver may also contribute to injury of the central nervous system, and/or substances produced by the liver, such as specific classes of amino acids, are needed for central nervous system health. For this reason, there is considerable interest in the development of artificial liver-support devices, consisting of hepatocytes grown on artificial matrices. Other machines incorporate artificial approaches to the detoxifying functions of the liver, such as those that provide for extracorporeal albumin dialysis (note that simple dialysis such as used in renal failure is not effective in liver failure due to the protein-bound nature of the toxins and metabolites that must be removed from the circulation). These systems might be used to mitigate the most serious effects of liver failure until an organ suitable for transplantation can be identified, and indeed, initial clinical trials with prototypes of such devices are encouraging that hepatic encephalopathy can be reversed, at least temporarily.

KEY CONCEPTS

 Ammonia in plasma is derived from protein degradation and deamination of amino acids, as well as from metabolism of urea by bacterial ureases.

 Excessive amounts of ammonia in the circulation are toxic to the central nervous system, so circulating levels are carefully regulated in health.

 The intestine supplies the majority of plasma ammonia.

 The liver is the site of ammonia catabolism via the Krebs–Henseleit, or urea cycle.

 The urea produced is mostly excreted by the kidneys.

 In the setting of liver disease, particularly if blood is shunted away from the liver, ammonia catabolism is decreased, which may increase plasma levels considerably.

 Increases in plasma ammonia, and perhaps other toxins, are associated with a condition known as hepatic encephalopathy, a serious condition.

 Treatments for hepatic encephalopathy focus predominantly on reducing the ammonia load coming from the colon.

 Currently, the only definitive treatment for hepatic encephalopathy is liver transplantation, but liver assisting devices may play a supportive role in the future.

 STUDY QUESTIONS

14–1. *In health, ammonia formed in the colon is partially excreted in the stool. Which of the following allows for this excretion?*
    A. *Limited diffusion of ammonia across colonocytes*
    B. *Short-chain fatty acid production*
    C. *Active secretion of ammonia by colonocytes*
    D. *Absorption of ammonium ions*
    E. *Uptake by bacteria*

14–2. *A 70-year-old man with long-standing alcoholic liver disease is noted to have progressively worsening confusion and disorientation. Loss of the function of which cell type accounts for his altered mental state?*

    A. *Kupffer cells*

    B. *Hepatocytes*

    C. *Colonocytes*

    D. *Vascular endothelial cells*

    E. *Stellate cells*

14–3. *A patient with severe portal hypertension is treated surgically by the placement of a shunt connecting the portal vein to the vena cava. Which of the following will pertain after the surgery compared to before?*

Risk of encephalopathy	Risk of variceal bleeding
A. *Increased*	*Decreased*
B. *Decreased*	*Decreased*
C. *Unchanged*	*Decreased*
D. *Increased*	*Increased*
E. *Decreased*	*Increased*
F. *Unchanged*	*Increased*

14–4. *Patients with advanced liver disease are at increased risk of sepsis due to bacteria derived from the colon. Which of the following treatments for hepatic encephalopathy would also reduce the risk for sepsis?*

    A. *Low-protein diet*

    B. *Lactulose*

    C. *Neomycin*

    D. *Passage of blood through a hepatocyte column*

    E. *Extracorporeal albumin dialysis*

14–5. *A patient with bladder cancer has his bladder removed, and his ureters surgically anastomosed to the colon. He subsequently develops liver disease. Which of the following outcomes of liver disease would he be particularly susceptible to, compared to a liver disease patient with an intact urinary system?*

    A. *Jaundice*

    B. *Hypoglycemia*

    C. *Ascites*

    D. *Encephalopathy*

    E. *Esophageal varices*

SUGGESTED READINGS

Brusilow SW, Horwich AL. Urea cycle enzymes. In: Scriver CR, Beaudet AL, Sly WS, Valle D, eds. *The Molecular and Metabolic Basis of Inherited Disease.* New York: McGraw-Hill; 1995:1187–1232.

Vaquero J, Blei A, Butterworth RF. Central nervous system and pulmonary complications of end-stage liver disease. In: Yamada T, Alpers DH, Kalloo AN, Kaplowitz N, Owyang C, Powell DW, eds. *Textbook of Gastroenterology.* 5th ed. Chichester: Wiley-Blackwell; 2009:2327–2351.

Olde Damink SW, Deutz NE, Dejong CH, Soeters PB, Jalan R. Interorgan ammonia metabolism in liver failure. *Neurochem Int.* 2002;41:177–188.

Rose CF. Ammonia-lowering strategies for the treatment of hepatic encephalopathy. *Clin Pharmacol Ther.* 2012;92:321–331.

Vaquero J, Chung C, Cahill ME, Blei AT. Pathogenesis of encephalopathy in acute liver failure. *Semin Liver Dis.* 2003;23:259–269.

Carbohydrate, Protein, and Water-Soluble Vitamin Assimilation

OBJECTIVES

- ▶ *Understand the barriers to assimilation of water-soluble macromolecules into the body*
- ▶ *Describe dietary sources of carbohydrates, and the pathways involved in the digestion and absorption of carbohydrate polymers, dietary disaccharides, and monosaccharides*
  - ▶ Define the relative roles of luminal and brush border digestion for each type of carbohydrate
  - ▶ Identify the membrane transporters involved in the uptake of monosaccharides
- ▶ *Describe how carbohydrate assimilation is regulated during development and by specific dietary components*
- ▶ *Compare and contrast protein assimilation with that of carbohydrates*
- ▶ *Identify essential amino acids, and understand why they must be provided in the diet*
- ▶ *Describe pathways involved in the digestion and absorption of proteins, peptides, and amino acids*
  - ▶ Define the relative roles of luminal, brush border, and cytosolic digestion for each substrate
  - ▶ Explain how the epithelium can transport a diverse set of peptides into the body
- ▶ *Understand how protein assimilation is regulated*
- ▶ *Define how key water-soluble vitamins are taken up into the body*
- ▶ *Describe conditions where the absorption of water-soluble components of the diet is abnormal*
- ▶ *Appreciate the basis of lactose intolerance, and why it is common in adults*

BASIC PRINCIPLES OF CARBOHYDRATE AND PROTEIN ASSIMILATION

It is perhaps ironic that it is only now, at the end of this volume, that we come to discuss in detail the processes that underpin what is arguably the most important physiologic function of the gastrointestinal system—namely, the assimilation of nutrients into the body. However, the author hopes that, by having provided thorough discussions of the secretory and motor functions of the gut, students will now be in a position to rapidly appreciate how these functions are ultimately integrated to respond to the ingestion of a meal.

Role and Significance

 Carbohydrates and proteins are water-soluble macromolecules of nutritional significance. Together with lipids, which will be discussed in the next chapter, they represent the major sources of calories in the diet, and each supplies specific building blocks for molecules needed for the physiologic function of the body as a whole. Dietary carbohydrates are the major exogenous source of glucose, which is utilized by cells as an energy source. Nutritionally significant carbohydrates include both large polymers and disaccharides consisting of two sugar molecules bound together (Table 15–1). Proteins supply amino acids, which are resynthesized into new proteins needed by the body. While the body can synthesize glucose *de novo* from a variety of substrates, as described earlier, some amino acids cannot be synthesized by the body. These are the so-called *essential amino acids*, which will be described in more detail later in this chapter.

Barriers to the Assimilation of Water-Soluble Macromolecules

 Due to their hydrophilicity, proteins and carbohydrates are "at home" in the aqueous environment of the intestinal lumen. However, neither they, nor the water-soluble end products of their digestion, can readily traverse the membranes of the epithelial cells that line the small intestine. Moreover, intact dietary polymers are too large to be transported into cells. Thus, a series of ordered chemical reactions, catalyzed by

Table 15–1. Nutritionally important carbohydrates

Starch
Amylose
Amylopectin
Disaccharides
Sucrose
Lactose
Monosaccharides
Glucose
Galactose
Fructose
Dietary fiber

specific hydrolase enzymes, break down both proteins and carbohydrate polymers to their component monomers or short oligomers thereof. Digestion of both carbohydrates and proteins takes place at two sites. First, enzymes secreted into the bulk contents of the intestinal lumen begin the digestive process. Second, membrane-bound hydrolases localized to the microvillous membrane ("brush border") of the epithelial cells lining the villus tips in the small intestine mediate the next stage of digestion. The epithelium is only capable of transporting monosaccharides and so even dietary disaccharides must be digested at the brush border before they can be absorbed. For proteins, on the other hand, the epithelium expresses transporters that can take up short peptides, as well as those specific for monomeric amino acids. Thus, peptides taken up into the enterocytes undergo a third stage of digestion in the cytosol, mediated by intracellular hydrolases.

CARBOHYDRATE ASSIMILATION

Sources of Carbohydrate in the Diet

Even in the era of the Atkins diet and the like, where those wishing to lose weight adhere to a diet very low in these compounds, carbohydrates continue to represent a major component of the human diet (typically 40–60% of total calories), and assume particular importance in specific populations (Table 15–1). In developing countries, where protein is scarce, carbohydrates may be the major caloric source. There are three main forms of carbohydrate that have nutritional significance—starch, sucrose, and lactose. The proportion of calories obtained from each varies among different populations. For example, those in developing countries ingest most of their carbohydrate in the form of starch, whereas infants obtain the majority of their carbohydrate calories from lactose, which is found in breast milk. Finally, "Western" diets in industrialized countries tend to be rich in refined sugar (i.e., sucrose).

Starch is the name given to a complex mixture of dietary polymers of glucose, and is derived from a variety of plant sources. Starch is found in cereals, in breads, and in starchy vegetables such as potatoes. There are two different types of glucose polymers in starch, which is significant because they require different enzymes to digest them fully. About 25% of starch consists of amylose, which comprises simple, straight-chain polymers of glucose (Figure 15–1). The remainder of the nutritional portion of starch consists of amylopectin, which comprises complex, branched polymers of glucose (Figure 15–1).

Sources of starch also supply other carbohydrate polymers, as well as noncarbohydrate polymers, that collectively are known as dietary fiber. Fiber is characterized by the fact that its constituent polymers cannot be degraded by luminal hydrolases, including those secreted by the pancreas, nor by those expressed on the surface of the enterocytes. Fiber is critical for intestinal health because, being indigestible in the small intestine, it remains in the lumen and provides bulk to the stool, retaining fluid and aiding passage of the fecal material through the colon. This is the basis for so-called "bulk-forming" laxatives, which add additional fiber to the diet and can be used to relieve constipation. It also explains why those who

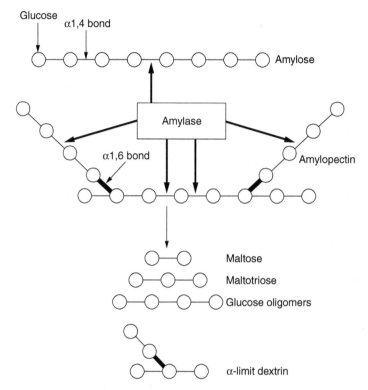

Figure 15–1. Structure of amylose and amylopectin, which are polymers of glucose (indicated by circles). These molecules are partially digested by the enzyme amylase, yielding the products shown at the bottom of the figure.

consume a diet rich in fruits, vegetables, and unrefined grains rarely suffer from such problems. Fiber has additional nutritional significance in that, although it is not subject to digestion by mammalian enzymes, it can be broken down by hydrolases expressed by certain colonic bacteria. These reactions generate short-chain fatty acids, which are important energy sources for colonocytes (you will recall that we also discussed this topic in Chapter 6).

Luminal Digestion of Carbohydrate

SALIVARY DIGESTION

Digestion of carbohydrates begins as soon as the meal is taken into the mouth. Saliva contains a 56-kDa amylase enzyme that is closely related to the 55-kDa amylase that is secreted into the pancreatic juice. As its name implies, salivary amylase is capable of digesting amylose, the straight-chain component of starch. Salivary amylase is not essential for the normal digestion of carbohydrates, since, as we have learned, all of the enzymes in the pancreatic juice are present in considerable excess of requirements. However, the salivary enzyme likely does assume an important role in specific situations. For example, in infants, there is a developmental delay in the production of pancreatic enzymes and so the salivary enzyme assumes a proportionately greater role. Salivary amylase is also an important backup in patients with pancreatic insufficiency, such as in the setting of cystic fibrosis.

Perhaps counterintuitively, salivary amylase is quite sensitive to acidic pH, and in theory its activity would be terminated as soon as the meal enters the stomach. However, it has been demonstrated that amylase activity can be protected if its substrate occupies the active site of the enzyme. Thus, while starch is present in the gastric lumen, it is likely that its digestion mediated by salivary amylase can continue, until the task is assumed by the pancreatic enzyme. The latter is also sensitive to acid, but acts in an environment where gastric juices have been neutralized by duodenal, pancreatic, and biliary bicarbonate secretion.

The synthesis and secretion of salivary amylase in the serous cells of the salivary glands are regulated by neurohumoral signals coincident with ingestion of a meal. Interestingly, in common with the pancreatic isoform, the synthesis of salivary amylase is upregulated by carbohydrate ingestion. Thus, the substrate controls the availability of the means of its digestion.

INTESTINAL DIGESTION

In health, the majority of starch digestion likely involves the 55-kDa amylase that is secreted as an active enzyme into the pancreatic juice by the pancreatic acinar cells (see Chapter 4). Both the pancreatic and salivary enzymes act rapidly to cleave starch into a mixture of products, depending on whether amylose or amylopectin is the substrate. The amylase enzymes target internal α-1,4 bonds of both molecules, but the terminal bonds, as well as the α-1,6 bonds that provide for the branched-chain structure of amylopectin, are resistant (Figure 15–1). This means that while the action of amylase is rapid, none of the products it generates can immediately be absorbed by the enterocytes, since we know that the epithelium can only transport monosaccharides. By the time the meal reaches the proximal small intestine, digestion of starch generates a mixture of maltose (a dimer of glucose), maltotriose (a trimer of glucose), and so-called α-limit dextrins, which are the simplest structures that can be derived from the branch points in amylopectin. Both maltose and maltotriose are resistant to amylase as they contain only terminal, and no internal, α-1,4 bonds.

Although the action of amylase is rapid, some sources of starch contain proteins and fiber components that may slow the action of this enzyme. This means that the rise in blood glucose that eventually follows the ingestion of starch will have differing kinetics depending on the food in which the starch is contained. Some nutritional supplement manufacturers have tried to take advantage of this by isolating so-called "starch blockers," which they claim can reduce the digestion of starch by inhibiting amylase activity and thereby are useful as aids to weight loss. However, your knowledge of gastrointestinal physiology should tell you that this is unlikely to be an effective approach, given the marked excess of pancreatic enzymes and the fact that the starch blockers are proteins, and therefore are themselves digested by mechanisms as we will discuss for dietary proteins later in this chapter. Further, any carbohydrate that escapes assimilation in the small intestine is rapidly broken down by bacterial hydrolases in the colon. Although this may carry the price of the generation of gas and bloating, it ultimately allows much of the caloric content of the starch to be reclaimed.

Brush Border Digestion of Oligo- and Disaccharides

The products of luminal starch digestion, as well as dietary disaccharides, are then acted upon by specific hydrolases localized to the enterocyte brush borders. Brush border digestion is an essential component of the pathways leading to assimilation of all dietary carbohydrates, with the exception of glucose (which accounts for the inclusion of the latter in energy drinks, and the like, because it can therefore be rapidly absorbed). Brush border hydrolysis of carbohydrates, as well as other dietary components, likely increase the efficiency of carbohydrate absorption because the monosaccharides generated are produced in close proximity to the transporters that are then required for their uptake. Likewise, this may also sequester digested monosaccharides from the limited numbers of small intestinal bacteria that might otherwise be stimulated to proliferate by the availability of this source of nutrition.

Brush border hydrolysis is catalyzed by a series of enzymes that are synthesized in the enterocytes as they differentiate along the crypt–villus axis. The enzymes are trafficked specifically to the apical membrane of these cells and anchored in the membrane by a single transmembrane segment. Brush border hydrolases are also heavily glycosylated as they are processed through the biosynthetic pathway. This may protect them, to some degree, from proteolysis catalyzed by the pancreatic proteases that are present in the lumen. The single polypeptide chains that constitute these hydrolases may be posttranslationally modified further to generate specific domains that may contain distinct or similar active sites. Finally, all of the carbohydrate hydrolases that have been described to date occur in the membrane as homodimers.

The enzymatic activities involved in brush border hydrolysis include sucrase, isomaltase, glucoamylase, and lactase (more properly referred to as lactase/ phlorizin hydrolase based on another enzymatic activity expressed by this specific protein). Sucrase and isomaltase activities are actually encoded in a single polypeptide chain with two distinct active sites, and thus the complete protein is referred to as sucrase-isomaltase. Overall, the brush border hydrolases cooperate to facilitate the complete digestion of dietary carbohydrates and the products derived from their luminal digestion.

Considerable information has been obtained about the structure and function of sucrase-isomaltase, which has provided a useful model of the gene regulatory events that accompany the differentiation of enterocytes from secretory cells in the crypt to the absorptive phenotype seen on the villus tips. This enzyme is expressed throughout the small intestine, but not in the stomach or colon, and complex regulatory factors govern its expression along both the vertical and horizontal axes of the intestine. Expression levels are higher in the villus than the crypt, and higher in the proximal than in the distal small intestine. Similar regulatory mechanisms likely also govern the expression of other brush border hydrolases, not only for carbohydrates, but also for peptides as will be discussed later. The sucrase-isomaltase proform is inserted into the apical plasma membrane of enterocytes where it becomes exposed to pancreatic trypsin, which cleaves the molecule to two segments that are then held together by noncovalent forces. The enzymatic activity of the two domains is quite distinct. Thus, while we will learn later that the isomaltase active site is critical for digesting the α-1,6 bonds contained in α-limit dextrins, it is incapable of digesting the α-1,2 bond that links the two monosaccharides contained in sucrose, namely glucose and fructose.

GLUCOSE OLIGOMERS AND α-LIMIT DEXTRINS

The final digestion of these products of amylose and amylopectin digestion involves the concerted action of several brush border enzymes (Figure 15–2). Glucoamylase, sucrase, and isomaltase activities are all capable of digesting the bonds contained in linear, short-chain (2–9 sugar units) oligomers of glucose, which include maltose and maltotriose. The relative contribution of each enzyme to digestion of these substrates is not known. However, isomaltase is critical for the full digestion of starch, since it is unique among the listed activities in being able to cleave not only the α-1,4 bonds of linear glucose oligomers, but also the α-1,6 bonds of the α-limit dextrins. Glucose released by the brush border hydrolysis of any of these substrates, however, uses a common mechanism to enter the enterocyte cytosol. Uptake is mediated by SGLT-1, a sodium–glucose cotransporter that we previously encountered in Chapter 5. This cotransporter takes advantage of the low intracellular sodium concentration established by the basolateral Na,K-ATPase to accumulate glucose in the cytosol against a concentration gradient (i.e., uphill transport). Additional discussion of the molecular characteristics of SGLT-1 and its regulation will be provided later.

SUCROSE

Sucrose, or table sugar, is a prominent carbohydrate in many western diets and requires no luminal digestion because it is a simple disaccharide consisting of glucose and fructose. Rather, it is digested exclusively at the level of the brush border by the enzyme sucrase, yielding the respective monosaccharides (Figure 15–3). As noted previously, sucrase represents one active site of the bifunctional hydrolase, sucrase-isomaltase. Expression of sucrase-isomaltase is usually significantly in excess of the requirements for this enzyme, at least in western populations that emphasize sucrose in the diet. This means that the rate-limiting step for sucrose assimilation is not its hydrolysis, but rather the uptake of the released products across the apical membrane of the enterocyte. This is particularly the case for fructose, which enters the cytosol not via the SGLT-1 transporter used by glucose, but rather a sodium-independent, facilitated diffusion pathway known as GLUT5.

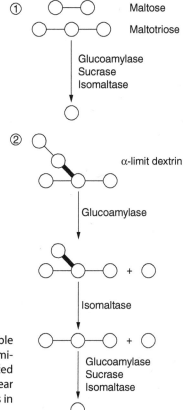

Figure 15–2. Brush border hydrolases responsible for the sequential digestion of the products of luminal starch digestion. Glucose monomers are indicated by circles. Panel 1 depicts the digestion of linear oligomers of glucose; panel 2 shows the final steps in digestion of alpha-limit dextrins.

LACTOSE

Lactose is an important nutrient in those who consume large quantities of milk, and thus its assimilation is predictably important in infants. Lactose is a disaccharide that consists of glucose and galactose, and provides an energy source for the developing infant that can easily be digested and absorbed. Lactose is broken down at the brush border by lactase, an enzyme that contains two identical active sites within a single polypeptide chain. The products of this hydrolysis reaction are, in turn, both substrates for SGLT-1 and thus can be accumulated against a concentration gradient (Figure 15–3).

Lactose assimilation is limited in two important ways. First, there is a developmental decline in lactase expression, meaning that levels of this enzyme in adulthood may be inadequate to hydrolyze all of the substrate presented to them. Thus, in contrast to the assimilation of sucrose, lactose hydrolysis, rather than transport of the products of this reaction, is usually rate-limiting for the assimilation of this disaccharide. Second, the activity of lactase is inhibited by glucose, in a process known as "end-product inhibition." If glucose levels rise in the vicinity of the

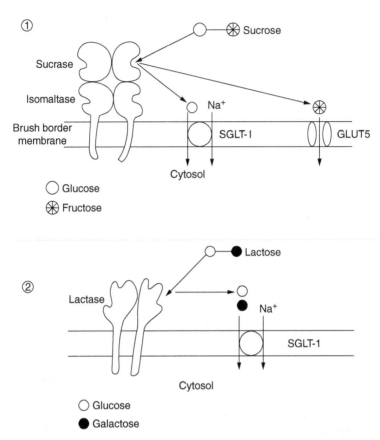

Figure 15–3. Brush border digestion and assimilation of the disaccharides sucrose (panel 1) and lactose (panel 2). SGLT-1, sodium–glucose cotransporter-1.

enzyme, breakdown of lactose will further be inhibited. These factors likely contribute to the relatively high prevalence of a condition known as "lactose intolerance," which will be discussed in more detail later.

FRUCTOSE

As a monosaccharide (as opposed to its presence in sucrose), fructose was previously not a common constituent of most diets. However, its consumption is increasing rapidly with the use of high-fructose corn syrups in food manufacturing. It is also included in so-called "sugar-free" candies prepared for diabetics, which are sweetened predominantly with this sugar. Such candies are not noncaloric, or even low in calories, but are useful because they avoid a rapid increase in plasma glucose that occurs when candies sweetened with either sucrose or glucose are eaten. However, ingestion of large quantities of fructose is likely to overwhelm the limited capacity of GLUT5 in the brush border membrane, meaning that the unabsorbed sugar continues into the large intestine where it is acted on by bacterial enzymes. The symptoms that occur in this setting are comparable to those encountered when a lactose-intolerant individual consumes dairy products.

Monosaccharide Uptake Pathways

The final steps in carbohydrate assimilation involve specific membrane transport pathways that permit uptake of these hydrophilic molecules across the enterocyte apical membrane, as well as mediating their transfer out of the enterocyte across the basolateral membrane and thence into the portal circulation. We have already discussed two of these transporters, SGLT-1 and GLUT5. SGLT-1 is of broader significance because it was the first mammalian transport protein to be cloned, by Ernest Wright at UCLA. It is synthesized by villus enterocytes but not by those in the crypts, likely as a result of transcriptional regulatory mechanisms that parallel those involved in establishing brush border hydrolase expression. It exists in the membrane as a homotetramer, which appears to be important for its function. The protein mediates the ordered transfer of both sodium and glucose across the membrane. Sodium binds first to an extracellular site on the transporter, followed by glucose, which triggers a conformational change in the protein (Figure 15–4). This transfers these substrates to the cytoplasmic face of the membrane, where

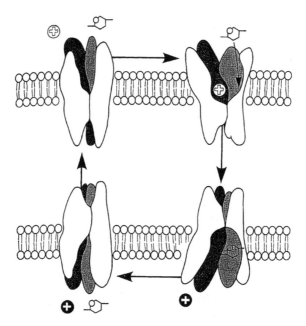

Figure 15–4. Conformational changes in the sodium–glucose cotransporter-1 (SGLT-1) homotetramer that provide for translocation of sodium (shown as a positive charge) and glucose across the apical plasma membrane of enterocytes. (From Wright et al. Molecular genetics of glucose transport. *J Clin Invest.* 1991;88:1435.)

first glucose, then sodium, can dissociate into the cytosol. Recent evidence suggests that the transport cycle of this protein likewise transfers significant numbers of water molecules along with the sodium and glucose, as discussed in greater detail in Chapter 5.

Transporters of the GLUT family also play important roles in carbohydrate assimilation. The portion of absorbed glucose that is not needed for immediate energy needs of the enterocyte exits the cell across the basolateral membrane via a facilitated diffusion pathway known as GLUT2. GLUT2 is sodium-independent, and thus the movement of glucose through this transporter will depend only on the relative concentrations of the sugar inside and outside the cell. Emerging evidence suggests that GLUT2 may also be recruited to the apical membrane of enterocytes to participate in the uptake of glucose and fructose when luminal concentrations of these sugars are high. The recruitment of this transporter apparently depends on the presence of SGLT-1, and thus GLUT2 cannot substitute for SGLT-1 in patients suffering from glucose–galactose malabsorption (a condition that arises from mutations in SGLT-1 that will be discussed at the end of the chapter). GLUT2 is also expressed in many other cell types throughout the body, where it participates in glucose uptake. A related molecule, GLUT5, provides for the brush border uptake of the fructose that is generated from the hydrolysis of sucrose (Figure 15–3). GLUT5 is also present in the basolateral membrane and thus can mediate transfer of fructose to the bloodstream, although there is evidence that fructose is additionally a substrate for GLUT2.

Regulation of Carbohydrate Assimilation

DEVELOPMENTAL

In humans, the machinery for brush border digestion and absorption of carbohydrates is all in place before birth, although this is not necessarily the case in other species, where certain hydrolases and transporters may not be expressed until the time of weaning. Even in humans, however, the capacity for luminal digestion of carbohydrates is regulated in the postnatal period. Expression of pancreatic amylase is low in infants below the age of 1 and is gradually induced as starch is added to the diet. Conversely, lactase levels in the brush border decline in the postweaning period. However, both of these responses likely do not reflect strict developmental regulation, but rather are appropriate adaptive responses to the appearance or disappearance of the relevant substrates in the normal diet.

DIETARY

Indeed, we know that the various components of the body's systems involved in carbohydrate assimilation are regulated by the diet both in the short- and long-term. Acutely, brush border hydrolases on the surface of enterocytes are degraded at the end of the meal, when dietary protein is no longer available to compete for the activity of pancreatic proteases. These enzymes are then resynthesized by the enterocyte to ready the epithelium to handle carbohydrates in the next meal.

This cycle of degradation and resynthesis is not specific for the enzymes involved in carbohydrate digestion, but rather impacts on the entire complement of brush border proteins needed for nutrient assimilation. On the other hand, and on a longer time scale, if carbohydrates are specifically withheld from the diet, there is a gradual decline in the expression of the hydrolases and transporters that are involved in the assimilation of this class of nutrients, and likely also in the expression of amylase. All of these components are, in turn, upregulated if carbohydrate is then returned to the diet. These long-term changes are specific for the nutrient withdrawn from the diet. If protein is retained, for example, there will be no corresponding effect on brush border peptidases, suggesting that transcriptional regulation of the digestive machinery can specifically respond to the availability of an individual class of nutrients.

There are also hormonal influences on the expression of brush border hydrolases and transporters that match the capacity for carbohydrate assimilation with the body's needs. Insulin, in particular, appears to suppress the levels of these molecules, meaning that glucose assimilation can be enhanced in the setting of type I diabetes. This has clinical implications for blood sugar control, since there may be an exaggerated response to glucose ingestion.

PROTEIN ASSIMILATION

Comparison with Carbohydrate Assimilation

We turn now to the pathways and mechanisms involved in the assimilation of proteins. The recommended daily intake of protein in adults is 0.75 g/kg body weight, with requirements increasing significantly in growing infants and those who are ill. Individuals, and particularly children, in many developing countries struggle to obtain these dietary amounts, and protein-energy malnutrition remains a major scourge worldwide, with lasting health consequences even if not fatal in childhood.

Since both are water-soluble macromolecules, the digestion and absorption of proteins and carbohydrates share many similar features, including a role for both luminal and brush border digestion and the presence of specific transporters in the apical membranes of enterocytes that take up the products of these digestion reactions. However, there are also important differences. First, the 20 naturally occurring amino acids, compared to the three nutritionally significant monosaccharides, mean that proteins represent a significantly more diverse set of substrates and require a broader spectrum of peptidases and transporters to mediate their digestion and uptake. Second, the intestine is capable of transporting not only single amino acids, but also short oligomers, encompassing di-, tri-, and perhaps even tetrapeptides. In fact, some amino acids are absorbed much more efficiently in the form of peptides than as the single molecules. Finally, the existence of peptide transport in the intestine implies that these molecules must eventually be digested to their component amino acids in order for these to be useful to other body tissues. This final stage of protein digestion takes place in the cytosol of the enterocyte.

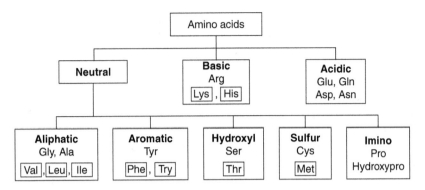

Figure 15–5. Naturally occurring amino acids organized on the basis of their physicochemical properties. Residues that are boxed are essential amino acids that must be obtained from dietary sources by humans.

ESSENTIAL AMINO ACIDS

Another important concept when considering protein assimilation is that of the essential amino acid. While the body (principally the liver) is quite ingenious in being able to convert one amino acid to another, seven of the naturally occurring amino acids cannot be synthesized *de novo*, and therefore must be obtained from the diet and absorbed either as the amino acid itself, or in peptide form (Figure 15–5). Proteins derived from animal sources are all considered to be "complete"—that is, they contain all of the essential amino acids. However, proteins from vegetable sources are "incomplete," meaning that they lack one or more of the essential amino acids. This has nutritional implications for those who chose to follow a vegetarian diet, and particularly for vegans, who consume no dairy products in addition to no meat or fish, and thus no animal proteins at all. The problem of incomplete proteins can be overcome without consuming proteins from animal sources by carefully combining different vegetable proteins with complementary sets of essential amino acids (e.g., rice and beans).

Luminal Proteolysis

Like carbohydrates, dietary proteins first undergo a series of luminal digestion events. These can be divided into events taking place either in the stomach or small intestine, and are mediated by distinct enzymes with properties that render them active in these two distinctive luminal environments.

GASTRIC

Digestion of dietary proteins begins in the stomach—there are no nutritionally significant proteolytic enzymes found in the saliva. As we learned in Chapter 3, on the other hand, the chief cells of the gastric glands synthesize and store pepsinogens, inactive precursors of pepsins, which are a group of related proteolytic enzymes specially suited to action in the stomach. At low pH, there is autocatalytic cleavage of an N-terminal peptide from pepsinogen which yields the active form. Pepsins preferentially cleave dietary proteins at neutral amino acids, with a preference for large aliphatic or aromatic side chains. Pepsins are also sensitive to the pH of their environment, and are inactivated at pHs above 4.5. This means that gastric pepsins are quickly inactivated once they enter the small intestine by bicarbonate coming from the duodenal epithelium, pancreatic ducts, and biliary system. This inactivation may be important to prevent digestion of the epithelium itself by pepsin, which is a rather "aggressive" protease.

Because of the relatively limited specificity of pepsins, gastric proteolysis results in quite incomplete digestion with only a few free amino acids; the products are mostly large, nonabsorbable peptides. In common with other aspects of the gastrointestinal system that are either redundant or present in excess, gastric proteolysis does not appear to be essential for normal levels of protein assimilation. Indeed, the efficiency of protein assimilation is not appreciably lessened by gastric reduction surgery for morbid obesity in the absence of other disease. In fact, when such surgery is successful in achieving weight loss, this likely results solely from causing the patient to eat only small meals (having lost the reservoir function of the stomach) rather than any loss in overall ability to digest and absorb nutrients.

INTESTINAL

The bulk of proteolysis, on the other hand, occurs in the small intestinal lumen. Small intestinal luminal proteolysis is a highly ordered process mediated by two families of pancreatic proteases, the secretion of which we discussed in Chapter 4. Endopeptidases cleave proteins and peptides at internal amide bonds. Ectopeptidases cleave at the terminal amino acid. It just so happens that all of the ectopeptidases secreted by the pancreas are carboxypeptidases—that is to say, they cleave off the amino acid located at the C-terminus of peptides derived from dietary sources. Despite their various specificities, however, all of the pancreatic peptidases have one important feature in common. They are all stored in the pancreatic acinar cells as inactive precursors, which apparently is important to prevent autodigestion of the pancreas in health.

How then are these inactive enzymes converted to their active forms only when they are in the correct location (i.e., the small intestinal lumen)? The answer lies in yet another proteolytic enzyme, this time expressed on the apical membrane of small intestinal epithelial cells and known as enterokinase. When the pancreatic juice is secreted into the intestine, it comes into contact with enterokinase, which specifically cleaves an N-terminal hexapeptide from the precursor of trypsin, trypsinogen, yielding the active form of the enzyme. Trypsin, in turn, can then activate additional trypsin molecules as well as all of the other inactive pancreatic peptidases only once they are in the intestinal lumen (Figure 15–6).

The pathways of luminal proteolysis are shown in diagrammatic form in Figure 15–7. Large peptides derived from gastric proteolysis are sequentially cleaved in the small intestinal lumen by the endoproteases that cut in the middle of peptide chains (trypsin, chymotrypsin, and elastase). These reactions yield shorter peptides with either neutral or basic amino acids at their C-terminus, which can be acted on in turn by carboxypeptidase A or carboxypeptidase B, respectively.

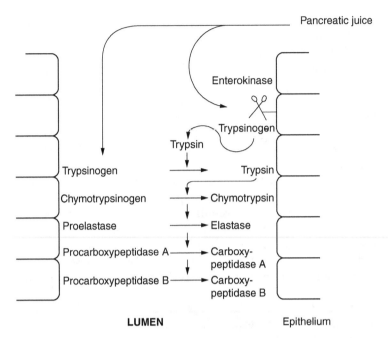

Figure 15–6. Mechanism to avoid activation of pancreatic proteases until they are in the duodenal lumen. Trypsinogen is cleaved by the enzyme enterokinase, which is expressed on the apical membrane of duodenal epithelial cells (depicted as the pair of scissors). The trypsin that is thereby liberated can activate all of the other pancreatic proteases.

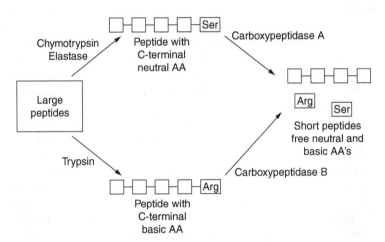

Figure 15–7. Luminal digestion of peptides resulting from partial proteolysis in the stomach. Individual amino acid residues are shown as squares.

Thus, the products of proteolysis in the intestinal lumen consist of free basic and neutral amino acids as well as short peptides that cannot be cleaved further due to the lack of an appropriate amino acid at their C-terminus. Approximately 60–70% of dietary protein is in the form of small oligopeptides following luminal hydrolysis; the remainder is in the form of amino acids.

Brush Border Hydrolysis

Like carbohydrate assimilation, the degradation of proteins in the lumen is incomplete and they also undergo a process of brush border hydrolysis. However, because of the diversity of possible substrates, there is the require- ment for a much larger number of brush border hydrolases. These membrane- bound enzymes comprise both endo- and ectopeptidases, and are expressed by villus, but not crypt, enterocytes. The activity of these enzymes yields free amino acids in the vicinity of the enterocyte apical membrane, although some peptides still remain relatively resistant to hydrolysis, and are taken up in their unhydrolysed form.

Uptake Mechanisms for Oligopeptides and Amino Acids

The next stage in protein assimilation involves the uptake of the products of protein digestion into the enterocyte. Again, the diversity of potential substrates derived from dietary proteins mandates a diverse assortment of membrane trans- porters to mediate their absorption.

PEPTIDE TRANSPORTERS

Perhaps the most fascinating aspect of protein assimilation is its dependence, in part, on a remarkable peptide transporter designated as PEPT1 (for peptide transporter-1) (Figure 15–8). This protein is expressed on the apical membrane of enterocytes, and mediates the proton-coupled uptake of a broad variety of di-, tri-, and possibly even tetrapeptides. In this respect, it takes advantage of the acidic microclimate that exists at the brush border, and its activity is therefore coupled to that of the sodium–hydrogen exchanger at this site, NHE3. What makes PEPT1 such an intriguing transport protein is its extremely broad sub- strate specificity, accommodating peptides of various sizes and charges. This stands in considerable distinction from other membrane transporters, which have quite restricted substrate specificities. Moreover, the stoichiometry of proton cou- pling can change, depending on the net charge of the peptide being transported. On the other hand, transport is strictly stereospecific—transport of peptides comprised of D-amino acids is negligible. It remains a puzzle to transport physi- ologists how the broad specificity of PEPT1 is possible. Perhaps only a portion of the peptide substrate is recognized by the transporter, or the substrate-binding pocket is in some way deformable. In any event, the activity of this transporter is nutritionally significant, because it mediates the uptake of peptides resistant to brush border hydrolysis and thus increases the efficiency of protein assimilation from the gut. Indeed, certain amino acids are much more effectively absorbed in

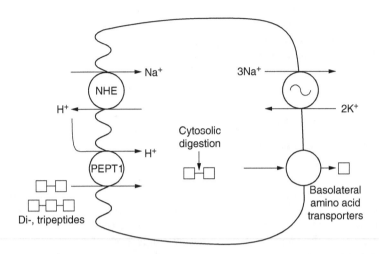

Figure 15–8. Disposition of short peptides in intestinal epithelial cells. Peptides are absorbed together with a proton supplied by an apical sodium–hydrogen exchanger (NHE) by the peptide transporter 1 (PEPT1). Absorbed peptides are digested by cytosolic proteases, and any amino acids that are surplus to the needs of the epithelial cell are transported into the bloodstream by a series of basolateral transport proteins.

peptide form than when presented as individual molecules, including especially glycine and proline.

PEPT1 also has significance for drug therapy, because some drugs have structures that resemble those peptides (peptidomimetics) and are therefore substrates for the transporter. This applies to several antibiotics, angiotensin-converting enzyme inhibitors, and amino-acid-coupled nucleoside analogues used in the therapy of human immunodeficiency virus infection. The ability to undergo uptake by PEPT1 is a property that may be exploited to improve the uptake of a given drug via the oral route. Likewise, a transporter related to PEPT1, PEPT2, is expressed in renal proximal tubule epithelial cells, and may recover peptides and peptidomimetic drugs that are filtered into the urine.

AMINO ACID TRANSPORTERS

Despite the significance of peptide uptake in the intestine, many amino acids are also absorbed in molecular form. The physiology of amino acid transport in the intestine was at one time a complex topic, given the diversity of transporters that had been defined only functionally as well as some overlapping specificities. Moreover, some, but not all, amino acid transporters are sodium-dependent, analogous to SGLT-1 that we considered earlier for glucose uptake, as well as the sodium-dependent bile acid transporter that recovers these molecules in the distal ileum. Others, analogous to PEPT1, may transport specific amino acids in concert with one or more protons. Finally, some amino acid transporters clearly have properties that classify them as facilitated diffusion pathways or even channels.

Table 15–2. Amino acid transporters

Transporter	Substrates	Ion dependence	Disease
SLC1A1	Anionic amino acids	Na^+, K^+, H^+	Dicarboxylic aciduria
SLC1A5	Ala, Ser, Cys, Gln, Asn	Na^+	
SLC6A6	Taurine	Na^+, Cl^-	
SLC6A14	Neutral and cationic amino acids	Na^+, Cl^-	
SLC6A19	Neutral amino acids	Na^+	Hartnup disease
SLC6A20	Imino acids	Na^+, Cl^-	
SLC7A9/SLC3A1*	Neutral and cationic amino acids, cysteine	None	Cystinuria
SLC36A1	Small neutral amino acids	H^+	

*Note: Heterodimer.

More recently, some clarity has been brought to this field by molecular cloning of a large number of amino acid transport proteins from the gut, and their organization into families. We now know that there are multiple transport systems for neutral, cationic and anionic amino acids, with each system being distinct but exhibiting overlapping specificity (Table 15–2). It is beyond the scope of a course in introductory physiology to discuss all of these transporters in detail. However, their activity clearly contributes to nutrition, as manifest by certain disease states associated with mutations in particular amino acid transporters, as will be discussed in more detail later.

Cytosolic Proteolysis

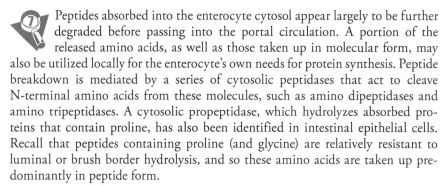 Peptides absorbed into the enterocyte cytosol appear largely to be further degraded before passing into the portal circulation. A portion of the released amino acids, as well as those taken up in molecular form, may also be utilized locally for the enterocyte's own needs for protein synthesis. Peptide breakdown is mediated by a series of cytosolic peptidases that act to cleave N-terminal amino acids from these molecules, such as amino dipeptidases and amino tripeptidases. A cytosolic propeptidase, which hydrolyzes absorbed proteins that contain proline, has also been identified in intestinal epithelial cells. Recall that peptides containing proline (and glycine) are relatively resistant to luminal or brush border hydrolysis, and so these amino acids are taken up predominantly in peptide form.

Regulation of Protein Assimilation

Many of the factors that regulate carbohydrate assimilation have analogous effects on protein assimilation. For example, brush border hydrolases, peptide transporters, and amino acid transporters can be degraded by proteolytic enzymes that remain in the intestinal lumen after dietary protein has been digested; these molecules are then resynthesized by the enterocyte to participate in the digestion and absorption of the next meal. Similarly, the membrane proteins involved in protein assimilation are expressed in gradients along the proximal to distal and crypt to villus axes. Likely because of the diversity of molecules required for protein assimilation, we do not have the level of detail as to how such gradients are established as is available for the regulation of carbohydrate hydrolases, and transporters. Nevertheless, the same general principles likely apply.

WATER-SOLUBLE VITAMIN ASSIMILATION

Vitamins are molecules that cannot be synthesized by the body, but which are essential to normal metabolism. Many act as cofactors for specific biochemical reactions, or play other critical roles in the body. Like nonessential amino acids, most vitamins must be obtained from dietary sources, and deficiencies can lead to disease. We will consider here the uptake of two key water-soluble vitamins, since this process is quite analogous to the assimilation of the end products of carbohydrate and protein digestion. Lipid-soluble vitamins will be discussed in the next chapter. However, it is beyond the scope of this text to consider all of the vitamins in detail, and indeed, the molecular basis of uptake is not fully understood for many such molecules.

Vitamin C

Vitamin C (ascorbic acid) acts as an antioxidant in the body as well as participates in a number of hydroxylation reactions. It is obtained from a variety of dietary sources, including citrus fruits and several vegetables. Having a pKa of 4.2, it is ionized at the pH of the small intestinal lumen and thus its passive diffusion across the epithelium is negligible. Thus, specific transport mechanisms exist in species incapable of synthesizing this compound (notably primates and guinea pigs) to ensure its assimilation.

Uptake of vitamin C is predominantly localized to the ileum—transport in the proximal small intestine is much less active and no active transport is thought to occur in the stomach or cecum. A series of studies conducted over the past 30 years or so have revealed that ascorbic acid is transported across enterocyte apical membranes via a family of sodium-coupled cotransporters referred to as SVCT1 and SVCT2. These transporters are stereospecific and transport vitamin C in conjunction with two sodium ions, therefore leading to electrogenic solute uptake. Both proteins possess 12 transmembrane segments as well as sites for glycosylation and phosphorylation by a variety of intracellular kinases, suggesting that transporter activity is likely controlled by intracellular signals. Vitamin C uptake is also regulated by the levels of this compound in the body. Thus, supplementation with this vitamin, either orally or via injection, leads to a decrease in intestinal capacity for its transport. This finding implies that, unlike nutrient uptake, the intestine displays a capacity to allow for "vitamin homeostasis," maintaining whole-body levels of vitamins at a relatively stable level, although this concept has not been completely evaluated at present and the underlying mechanisms are unknown.

Vitamin B$_{12}$ (Cobalamin)

Another water-soluble vitamin of note is vitamin B$_{12}$, which is utilized by all cells in its coenzyme form in various metabolic reactions. Unlike vitamin C, whose uptake occurs via a simple, sodium-coupled mechanism, the uptake of cobalamin is more complex, and requires the participation of a specific binding factor secreted by the parietal cells of the stomach, known as intrinsic factor. You will recall from Chapter 3 that intrinsic factor secretion is triggered in the stomach by the same neurohumoral cues that result in gastric acid secretion coincident with the ingestion of a meal. Thus, intrinsic factor becomes available in the gastric lumen where it binds to dietary cobalamin and later provides for the uptake of this vitamin. In an analogous fashion, cobalamin in the circulation is bound to a separate protein, plasma transcobalamin II (TC II). Specific receptors exist to mediate the endocytosis of cobalamin bound to each of these carrier proteins, although transport of cobalamin as a free molecule likely can also occur to a limited extent (via diffusion) if large enough doses are given orally. This is exploited in children with defects in cobalamin transport to avoid the complications of deficiencies of this vitamin (see later).

Here, of course, we are chiefly concerned with the processes mediating cobalamin uptake from the intestinal lumen (Figure 15–9). In the gastric lumen, cobalamin is released from binding to dietary proteins and binds initially to the so-called R-binding protein (also known as haptocorrin), forming a complex that is stable at the acidic pH that pertains at this site. R-binding protein likely derives predominantly from the salivary glands. Intrinsic factor, on the other hand, is a glycoprotein with an approximate molecular mass of 50 kDa, and one high-affinity binding site for cobalamin. However, intrinsic factor cannot bind to cobalamin at low pH. Rather, it follows the cobalamin-R-binding protein complex into the duodenum, where the R-binding protein is degraded by pancreatic proteases and the cobalamin is transferred to intrinsic factor at the increased pH that is brought about as gastric secretions are neutralized. The N-terminus of intrinsic factor also contains a binding sequence recognized by an apical receptor for this molecule that is expressed by enterocytes, known as the intrinsic factor-cobalamin receptor (IFCR). Intrinsic factor-cobalamin receptor is highly expressed in the distal small intestine (particularly the terminal ileum), as well as in a few additional epithelial sites, including the kidney. When the complex of intrinsic factor and cobalamin binds to IFCR, the receptor plus the bound ligand is internalized, and these are then directed to a vesicular pathway for sorting and trafficking. Intrinsic factor is degraded, and the released cobalamin is then bound to TC II, synthesized by the enterocyte. In turn, this new complex is trafficked to the basolateral membrane, and released

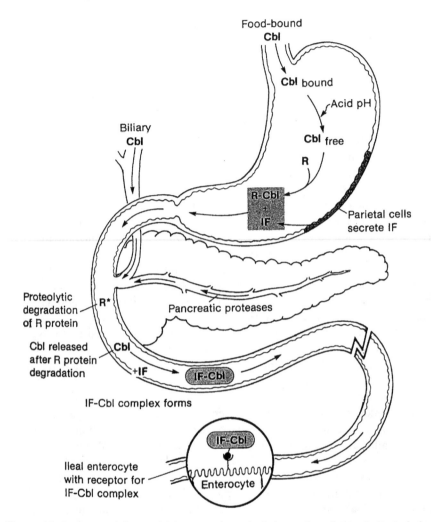

Figure 15–9. Sequential steps in the gastrointestinal absorption of vitamin B_{12} (cobalamin, Cbl). In the stomach, Cbl binds salivary R protein and intrinsic factor (IF) secreted by parietal cells. Proteolytic degradation of the R protein in the intestinal lumen yields a complex of only Cbl and IF, which then binds to a specific receptor located in the apical membrane of epithelial cells lining the terminal ileum. (From Halsted CH, Lonnerdal BL. Vitamin and mineral absorption. In: Yamada T, Alpers DH, Kaplowitz N, Laine L, Owyang C, Powell DW, eds. *Textbook of Gastroenterology.* 4th ed. Philadelphia: Lippincott Williams and Wilkins; 2003.)

into the circulation in this form via vesicular fusion events. Cobalamin bound to TC II can in turn be taken up via the specific receptor for this complex that is ubiquitously expressed throughout the body, including on the basolateral membrane of enterocytes where it mediates the uptake of cobalamin needed for normal enterocyte function.

PATHOPHYSIOLOGY AND CLINICAL CORRELATIONS

While most of the components needed for the assimilation of carbohydrates, proteins, and water-soluble vitamins are present in excess, there are specific conditions where defective uptake can occur, resulting in disease states. Altered assimilation can result from deficiencies in hydrolysis and/or transport, as will be summarized in greater detail later.

Malabsorption

Carbohydrate or protein malabsorption refers to conditions where these dietary components are not fully assimilated during their passage through the small intestine. For reasons that we will discuss in the next chapter, malabsorption of these substances is less likely to occur in general than that of lipids. However, malabsorption of specific substrates can be quite common, particularly in the case of lactose intolerance to which we have already alluded. On the other hand, other malabsorption syndromes are rare disorders, but are important to know about because of the way in which they have provided an understanding of the molecular basis of carbohydrate or protein transport in the intestine.

LACTOSE INTOLERANCE

A deficiency in the ability to assimilate dietary lactose is a common disorder, particularly in specific ethnic groups such as African-Americans and Asians who have not traditionally emphasized milk as a component of the adult diet. Lactose intolerance arises secondary to the normal developmental decline in lactase-phlorizin hydrolase levels that occurs after weaning, which occurs to a greater extent in some people than in others. Some genetic variants of lactase-phlorizin hydrolase have been identified that permit persistence of expression of the enzyme even into adulthood, but it is not known whether these have been selected for in populations that emphasize dairy products in the diet, or *vice versa*. In susceptible individuals, ingestion of lactose in dairy products overwhelms the capacity of the brush border lactase-phlorizin hydrolase to digest this disaccharide, leaving the undigested material in the small intestinal lumen from where it passes to the colon. In the colon, commensal bacteria, on the other hand, are highly active in degrading lactose as an energy source, leading to symptoms of abdominal pain and bloating from the hydrogen and CO_2 gas that is produced. The delayed production of hydrogen (or labeled CO_2) in the breath following lactose ingestion can accordingly be used as a test for the presence of lactose intolerance.

Patients with lactose intolerance who wish to consume dairy products can do so without major discomfort if they also take oral supplements of a lactase enzyme derived from bacteria, which are available over the counter under a variety of brand names. This supplemental lactase is resistant to degradation by gastric acid, and thus is available in the small intestinal lumen to cleave dietary lactose into its component monosaccharides, than can then be absorbed by the small intestine.

BACTERIAL OVERGROWTH

We encountered the concept of inappropriate overgrowth of bacteria in the small intestine in Chapter 6. To reiterate briefly, an increase in the number of bacteria in the small intestine, most often caused by stasis or obstruction, can have several consequences for the assimilation of water-soluble nutrients. First, the bacteria may rapidly ferment carbohydrates, leading to bloating and abdominal cramps. This can be exploited diagnostically, since oral administration of a disaccharide that is not normally broken down by mammalian enzymes, such as lactulose, will result in a prompt increase in breath hydrogen if large numbers of anaerobic bacteria are present in the small intestinal lumen (recall that anaerobes responsible for fermentation reactions are normally essentially wholly restricted to the colon). Second, the bacteria may compete with enterocytes for uptake of the products of protein and carbohydrate digestion if overgrowth is severe, resulting in the possibility of impaired absorption of these substances into the host, at least in theory. A more significant possibility for malabsorption, however, is for vitamins since these are normally present in the diet in trace amounts. For cobalamin in particular, bacteria may avidly absorb this substance, which can result in deficiencies and resulting anemia, even in the presence of adequate dietary intake. Treatment of the consequences of bacterial overgrowth should center on reversing the root course of the stasis of intestinal contents.

PANCREATIC INSUFFICIENCY

Loss of adequate production of pancreatic enzymes can lead to malabsorption of dietary components if particularly severe, such as in the case of cystic fibrosis, pancreatitis, or pancreatic obstruction such as secondary to a tumor. Abnormal absorption in this case can result from two problems—both an actual deficiency in the enzymes themselves, and the failure to appropriately alkalinize the small intestinal contents, leading to inactivation of the pancreatic hydrolases, which all have pH optima in the neutral range. In general, levels of pancreatic enzymes must be reduced to below 10% of normal output before effects on nutrient assimilation are seen. This again underscores the marked surplus of the materials needed for digestion and absorption that characterizes the workings of the gastrointestinal system. On the other hand, because levels of pancreatic proteases are diminished, those of brush border hydrolases may be increased because they are subject to less degradation in the postprandial period. Pancreatic insufficiency can be treated by administration of pancreatic extracts containing digestive enzymes along with antacids to preserve their activity, and may be critical to provide for appropriate growth and development particularly in children afflicted with cystic fibrosis.

CELIAC DISEASE

Protein and carbohydrate assimilation may also be adversely impacted by disease states that reduce the absorptive surface area of the small intestine, usually as a result of a selective loss of mature villus enterocytes. Perhaps the most common disorder in which such a change occurs is that of celiac disease, which results from an inappropriate immune response to a dietary constituent known as α-gliadin, which is a constituent of gluten that is a key structural component of wheat and some other grains. Patients with this disorder, which is now known to be much more common than was previously thought, particularly in Caucasian populations, may display, in the severest forms of the disease, a characteristic "flat" mucosa on biopsy of the small intestine, which results from the total loss of intestinal villi. Because the villi are the site to which both brush border hydrolases and nutrient transporters are localized, patients with untreated celiac disease may present with symptoms of impaired nutrient uptake (such as failure to thrive in children) as well as evidence that undigested and/or unabsorbed nutrients remain in the lumen to be acted on by colonic bacteria, resulting in abdominal cramps and bloating much the same as experienced by patients with lactose intolerance. Some patients may display symptoms starting shortly after weaning to solid foods containing wheat products, whereas others may only develop the disease later in life, perhaps as the result of an infection or other insult that primes the mucosal immune system.

The treatment for celiac disease is strict avoidance of foods containing α-gliadin, including bread, some cereals, and a large number of processed foods. Within a short time, exclusion of these substances from the diet results not only in the resolution of symptoms, but also restoration of the normal structure of the intestinal mucosa. In some patients, it may be possible to cautiously reintroduce gluten-containing foods into the diet after a period of time has elapsed, whereas others remain sensitive to this substance throughout their lives. The reasons for this diversity are not yet understood, but may relate to variations in regulation of the mucosal immune response.

Glucose–Galactose Malabsorption

Glucose–galactose malabsorption is an extremely rare pediatric condition where infants present with severe diarrhea shortly after birth. However, the condition has proved important in understanding the basis of hexose transport in the intestine. We now know that this condition is caused by a variety of missense mutations in SGLT-1 that result either in the production of a protein that is defective in transport function, or one that does not traffic appropriately to the apical membrane of small intestinal enterocytes. In either case, when glucose or galactose are present in the diet (such as in the form of the disaccharide, lactose, that is present in breast milk), neither can be transported into the enterocyte and thus they remain in the intestinal lumen to cause an osmotic diarrhea as well as bloating and abdominal pain secondary to bacterial fermentation. Likewise, if left untreated, glucose–galactose malabsorption will result in severe malnutrition due to the failure to absorb sufficient glucose. Fortunately, once diagnosed, such infants can be fed with formulas lacking complex carbohydrates, and containing sufficient fructose to meet energy requirements. As predicted from the molecular specificity of this disorder, assimilation of other nutrients, such as fructose or indeed peptides and amino acids, is normal.

Protein-Losing Enteropathy

In contrast to the foregoing discussion, where malabsorption of water-soluble nutrients arises from their maldigestion and/or impaired transport across the small intestinal epithelium, the condition of protein-losing enteropathy apparently results from defects beyond the level of the epithelium. Damage to or obstruction of the mucosal lymphatics and/or portal circulation apparently causes the products of protein digestion to "back-up" into the lumen, although why this should be specific for protein is not known. Nevertheless, such patients can display signs of protein malnutrition if the condition is severe, including hypoalbuminemia that results in edema of the lower extremities. The condition of protein-losing enteropathy can result from congenital defects in lymphatic formation, or from local damage to lymphatics and capillaries provoked by an immune response to infection, or inappropriate immune responses to dietary constituents, such as cow's milk in children allergic to this substance.

Selective Defects in Amino Acid Transport

With increasing knowledge about the molecular basis of peptide and amino acid transport in the intestine, we are also developing a greater understanding of conditions where such transport is abnormal. Specific deficiencies in the ability of the intestine to transport specific amino acids have long been known, and can now be ascribed in many cases to genetic mutations (Table 15–2). However, note that in most cases, even the total absence of an uptake system for a particular amino acid, even if an essential one, does not lead to deficiencies in this molecule in the body. This is because the needed amino acid can usually be assimilated in the form of a peptide rather than as the individual molecule. We will, however, discuss two amino acid transport disorders that can present with symptoms, not because of a lack of uptake of the amino acid(s) in question from the diet, but likely because transport is also defective in other critical sites in the body.

HARTNUP DISEASE

Hartnup disease is a condition where intestinal and renal transport of neutral amino acids, including tryptophan, is abnormal. It is noted for its clinical variability, with most patients having no clinical manifestations, while others display a skin rash and/or neurologic symptoms, such as mental retardation. The phenotypic manifestations are thought to result from the lack of nicotinamide, which is a metabolite of tryptophan, and symptomatic patients can be treated by supplementing the diet with this substance. The disease is diagnosed by the finding of high levels of neutral amino acids in the urine. The disease has been attributed to mutations in SLC6A19, a sodium-dependent neutral amino acid transporter expressed predominantly in the small intestine and kidney. In the latter site, the transporter is responsible for recovery of filtered neutral amino acids from the urine. Presumably, in patients who fail to develop symptoms of this genetic mutation, other transporters, including PEPT1 and its relatives, are sufficient to meet the body's needs both for intestinal uptake of neutral amino acids, and to avoid renal wasting of these molecules.

Cystinuria

As the name implies, cystinuria is defined as the excessive loss of cystine to the urine. In fact, other dibasic amino acids such as lysine and arginine are also lost, and all three amino acids display absent or diminished intestinal absorption in their molecular forms, while they continue to be absorbed in the form of short peptides. Because of peptide transport, nutritional deficiencies in these amino acids do not occur in patients with cystinuria. Rather, the main symptom of this disease is the increased incidence of kidney stones, since cystine is poorly soluble. Indeed, it has been estimated that 10% of kidney stones in children arise as a result of cystinuria.

Cystinuria is also a complex disorder at the genetic level. While many cases are attributable to mutations in the SLC3A1 cystine and dibasic amino acid transporter, abnormalities in other gene products can also result in similar disease manifestations. This reflects the overlapping specificities of intestinal amino acid transporters and the redundancies inherent in the intestinal absorption of nutrients. Treatment of the disease mostly centers around management of the renal manifestations, including paying careful attention to hydration to limit stone formation and limiting ingestion of dietary sodium and methionine.

Vitamin B$_{12}$ Deficiency

Lastly, we consider mechanisms and consequences of defects in cobalamin uptake by the intestine. As should be apparent from the foregoing discussion of cobalamin uptake, inherited defects in cobalamin assimilation can result from defects in R-binding protein, intrinsic factor, transcobalamin II, or IFCR. Mutations in each of these genes have been described and each results in abnormal cobalamin delivery to the systemic circulation. Interestingly, at least one mutant form of intrinsic factor is a gene product that has increased susceptibility to degradation by acid and pepsin, reducing luminal levels that would otherwise serve as a carrier for cobalamin and thus reducing its uptake. Cobalamin deficiencies may also be acquired, either as a result of autoimmune damage to parietal cells as seen in pernicious anemia (also discussed in Chapter 3) or injury to the absorptive mucosa. Likewise, during the normal process of aging, gastric secretory capacity declines, and this may reduce the normal sequence of cobalamin binding to its carrier proteins and thus reduce the efficiency of its uptake. Conversely, if gastric acid is excessive, such as in Zollinger–Ellison syndrome (gastrinoma), cobalamin may not be transferred effectively from haptocorrin to intrinsic factor.

The manifestations of severe cobalamin deficiency include anemia and symptoms caused by injury to peripheral nerves. As noted earlier, in the case of inherited disorders of cobalamin transport, large doses of the vitamin can be given to bypass the transport deficiency. Acquired disorders are best treated by addressing the underlying cause. It is also recommended that persons over the age of 50 take supplements of vitamin B$_{12}$ or ingest food that is fortified with this vitamin (such as many breakfast cereals).

KEY CONCEPTS

 Carbohydrates and proteins are water-soluble polymers that are important sources of nutrition.

 The end-products of digestion are hydrophilic, and thus specific transporters are needed to translocate them across the plasma membrane of enterocytes.

 Both carbohydrates and proteins, with the exception of glucose monomers, must be digested to allow for their uptake across the intestinal epithelium.

 Only monosaccharides can be absorbed by the intestine, whereas the intestine can assimilate short peptides in addition to free amino acids.

 Digestion of both carbohydrates and proteins occurs in an ordered series of distinct stages.

 Both luminal and brush border hydrolysis are important; the latter may increase efficiency.

 Absorbed peptides also undergo cytosolic digestion in the enterocyte.

 Water-soluble vitamins also undergo selective transport across the intestinal epithelium.

 Transport of cobalamin requires sequential interactions with binding proteins, especially intrinsic factor, which mediates uptake of this vitamin in the terminal ileum.

 Failures in the uptake of carbohydrates, proteins and water-soluble vitamins are rare because the components of the various systems for digestion and absorption are generally present in excess. Lactose intolerance is a notable exception to this generalization.

15–1. Digestive enzymes can be secreted by the pancreas in active or inactive forms. Enzymes capable of digesting which of the following nutrients are only secreted as inactive precursors?

A. Starch

B. Nucleic acids

C. Proteins

D. Triglyceride

E. Cholesterol esters

15–2. An infant with diarrhea is given a glucose and electrolyte solution orally. What membrane protein accounts for the ability of this solution to provide rapid hydration?

A. Sucrase-isomaltase

B. SGLT-1

C. CFTR

D. Chloride-bicarbonate exchanger

E. Lactase-phlorizin hydrolase

15–3. Glucose-galactose malabsorption is a rare disorder caused by mutations in SGLT-1. Infants with this disorder develop severe osmotic diarrhea if they consume certain carbohydrates. Of the following, which would not be expected to cause symptoms in these patients?

A. Sucrose

B. Glucose

C. Amylopectin

D. Lactose

E. Fructose

15–4. A child is brought to the pediatrician because of severe failure to thrive, diarrhea and edema of the extremities. Blood tests reveal that he has hypoproteinemia. Duodenal aspirates are obtained at endoscopy after intravenous administration of cholecystokinin, and are found to be incapable of protein hydrolysis at neutral pH unless a small amount of trypsin is added. The patient is likely suffering from a congenital lack of which of the following?

A. Pepsinogen

B. PEPT1

C. Trypsinogen

D. Carboxypeptidases

E. Enterokinase

15-5. A 75-year-old woman comes to her physician complaining of progressively worsening fatigue and numbness in her fingers. A blood test reveals that she is anemic, despite adequate iron intake. Her symptoms resolve once she begins taking a daily multivitamin. Her symptoms are consistent with an age-related decline in synthesis of which of the following proteins?

A. Haptocorrin

B. Intrinsic factor

C. Transcobalamin

D. SVCT1

E. PEPT1

SUGGESTED READINGS

Daniel H. Molecular and integrative physiology of intestinal peptide transport. *Annu Rev Physiol.* 2004;66:361–384.

Ganapathy V, Ganapathy ME, Leibach FH. Protein digestion and assimilation. In: Yamada T, Alpers DH, Kalloo AN, Kaplowitz N, Owyang C, Powell DW, eds. *Textbook of Gastroenterology.* 5th ed. Chichester: Wiley-Blackwell; 2009:464–477.

Kagnoff MF. Overview and pathogenesis of celiac disease. *Gastroenterology.* 2005;128:S10–S18.

Martin MG, Wright EM. Disorders of epithelial transport in the small intestine. In: Yamada T, Alpers DH, Kalloo AN, Kaplowitz N, Owyang C, Powell DW, eds. *Textbook of Gastroenterology.* 5th ed. Chichester: Wiley-Blackwell; 2009:1259–1283.

Said HM. Recent advances in carrier-mediated intestinal absorption of water-soluble vitamins. *Annu Rev Physiol.* 2004;66:419–446.

Sibley E. Carbohydrate assimilation. In: Yamada T, Alpers DH, Kalloo AN, Kaplowitz N, Owyang C, Powell DW, eds. *Textbook of Gastroenterology.* 5th ed. Chichester: Wiley-Blackwell; 2009:429–444.

Swallow DM. Genetics of lactase persistence and lactose intolerance. *Annu Rev Genet.* 2003;37:197–219.

Thwaites DT, Anderson CMH. The SLC36 family of proton-coupled amino acid transporters and their potential role in drug transport. *Br J Pharmacol.* 2011;164:1802–1816.

Lipid Assimilation

16

OBJECTIVES

- ▶ *Understand the special barriers to absorption of lipids supplied in the diet*
- ▶ *Describe the phases of lipid digestion*
  - ▶ Understand how lipid digestion is facilitated by gastric events
  - ▶ Define the mechanisms of lipid digestion in the intestinal lumen
  - ▶ Identify how bile acids and micelles participate in the process of lipid assimilation
- ▶ *Describe events at the level of the intestinal epithelium that govern uptake of different classes of lipids*
  - ▶ Understand how the products of lipolysis cross the brush border
  - ▶ Delineate pathways for lipid processing in the enterocyte
  - ▶ Describe how chylomicrons are formed and their eventual disposition
- ▶ *Define how lipid digestion and/or absorption can be altered in the setting of disease*

GENERAL PRINCIPLES OF LIPID ASSIMILATION

Role and Significance

Lipids are defined as organic substances that are hydrophobic, and thus are more soluble in organic solvents (or cell membranes) than in aqueous solutions. Lipids form an important part of most human diets. First, they are denser in calories than either proteins or carbohydrates, increasing the nutritional content of a given meal. Second, several vitamins are lipids (the so-called *fat-soluble vitamins*). Third, many of the compounds that account for the flavor and aroma of foods are volatile hydrophobic molecules, meaning that lipids serve as an important vehicle to render food palatable. In short, dietary lipids are tasty!

Barriers to Assimilation of Hydrophobic Molecules

In the last chapter, we considered the barriers to assimilation of the water-soluble nutrients, carbohydrate, and protein. These molecules are readily soluble in the aqueous environment of the gut lumen, but, following digestion, they require special mechanisms to facilitate their transport across the hydrophobic domain of the enterocyte apical membrane. Conceptually, when considering the assimilation of dietary lipids, the opposite problems pertain. The products of lipid digestion—*lipolysis*—are, in a large part, readily able to cross cell membranes to allow for absorption into the body. However, lipids are not "at home" in the aqueous milieu of the intestinal contents. Likewise, they must interact with lipolytic enzymes that are themselves soluble proteins. Finally, the products of lipolysis must arrive at the brush border at a sufficient rate to allow for uptake before being propelled along and out of the gut. Systems therefore exist to maintain lipids in suspension in the gut contents with a sufficiently dispersed surface area to allow for lipolysis at the oil–water interface. Additional phase transitions allow for efficient trafficking of lipids to the enterocyte surface, where they can be absorbed.

Dietary and Endogenous Sources of Lipids in Intestinal Content

Lipids represent a major source of calories in most Western diets, with an average of 120–150 g consumed on a daily basis by a typical adult. Despite their hydrophobicity, the process of lipid assimilation has evolved to be highly efficient, with significant reserve capacity also present in the system. The ready availability of lipid-rich foods in developed countries may therefore be an important contributor to the burgeoning problem of obesity. Indeed, the intestine is also an active participant in lipoprotein metabolism and homeostasis, with implications for the health of the cardiovascular and other body systems. On a daily basis, the intestine is also presented with 40–50 g of endogenous lipid arising from the biliary system.

Lipid in the diet as well as in endogenous pools comprises several distinct molecular classes. This has implications for the absorption of these substrates since greater or lesser degrees of hydrophobicity may govern the precise pathways by which such molecules are taken up by the body. The majority of lipid in the diet is in the form of long-chain triglycerides (i.e., 3 fatty acids with at least 12 carbon atoms each, esterified to glycerol). Phospholipids, which are components of cell membranes, are also significant contributors. Note also that one phospholipid, phosphatidylcholine, is additionally an important constituent of the mixed micelles present in the bile, as we discussed in Chapter 11. Other, more minor sources of dietary lipids include plant sterols (whose absorption may be inefficient) and cholesterol, another membrane constituent that is present in the diets of all except vegans, who consume no meat or dairy products. However, even vegans will encounter cholesterol in the intestinal contents because, like phosphatidylcholine, cholesterol is secreted into the bile. In fact, the endogenous secretion of cholesterol of 1–2 g/day usually exceeds dietary intake of 200–500 mg that is typical of most individuals. The lipid fraction of oral intake may also include hydrophobic xenobiotics and plant waxes.

A special class of dietary lipids is the fat-soluble vitamins. While these are only present in trace amounts, like other vitamins, their absorption is critical for a variety of body processes. The fat-soluble vitamins are A, D, E, and K. Vitamin A (retinoic acid) is an important regulator of gene transcription. Vitamin D regulates calcium absorption by the intestine, and homeostasis of this ion throughout the body. Vitamin E (tocopherol) is a vital antioxidant. Finally, vitamin K is utilized by the liver to catalyze the posttranslational modification of several blood-clotting factors. The fat-soluble vitamins, as a group, have negligible aqueous solubility. Thus, their absorption depends critically on mechanisms designed to enhance their diffusion across aqueous barriers, as will be discussed in more detail later.

INTRALUMINAL DIGESTION

As for assimilation of protein and carbohydrate, the initial stages of lipid assimilation take place in the intestinal lumen. Luminal events include dispersion of the lipid phase, which is liquid at body temperature, into an emulsion, thereby maximizing the area of the oil–water interface at which lipolysis occurs. Luminal events also include lipolysis, mediated by a series of pancreatic and other enzymes, and uptake of the products of lipolysis into micelles, which can then transfer these molecules to the epithelial surface. Indeed, there is an ordered series of phase transitions that facilitate lipid assimilation. Oil droplets are converted to lamella, vesicular, and liquid crystalline product phases, and finally to micelles that contain the products of lipolysis together with bile acids.

Gastric Digestion

Digestion of the lipid components of the diet begins in the stomach. Gastric peristalsis and mixing patterns provide a shearing action that disperses triglyceride and phospholipids into a fine emulsion. The oil droplets within this emulsion can then be acted upon by gastric lipase, a product of chief cells in the gastric glands that is released in response to neurohumoral triggers coincident with meal intake, and which also promotes gastric acid secretion (see Chapter 3). The lipase binds to the surface of the oil droplets where it can act on triglyceride molecules to generate free fatty acids and diglycerides. However, at the low pH that pertains in the gastric lumen, the fatty acids become protonated and therefore move into the center of oil droplets. Thus, overall, gastric lipolysis is both incomplete, and fails to generate products that are free to diffuse to the mucosal surface where they might be absorbed. In general, 10–30% of overall lipolysis takes place in the stomach in a healthy adult, and gastric digestion of lipids is not essential to their normal uptake. On the other hand, gastric lipolysis may assume a more pronounced role in neonates, where there is a developmental delay in the full expression of pancreatic enzymes, as well as in adults suffering from disease states that impair the production or outflow of pancreatic juice.

Gastric lipase, the enzyme that initiates digestion in the lumen of the stomach, is specialized for activity in the unique conditions that pertain to this segment of the gastrointestinal tract. Most notably, the enzyme displays a pH optimum consistent with that of the gastric contents: 4.0–5.5. The enzyme is also relatively resistant to the action of pepsin, the proteolytic enzyme that is also produced by chief cells. Further, gastric lipase is independent of the presence of any specific cofactors, but is inhibited by bile acids. Finally, gastric lipase acts preferentially to

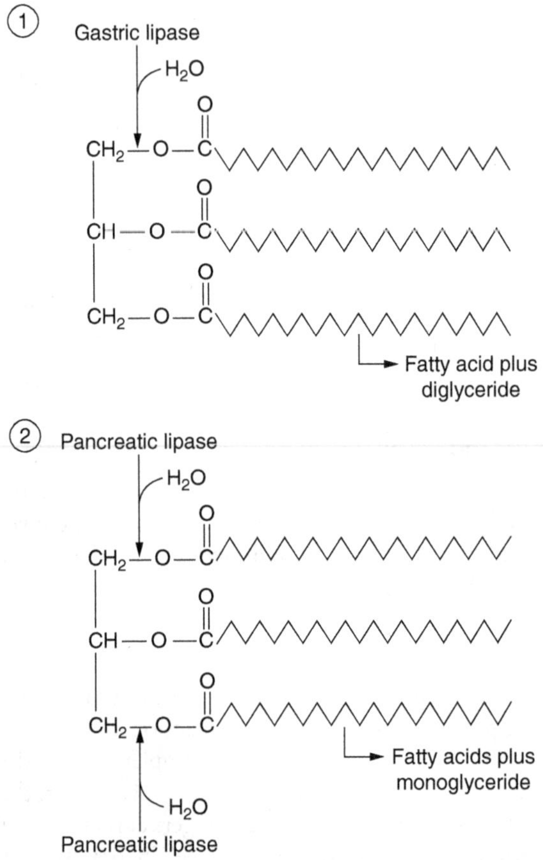

Figure 16–1. Positional specificity of gastric (1) and pancreatic (2) lipases. Both enzymes can digest triglycerides but the products differ.

hydrolyze the fatty acid linked to the first position of triglyceride (Figure 16–1) and is subject to end-product inhibition such that gastric lipolysis is largely incomplete from the standpoint that the triglyceride molecule is not fully broken down to its component parts.

Intestinal Digestion

The meal moves from the acidic gastric environment to that of the small intestine. As the pH rises secondary to pancreatic, biliary, and duodenal bicarbonate secretion, the fatty acids that were liberated by gastric lipase become ionized and orient themselves to the outside of the oil droplets in the intestinal content. This surrounds the droplet with a layer of ionized fatty acids that serves to stabilize the fat emulsion. Because even long-chain fatty acids have measurable solubility in water, some will dissociate from the droplet and traverse the lumen to meet with the intestinal epithelium. Fatty acids are potent stimuli of cholecystokinin (CCK) release, likely acting via the initial release of the CCK-releasing peptide that we discussed in Chapter 4. Cholecystokinin has a number of actions that are pertinent to lipid digestion and absorption. First, it causes an increase in secretion of pancreatic enzymes. Second, it relaxes the sphincter of Oddi, allowing outflow of the pancreatic juice into the intestinal lumen, and finally, it contracts the gallbladder, providing a bolus of concentrated bile that contains the bile acids needed eventually to dissolve the products of lipolysis in mixed micelles.

ENZYMES AND OTHER FACTORS INVOLVED IN DIGESTION

Pancreatic acinar cells secrete a number of proteins that are important in fat digestion (Table 16–1). The first of these is pancreatic lipase. This enzyme is functionally related to the gastric lipase we considered above, but it displays a number of important differences. First, it has a different positional specificity, acting on both the 1 and 3 positions of the glycerol molecule to liberate esterified fatty acids (Figure 16–1). Thus, the products of pancreatic lipase are fatty acids and monoglycerides. Second, it displays a pH optimum in the neutral range, more suited to the conditions that pertain once gastric acid has been neutralized. Indeed, among all of the pancreatic enzymes, lipase is the most susceptible to acid inactivation, meaning that malabsorption of lipid (detected as fat in the stool, or *steatorrhea*) is often the earliest symptom of pancreatic dysfunction. However, both gastric and pancreatic lipases share the property of being inhibited by bile acids. This is not a major issue in the stomach, which is

Table 16–1. Mediators of intestinal lipolysis

Protein	Source	Activity	Comments
Pancreatic lipase	Pancreatic acinar cells	Hydrolyzes 1 and 3 positions of triglyceride	Inhibited by bile acids
Colipase	Proform secreted by pancreatic acinar cells	Cofactor for lipase	Binds to lipase and to bile acids
Secretory phospholipase A_2	Proform secreted by pancreatic acinar cells	Hydrolyzes fatty acid in 2 position of phospholipids	Requires calcium for activity
Cholesterol esterase	Pancreatic acinar cells	Broad substrate specificity— cholesterol and vitamin esters; 1, 2, and 3 positions of triglyceride	Requires bile acids for activity
Breast milk lipase	Mammary gland	Related to cholesterol esterase	Important in neonates

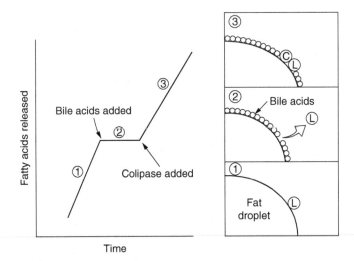

Figure 16–2. Role of colipase in promoting lipase activity in the intestinal lumen. Lipase (L) can absorb to the surface of fat droplets (1), but is displaced by the binding of amphipathic bile acids that arrange themselves around the exterior of the oil droplet (2). Colipase (C) can bind to both bile acids and to lipase, again bringing lipase in proximity to its substrates in the oil droplet (3).

proximal to the entry of bile. Thus the stomach should contain few bile acids in health. How to solve this conundrum, on the other hand, for pancreatic lipase? The answer lies in the presence of a second product of pancreatic acinar cells, colipase. Colipase is synthesized as an inactive precursor (procolipase) that is secreted in approximately equimolar amounts with lipase, and is activated by proteolytic cleavage when it reaches the intestinal lumen. Colipase is capable of binding to both bile acids and lipase, which stabilizes the presence of lipase on the surface of luminal oil droplets. The significance of this interaction is shown in Figure 16–2, which depicts the rate of lipolysis of an oil emulsion under various experimental conditions. If lipase alone is present, it adsorbs to the surface of the oil droplets and generates free fatty acids. With addition of bile acids, however, these array themselves on the surface of the oil droplets and displace lipase, halting its enzymatic activity. However, if colipase is also present, the binding specificities of this molecule can therefore anchor lipase to the oil droplet, and thus its lipolytic action is restored.

Additional pancreatic exocrine products also contribute to lipid digestion. One important enzyme is phospholipase A_2, which is also stored in pancreatic acinar cells as an inactive proform that is activated by proteolytic cleavage once it reaches the intestinal lumen. Because phospholipids are the major constituent of cell membranes, including those of pancreatic duct cells, this delayed activation of the enzyme is likely important in the prevention of autodigestion of the pancreas. Phospholipase A_2 breaks down dietary phospholipids by cleaving the fatty acid located at the 2-position of glycerol, as well as degrading (and thereby reclaiming) the phosphatidylcholine that is present in biliary secretions. The activity of this enzyme is dependent on luminal calcium. It is also important to distinguish the secretory phospholipase A_2, which is of low molecular weight and is synthesized and stored as a proform, from the cytosolic phospholipase A_2 that is present in many cells, and is involved in cellular signaling events that involve the liberation of arachidonic acids from cellular phospholipids.

A final lipolytic enzyme in the pancreatic juice is cholesterol esterase, also referred to as nonspecific esterase. This enzyme is capable of degrading not only esters of cholesterol derived from dietary sources, but also the esters of vitamins A, D, and E. Likewise, the broad specificity of this enzyme renders it capable of complete digestion of triglycerides, since it is capable of hydrolyzing the 2-position fatty acid that is left untouched by both the gastric and pancreatic lipases. Cholesterol esterase acts in the lumen as a tetramer, and interestingly, the formation of this complex depends on the presence of bile acids, distinguishing this enzyme from both acid (i.e., gastric) and pancreatic lipases. It is also important to note that an enzyme closely related to cholesterol esterase, known as breast milk lipase, is produced in the mammary gland of lactating females. This enzyme may "predigest" the lipid components of breast milk, increasing the efficiency of their uptake in the neonatal period. Breast milk lipase shares the broad specificity of cholesterol esterase.

PHASE TRANSITIONS INVOLVED IN PRODUCT SOLUBILIZATION

Not only do dietary and endogenous lipids need to be digested by enzymes to allow for their assimilation into the body, but they must also be trafficked across the intestinal lumen. This is accomplished in the first instance by so-called "phase transitions" that move the products of lipolysis from the oil droplets where they are generated eventually to the epithelial surface.

The phases involved in lipid absorption can actually be visualized by mixing an emulsion of fat with lipase, colipase, and bile acids on a microscope slide. The products of lipolysis that are released from the surface of the oil droplet form a *lamellar* phase somewhat akin to the lipid bilayer that surrounds cells. Vesicles bud off from this lamellar phase, which can be observed under the microscope as a liquid crystalline phase that is clearly distinct from the oil droplets. If calcium is present, this phase is also transiently stabilized as a calcium "soap," although this appears, at least in vivo, to be simply a transition to the eventual formation of micelles, as discussed later. The details of the physical chemistry aside, however, the phase transitions that can be observed microscopically as lipids undergo digestion under conditions designed to model those in the small intestine are directed to a single end—to transfer the products of lipolysis ultimately to the absorptive epithelium.

ROLE OF BILE ACIDS/MICELLES

 As the gallbladder contracts, the meal encounters a bolus of concentrated bile. The bile acids contained therein have an important role in solubilizing the end products of lipolysis and promoting their transfer to the absorptive epithelium. In essence, as the ratio of bile acids to lipolytic products increases, the relatively insoluble lipids are incorporated into structures known as mixed micelles. The formation of these structures is dependent on the physico-chemical properties of bile acids. Likewise, micelle formation depends on the concentration of bile acids in the lumen, since these structures cannot form unless bile acid concentrations exceed the "critical micellar concentration," or CMC (recall that we introduced this concept in Chapters 11 and 12). Finally, it is important to recognize that lipolytic products that are captured in micelles are truly in solution, compared with the emulsion of oil droplets that has been their physical form hitherto. This can be seen experimentally by adding sufficient quantities of bile acids to an emulsion of fat in water. A turbid (cloudy) suspension is thereby converted to a clear solution, demonstrating that the lipid molecules have been incorporated into structures that are no longer large enough to refract light.

Physical techniques have also elucidated the basic structure of the micelles that form in small intestinal content. These are pivotally dependent on the amphipathic nature of bile acids, with both a hydrophilic and hydrophobic face. The structure of the mixed micelles in the intestine is analogous to that of the biliary mixed micelles we discussed in Chapter 11 (Figure 11–3). The bile acids assemble such that their hydrophilic faces are opposed to the aqueous environment. At the same time, the hydrophobic faces of the bile acid molecules can sequester the products of lipolysis such that their solubility is measurably increased. The resulting mixed micelles carry fatty acids and other lipolytic products through the aqueous lumen, and especially through the unstirred aqueous layers that are adjacent to the enterocytes, markedly increasing their rate of diffusion. Indeed, the rate-limiting step for lipid assimilation is the ability to present lipid molecules at a sufficient concentration at the brush border to provide for uptake. It is this step in the process of lipid assimilation that bile acids are designed to promote.

While bile acids increase the efficiency of uptake of the products of lipolysis, it is important to appreciate that the majority of such products are not dependent on micellar solubilization for their assimilation into the body. Thus, fatty acids and monoglycerides have measurable aqueous solubility and can diffuse in molecular form to the brush border, where they can then be absorbed. This raises the concept of the "anatomic reserve" of the small intestine. The normal surface area of the small intestine, and its length, are sufficient to provide for molecular uptake of fatty acids and monoglycerides even if micelles are absent—one simply recruits a greater length of intestine to mediate lipid uptake, and transport rates are slower. Thus, micelles are not essential to lipid assimilation overall. On the other hand, some dietary lipids have such limited aqueous solubility that they are essentially incapable of absorption unless dissolved in micelles. This is the case for cholesterol, fat-soluble vitamins, and plant sterols. Indeed, a patient who cannot generate adequate bile acid concentrations in the lumen of the small intestine to promote micelle formation will also become deficient in fat-soluble vitamins.

EPITHELIAL EVENTS IN LIPID ASSIMILATION

Brush Border Events

Micelles transfer the products of lipolysis to the epithelial brush border, where they can be absorbed. Alternatively, in the absence of micelles, "soluble" products such as free fatty acids will also eventually arrive at the epithelial surface. In this section, therefore, we will consider the mechanisms that provide for uptake of these nutrients across the apical membrane of the enterocyte.

MECHANISMS OF ABSORPTION OF LIPOLYTIC PRODUCTS

In theory, the products of lipolysis have sufficient hydrophobicity that they should be able to passively "flip" across the enterocyte apical membrane by simply partitioning into the lipid bilayer. Such a mechanism may indeed contribute to the intestinal uptake of the various products of the mixed micelle, with the exception of conjugated bile acids, which are exclusively absorbed via an active transport mechanism localized to the terminal ileum, as we discussed in Chapter 11. However, data that have emerged over the past 20 years suggest that there are likely also to be carrier-mediated mechanisms that assist in transporting the products of lipid digestion across the microvillous membrane. Evidence for a proteinaceous carrier for fatty acids, at least, derived originally from studies showing that the uptake of long-chain fatty acids into vesicles prepared from brush border membranes was saturable, competitive, and sensitive to heat and trypsin. This suggests that at least part of the uptake of long-chain fatty acids occurs via facilitated diffusion that is mediated by a proteinaceous carrier or carriers. The molecule CD36, which mediates the uptake of long-chain fatty acids into cells elsewhere in the body, has emerged as one candidate for this carrier, although its capacity is limited and its transport function may not be quantitatively important for overall lipid assimilation. However, it has become clear that CD36 is critically involved in directing long-chain fatty acids to the intracellular machinery that packages them into chylomicrons. CD36 is also important in the perception of fatty acids in the taste buds and possibly in the gut itself. No protein carrier has been identified to enhance the uptake of monoglyceride, although this does not exclude the possibility that such a protein exists.

We discussed earlier that the uptake of plant sterols from the diet is inefficient. At least part of the reason for this was revealed by studying the disease known as *sitosterolemia*, where patients accumulate abnormally high levels of plant sterols in the plasma. We now know that this disease is caused by mutations in two ATP-binding cassette (ABC) transporters, ABCG5 and ABCG8. Together, these proteins normally come together to form an efflux pump that transports any plant sterols that are taken up into the enterocyte back out into the intestinal lumen. The transporter so formed can also export cholesterol, albeit with less efficiency, explaining why the absorption of either dietary or biliary cholesterol is incomplete. However, enterocytes also express at least one specific pathway for the uptake of cholesterol from the intestinal lumen, known as the Niemann Pick C1 Like 1 (NPC1L1) gene product. This protein is the target for a drug, ezetimibe,

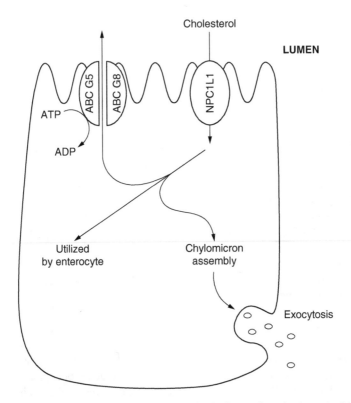

Figure 16–3. Intestinal handling of cholesterol. Cholesterol in the intestinal lumen is taken up via the NPC1L1 transporter. Absorbed cholesterol can be effluxed back out of the cell via the ABCG5/ABCG8 efflux pump at the expense of ATP hydrolysis, can be retained for use in the enterocyte, or can be packaged with other absorbed lipids into chylomicrons, which leave the epithelial cell via exocytosis.

which is useful in treating patients with hypercholesterolemia by reducing uptake of this lipid from the intestinal lumen (Figure 16–3).

In summary, therefore, uptake of the products of lipolysis appears to involve a combination of passive transfer across the brush border membrane, as well as facilitated diffusion for some lipids that is mediated by specific protein carriers. Intestinal absorption of at least some lipids is additionally compromised by the existence of apical membrane pumps that can efflux lipid substrates from the enterocyte cytosol, limiting their ability to enter the body. Additional understanding of the basis of lipid uptake across the intestinal epithelium may offer the hope of new treatments for abnormal cholesterol homeostasis as well as, perhaps, obesity.

Special Considerations for Medium-Chain Fatty Acids

Fatty acid chain length, likely via effects on aqueous solubility, also appears to have an important influence on the molecular mechanisms that govern uptake of these molecules. Importantly, medium-chain fatty acids, with 6–12 carbon atoms, have increased water solubility, and this means that they have measurable absorption via the paracellular route. They are also absorbed transcellularly, but they are not substrates for the acyl CoA synthetase enzymes that are involved in re-synthesis of triglyceride from absorbed long-chain fatty acids and monoglycerides, and thus they bypass these intracellular processing events. As a result, medium-chain fatty acids also follow a different route out of the gut, being exported chiefly via the portal circulation rather than the lymphatic route used by other lipids.

These differences have therapeutic implications. Thus, patients lacking adequate concentrations of conjugated bile acids in the small intestinal lumen (usually as a consequence of an interruption in the enterohepatic circulation) may suffer from fat malabsorption and steatorrhea. This can be alleviated to a considerable degree by feeding diets rich in medium-chain rather than long-chain triglycerides The former compounds are digested more rapidly, and the resulting fatty acids can readily be absorbed in molecular form and they enter the portal circulation directly, which makes them more available to other body tissues. They are often used in infant formulae for similar reasons.

Intracellular Processing

ROLE OF FATTY ACID BINDING PROTEINS

The small intestinal epithelium expresses a family of low molecular weight binding proteins that are capable of binding fatty acids and other dietary lipids. The most well-studied of these are the ileal-fatty acid binding protein (I-FABP) and the liver-type FABP, with the latter, as its name implies, also expressed in hepatic tissue. These and related proteins are assumed to participate in the directed trafficking of absorbed lipids across the enterocyte cytosol, specifically to the smooth endoplasmic reticulum which is the site of intracellular lipid processing. Despite intense investigation, the relative physiologic roles of the various members of this family remain unknown, although a mouse engineered to lack I-FABP displayed a normal capacity to assimilate dietary lipids. This presumably underscores the functional redundancy among these various intracellular lipid chaperones.

CHYLOMICRON FORMATION

Unlike the products of protein and carbohydrate digestion, which are exported to the body in their digested forms (amino acids and monosaccharides, respectively), the products of lipid digestion are unique in that they are reassembled in the enterocyte prior to export to the systemic circulation. Indeed, absorbed fatty acids are prevented from refluxing back out of the epithelium by a process known as "metabolic trapping." Thus, they are rapidly converted to their acyl-CoA derivatives, in which form they can be re-esterified into triglyceride molecules. Long-chain fatty acids and monoglycerides are reesterified into triglyceride in the smooth endoplasmic reticulum; phospholipids, cholesterol, and fat-soluble vitamins are also selectively trafficked and reesterified.

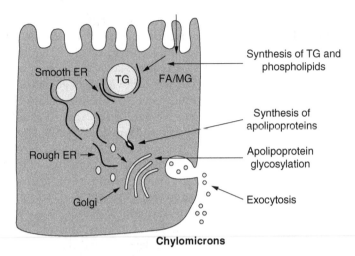

Synthesis of TG and phospholipids

Synthesis of apolipoproteins

Apolipoprotein glycosylation

Exocytosis

Smooth ER

TG

FA/MG

Rough ER

Golgi

Chylomicrons

Figure 16–4. Secretion of chylomicrons by intestinal epithelial cells. Absorbed fatty acids (FA) and monoglycerides (MG) are reesterified to form triglyceride (TG) in the smooth endoplasmic reticulum. Apolipoproteins are synthesized in the rough endoplasmic reticulum and glycosylated, then coated around lipid cores and secreted from the basolateral pole of the enterocyte via a mechanism of exocytosis.

Approximately 75% of absorbed fatty acids are reassembled into triglyceride; the remainder are retained within the enterocyte for local needs.

The various reassembled lipids are then coated with proteins known as apoproteins for export from the enterocyte (Figure 16–4). Apoproteins are synthesized in the rough endoplasmic reticulum, and undergo glycosylation in the Golgi apparatus where they also encounter the reesterified lipids taken up from the intestinal lumen. The particles that are formed via this process are referred to as *chylomicrons*, and have a core of triglyceride surrounded by phospholipids, cholesterol esters, and the apoproteins. The chylomicron is the structure that is used to transport the various dietary lipids to other locations in the body. Approximately 80–90% of the chylomicron by weight is comprised of triglyceride, with 8–9% phospholipids and trace amounts of cholesterol, fat-soluble vitamins, and protein. The resulting structure is exported across the basolateral membrane of the enterocyte by a process of exocytosis. Note that apoprotein synthesis is vital for chylomicron formation and export, and if this process is interrupted, large quantities of triglyceride accumulate in the cytosol of the enterocyte.

Lymphatic Uptake of Absorbed Lipid

The physical form of lipid exported from the enterocyte determines the subsequent route this nutrient can take to leave the gut. As we have discussed, medium-chain fatty acid molecules can enter the portal circulation in common with other absorbed nutrients. However, chylomicrons range in size from 750–5000 Å in diameter. They are therefore too large to cross the intercellular junctions linking capillary endothelial cells. This means that the only way for remaining dietary lipids, incorporated into chylomicrons, to leave the intestine is via the lymphatics, which have leakier junctions. However, eventually these chylomicrons will enter the systemic circulation via the thoracic duct. As a consequence, blood samples obtained from a subject who has recently consumed a fatty meal will exhibit a "milkiness" of the plasma, reflecting the presence of chylomicrons.

The lipid-bearing chylomicrons serve to carry lipids to various body tissues. They are too large to exit the bloodstream across the fenestrae of hepatic endo-thelial cells, and thus are retained in the plasma, although components may leave the chylomicron as needed at this and other body sites. Specifically, their triglyceride content is reduced secondary to the action of lipoprotein lipase, an enzyme expressed by endothelial cells. Eventually, the chylomicrons are reduced to remnants that are small enough to pass into the space of Disse, and can finally have their remaining components recycled by hepatic metabolism.

ABSORPTION OF FAT-SOLUBLE VITAMINS

Despite their importance, relatively little is understood about the specific molec-ular basis of the absorption and handling of fat-soluble vitamins by intestinal epithelial cells. It is known that such vitamins are reesterified in the enterocyte, and incorporated into the developing chylomicron. Presumably this is the form in which they are trafficked to sites of need—additionally, several cell types may act as reservoirs for specific fat-soluble vitamins (e.g., resting hepatic stellate cells for vitamin A). However, the details of these processes have yet to be elucidated. What is known, however, is the essentially absolute dependence of fat-soluble vitamins on micelles to allow them to be presented to the brush border mem-brane. A failure to form micelles in the intestinal lumen will almost inevitably be followed by deficiencies in fat-soluble vitamins in the body as a whole, which may manifest clinically as rickets, night blindness, or an inability to effectively clot the blood, among others. Many fat-soluble vitamins are now available in more water-soluble forms that can be used to treat such problems, such as prior to elective surgery.

PATHOPHYSIOLOGY AND CLINICAL CORRELATIONS

Overall, the normal process of lipid digestion and absorption is highly efficient. A significant portion persists even in the absence of pancreatic secretions or bile. Likewise, it has been calculated that pancreatic output must be reduced by approximately 90% before effects on lipid assimilation are observed. Nevertheless, abnormalities of lipid assimilation can be seen, and these can be subdivided broadly into those ascribable to decreased digestion of dietary lipids, versus those that can be attributed to abnormal absorption. The most com-mon causes of such conditions are summarized briefly here.

Decreased Digestion

PANCREATIC INSUFFICIENCY

If the output of pancreatic enzymes is grossly reduced, the ability to digest lipids will eventually be impaired. This results not only from a failure to secrete enzymes capable of lipid hydrolysis, but also from the lack of active colipase, which is required for the activity of pancreatic lipase in the presence of bile acids as discussed earlier. The most common causes of pancreatic insufficiency include chronic pancreatitis, a frequent sequela of alcohol abuse, and cystic fibrosis, where the lack of pancreatic enzymes may occur even prior to birth. Pancreatic tumors can also result in pancreatitis secondary to an obstruction to the outflow of pancreatic juice. Treatment for such patients often includes the provision of pancreatic supplements, which are dried extracts of (usually) hog pancreata that are enteric-coated to protect the enzymes during gastric passage.

CONGENITAL LIPASE DEFICIENCY

A rarer cause of impaired lipid assimilation is a congenital deficiency of pancreatic lipase, usually in the absence of effects on other products of pancreatic acinar cells. Patients with this abnormality usually present during childhood with a history of passing oily stools, that is, evidence of steatorrhea. Despite this, there remains an appreciable degree of fat absorption that can be enhanced further by the administration of pancreatic enzyme supplements. Such patients also do not suffer from deficiencies in fat-soluble vitamins unless there is another underlying condition that results in impaired micelle formation. Presumably, in such patients, lipid digestion relies on the activity of gastric lipase and cholesterol esterase.

ENZYME INACTIVATION

Among the pancreatic enzymes, pancreatic lipase is particularly sensitive to inactivation by a low pH and thus, under circumstances where the small intestinal pH is reduced, relative lipid malabsorption may be seen prior to deficiencies in protein or carbohydrate digestion. Because luminal pH reflects a balance between gastric acid delivery and secretion of bicarbonate by the pancreatic and biliary ducts, as well as by the duodenum itself, both factors can contribute to the inactivation of lipase. Thus, when the outflow of pancreatic juice is reduced, not only are pancreatic lipase concentrations reduced in the lumen, but those lipase molecules that are present also may not be active if there is inadequate bicarbonate secretion to neutralize gastric acidity. Conversely, in patients with a secreting gastrinoma (Zollinger–Ellison syndrome), enhanced rates of gastric acid secretion may overcome the capacity for neutralization, again impairing lipolysis. If luminal pH remains low, not only will the activity of pancreatic lipase be impaired, but also any fatty acids released by the gastric lipase will be protonated, and retained in the center of oil droplets where they will be less available to diffuse in molecular form to the absorptive epithelium.

Interestingly, there are also reports of children with congenital defects in colipase expression. This condition can be predicted to have the same symptoms as pancreatic lipase deficiency because this enzyme cannot act in the presence of bile acids without the cooperation of colipase. Finally, in some rare kindreds, both lipase and colipase are selectively absent.

Decreased Absorption

BILE ACID MALABSORPTION

 Lipid assimilation, particularly for components with negligible water solubility, will also be impaired in the setting of a fall in luminal bile acid concentrations below the critical micellar concentration. This occurs in two main conditions. First, if outflow of bile is obstructed, such as in the case of a stone blocking the biliary ducts at some level, bile acids will not be available to solubilize the products of lipolysis. Second, in the case of injury to, or resection of, the terminal ileum, the enterohepatic circulation of bile acids is interrupted. While hepatic synthesis of bile acids is markedly upregulated under these conditions, it may not be sufficient to keep pace with fecal losses, and impaired lipid assimilation can accordingly result. Predictably, deficiencies in fat soluble vitamins are seen before overall lipid absorption is affected, since fatty acids and monoglycerides can be absorbed in molecular form by taking advantage of the anatomic reserve.

SHORT BOWEL SYNDROME

Short bowel syndrome is defined as being present in a patient who no longer has sufficient mucosal area for the adequate uptake of nutrients, water, or electrolytes via the enteral route, and thus requires parenteral nutritional support. If the segment of missing bowel includes the terminal ileum, the situation will be complicated further by a decrease in the bile acid pool, in the absence of an anatomic reserve that might otherwise compensate for this. Short bowel syndrome is usually the consequence of surgery—either to remove segments of necrotic bowel in a pediatric condition known as necrotizing enterocolitis, which may have an infectious pathogenesis in some cases, or in patients who have undergone resections for extensive Crohn's disease. Eventually, small bowel transplantation may offer hope that such patients will be able to dispense with parenteral nutrition, although problems with conserving the bowel in a viable state prior to transplantation, as well as the usual problems of rejection, have not yet fully been resolved. Likewise, some exciting experimental treatments that employ growth factors to increase mucosal mass may hold promise, but concerns that these therapies might predispose to intestinal malignancies would need to be resolved.

KEY CONCEPTS

 Lipids are important constituents of most diets, make food more palatable, and are energy-dense.

 Lipid digestion and absorption involves a complex series of events designed to emulsify, digest, and solubilize these hydrophobic dietary constituents.

 The intestine is presented with a significant load of biliary lipids on a daily basis.

 Biliary excretion of cholesterol may substantially exceed dietary intake.

 Micelles increase the efficiency of absorption of the products of triglyceride digestion, but they are not required for this process in healthy individuals.

 Absorption of fat-soluble vitamins and cholesterol are entirely dependent on micellar solubilization.

 Absorbed lipids are esterified and repackaged in the enterocyte into a structure known as a chylomicron, which then traffics absorbed lipids around the body, initially bypassing the portal circulation.

 Chylomicrons consist predominantly of resynthesized triglyceride, but apoproteins are essential components.

 Lipid digestion is a highly efficient process and significant excess capacity exists in the system.

 Failure of lipid digestion and/or absorption manifests clinically as steatorrhea, and may involve specific vitamin deficiencies.

STUDY QUESTIONS

16–1. A patient with obstructive jaundice who is scheduled for gallbladder surgery is found to have an elevated prothrombin time. This laboratory finding is most likely due to malabsorption of which of the following vitamins?

A. A

B. B12

C. D

D. E

E. K

16–2. A patient is treated for hypercholesterolemia with cholestyramine, a resin that binds bile acid molecules. Absorption of which of the following is likely to be abnormal in this patient?

A. Long-chain triglyceride

B. Medium-chain triglyceride

C. Starch

D. Vitamin D

E. Vitamin C

16–3. A mouse was constructed in which the expression of NPC1L1 was knocked out by genetic targeting. Assimilation of which of the following substances from the diet would be expected to be abnormal in these animals?

A. Triglyceride

B. Vitamin D

C. Vitamin E

D. Cholesterol

E. Phospholipids

16–4. A patient with a long-standing history of mild cystic fibrosis notices that his stools are becoming bulky and oily. Laboratory tests confirm steatorrhea. Which of the following is not involved in the apparently decreased fat assimilation in this patient?

A. Lipase inactivation

B. Decreased pancreatic lipase output

C. Reduced pancreatic bicarbonate secretion

D. Loss of the anatomic reserve

E. Decreased colipase synthesis

16-5. *An otherwise healthy child is found to have mild, intermittent steatorrhea but no evidence of malabsorption of fat-soluble vitamins. There are also no defects in protein or carbohydrate assimilation. His brother was similarly affected. Lack of which of the following is most consistent with the clinical picture?*

    A. Bile acid micelles

    B. Cholesterol esterase

    C. CD36

    D. Gastric lipase

    E. Pancreatic lipase

SUGGESTED READINGS

Abumrad NA, Davidson NO. Role of the gut in lipid homeostasis. *Physiol Rev.* 2012;92:1061–1085.

Lowe ME. The triglyceride lipases of the pancreas. *J Lipid Res.* 2002;43:2007–2016.

Storch J, Thumser AE. The fatty acid transport function of fatty acid binding proteins. *Biochim Biophys Acta.* 2000;1486:28–44.

Sudhop T, Lutjohann D, von Bergmann K. Sterol transporters: targets of natural sterols and new lipid lowering drugs. *Pharmacol Ther.* 2005;105:333–341.

Sun W, Lo C, Tso P. Intestinal lipid absorption. In: Yamada T, Alpers DH, Kalloo AN, Kaplowitz N, Owyang C, Powell DW, eds. *Textbook of Gastroenterology.* 5th ed. Chichester: Wiley-Blackwell; 2009:445–463.

Turley SD, Dietschy JM. Sterol absorption by the small intestine. *Curr Opin Lipidol.* 2003;14:233–240.

Williams KJ. Molecular processes that handle—and mishandle—dietary lipids. *J Clin Invest.* 2008; 118:3247–3259.

Answers to Study Questions

Chapter 1

1–1.	A
1–2.	B
1–3.	C
1–4.	E
1–5.	D

Chapter 2

2–1.	E
2–2.	A
2–3.	B
2–4.	B
2–5.	E
2–6.	A

Chapter 3

3–1.	A
3–2.	E
3–3.	E
3–4.	D
3–5.	B

Chapter 4

4–1.	A
4–2.	E
4–3.	C
4–4.	C
4–5.	D

Chapter 5

5–1.	A
5–2.	A
5–3.	D
5–4.	E
5–5.	A

Chapter 6

6–1.	B
6–2.	C
6–3.	C
6–4.	E
6–5.	D

Chapter 7

7–1.	D
7–2.	C
7–3.	A
7–4.	E
7–5.	E

Chapter 8

8–1.	A
8–2.	B
8–3.	C
8–4.	E
8–5.	A

Chapter 9

9–1.	C
9–2.	E
9–3.	E
9–4.	E
9–5.	C

Chapter 10

10–1.	E
10–2.	C
10–3.	D
10–4.	C
10–5.	B

Chapter 11

11–1.	A
11–2.	E
11–3.	E
11–4.	D
11–5.	A

Chapter 12

12–1.	A
12–2.	C
12–3.	E
12–4.	A
12–5.	D

Chapter 13

13–1.	C
13–2.	B
13–3.	E
13–4.	D
13–5.	A

Chapter 14

14–1.	B
14–2.	B
14–3.	A
14–4.	C
14–5.	D

Chapter 15

15–1.	C
15–2.	B
15–3.	E
15–4.	E
15–5.	B

Chapter 16

16–1.	E
16–2.	D
16–3.	D
16–4.	D
16–5.	E

Index

Page numbers followed by *f* and *t* indicate figures and tables, respectively.

CPSIA information can be obtained
at www.ICGtesting.com
Printed in the USA
LVHW081811090922
728007LV00003B/44

9 780071 774017